THE NEW WEBSTER'S MEDICAL DICTIONARY

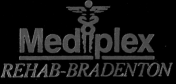

THE NEW WEBSTER'S MEDICAL DICTIONARY

PUBLISHED BY
THE LEWTAN LINE ®
HARTFORD, CONN., U.S.A.
Printed in U.S.A.   All Rights Reserved
Latest Printing 1991

THE NEW WEBSTER'S MEDICAL DICTIONARY

Prepared by
Alyce Bolander, R.N., M.Ed.
Editor
Donald O. Bolander, M.A., Litt. D.

MEDICAL ABBREVIATIONS and TERMINOLOGY

MEDICAL ABBREVIATIONS
and TERMINOLOGY

ABD, abdominal
a.c., before meals
ad, to; up to
a.d., right ear
ad lib., at pleasure
AF, atrial fibrillation
agit., shake; stir
AI, Aortic insufficiency
alt. dieb., every other day
ante, before
aq., water
a.s., left ear
AS, aortic stenosis
a.u., each ear; both ears together

BE, barium enema
bib., drink
b.i.d., twice daily
BMR, basal metabolism rate
BUN, blood urea nitrogen

c̄, c, with
c., cal., calorie
Ca, carcinoma
cap., let him/her take
caps., a capsule
CBC, complete blood count
C.C., chief complaint
c.c., cubic centimeter
c.m., tomorrow morning
c.n., tomorrow night

CNS, central nervous system
C.V.A., cerebrovascular accident; a stroke

DD., differential diagnosis
DIFF., differential blood count
dil., dilute
DPT, diptheria, pertussis, tetanus
D & C, dilation and curettage
D & E, dilation and evacuation
divid., divide

EKG, ECG, electrocardiogram
EEG, electroencephalogram
EENT, eye, ear, nose and throat
EMG, electromyogram
elix., an elixir
en., enem., an enema
ENT, ear, nose and throat
et, and

F, fahrenheit
f., ft., make
FBS, fasting blood sugar
fldxt., fluidextract
FSH, follicle stimulating hormone

GB viz., gall bladder visualization
GC, gonorrhea, gonoccocal
GI, gastrointestinal
Gm., gm., gram
gran, gr., grain
gt., gutt., drop, drops
GU, genitourinary

h.d., at bedtime

Hgb., hemoglobin

I^{131}**,** radioactive iodine uptake
id., the same
IM, intramuscular
inj., injection
IP, intraperitoneal
IV, intravenously; intravenous
IVP, intravenous pyelogram

LE, lupus erythematosus
LH, luteinizing hormone

mEq, milliequivalent
MI, mitral insufficiency
MLD, minimal lethal dose
MOM, milk of magnesia
MONO, mononucleosis
MS, mitral stenosis; multiple sclerosis

N, normal
noct., at night
non rep., do not repeat

OB-GYN, obstetrics and gynecology
O.D., right eye
O.S., O.L., left eye
o.u., both eyes

pa, percussion and auscultation
PAT, paroxysmal atrial tachycardia
PCI, protein-bound iodine
p.c., after eating
Ped., pediatrics, pediatrician

pH, expression of acidity or alkalinity. pH 7 is neutral.
prand., dinner

q.d., every day
q.h., q.q.h., each hour; every hour
q.i.d., 4 times a day
q.q.h., q.q.hor., every four hours
q.v., as much as you wish

R., take
RBC, red blood count
rep., repeat; let it be repeated

s.c., subcataneous
sig., write; let it be written
sine, without
Stat., immediately

T & A, tonsillectomy and adenoidectomy
TB, tuberculosis
temp., temperature
t.i.d., 3 times a day
tus., a cough

ung., an ointment
ut dict., as directed
VD, veneral disease
VDRL, serology

WBC, white blood count

A

abarticulation, joint dislocation.

abasia, inability to walk due to incoordination.

abatement, decrease in severity of pain or other symptom.

abdomen, area of body between thorax and pelvis.

abdominoscopy, examination of the abdominal cavity by an instrument.

abduct, to draw an extremity away from the body.

aberration, deviation from normal state or action.

ablation, removal or separation by surgery.

abnormal, variation from normal.

abortion, the termination of pregnancy, spontaneous or induced.

abrade, chafing of skin by friction.

abrasion, a scraping injury to the outer layer of skin.

abscess, a localized collection of purulent matter in any part of the body that may cause pain or swelling.

abscission, the removal of a growth by surgical means.

absolute, pure or perfect.

absorb, to take in by soaking up.

abuse, improper use, frequently cited in connection with drugs or alcohol misuse or mistreatment of children.

acariasis, a skin disease caused by a mite or acarid. See scabies.

acclimation, becoming accustomed to a different climate or situation.

accomodation, adjustment of the eye for seeing varied distances.

accouchement, act of delivery in childbirth or confinement.

acetabulum, the cavity in the hip bone which receives the head of the femur or thigh bone.

acetic, having properties of vinegar.

acetic acid, used as a reagent. An aqueous solution containing alcohol.

acetone, a volatile, colorless and inflammable liquid useful as a solvent; found in the blood and urine of diabetics.

acetylcholine, an acid found in various organs and tissues necessary for the transmission of nerve impulses.

acetylicysalic acid, used to relieve symptoms of pain and fever. Syn: aspirin.

achalasia, inability of muscles or sphincters to relax.

ache, a continued dull or severe pain.

Achilles tendon, connects the muscles of the calf of the leg to the heel bone.

achlorhydria, abscence of hydrochloric acid in stomach.

acholic, absence of bile.

achondroplasia, dwarfism caused by a defect in the formation of cartilage in which the trunk of the body is of normal size but the limbs are abnormally short.

acroma, an absence of normal pigmentation; albinism.

achromatin, found in a cell nucleus which lacks staining properties.

acid, a sour tasting compound containing hydrogen that easily combines with metals; also, informal term for the hallucinogenic drug LSD.

acid-fast, pertaining to bacteria which are not easily decolorized after staining but retain the red dyes.

acidity, a sour stomach due to an excess of hydrochloric acid.

acidosis, an accumulation of acids causing a disturbance in the acid-base balance of the body often seen in diabetic acidoses or renal disease.

acne, a disease of the sebaceous glands and hair follicles of the skin characterized by blackheads and pimples which usually occurs during adolescence.

acoria, ingestion of large amounts of food; gluttony.

acoustic, relating to hearing or sound.

acoustics, the science of sound.

acquired, originating outside the organism.

acrid, biting or irritating.

acriflavine, an orange granulated powder used as an antiseptic.

acromegaly, excessive growth of the extremities -- fingers, toes, jaw and nose; caused by an overactive pituitary gland.

acromion, the highest extension of the shoulder.

acrophobia, an abnormal fear of high places.

ACTH, a pituitary hormone; adrenocorticotropic hormone that stimulates a specific area of the adrenal glands.

actin, a muscle protein.

actinodermatitis, an inflammation to the skin caused by excessive exposure to the sun or X-rays.

actinomcete, a parasite that causes a fungus disease in animals; sometimes communicated to man.

actinomycin, an anti-bacterial substance effective against gram-positive organisms.

acuity, clarity of vision; sharpness.

acupuncture, method of treatment used for a variety of disorders by puncturing specific points on the body with long needles; a technique first used by the ancient Chinese.

acute, a sudden onset of an illness that is attended by a brief course and severe symptoms.

adactyly, congenital absence of digits of hands or feet.

Adam's apple, prominence on the front of throat produced by the thyroid cartilage.

adaptation, ability of an organism to adjust to its environment for survival.

addict, one who exhibits addiction.

addiction, the state of being physically or psychologically dependent on some agent such as drugs or alcohol.

Addison's Disease, a condition caused by underactive adrenal glands characterized by pigmentation of skin, weakness, fatigue, and digestive disturbances.

additive, a substance added to another to enhance its appearance, or nutritional value.

adduct, the movement of an extremity toward the body's main axis.

adduction, the movement of a limb, the trunk, or head toward the median axis of the body.

adductor, the muscle that adducts.

adenalgia, pain in a gland.

adenectomy, surgical removal of a gland.

adenine, white, crystaline substance found in plant and animal tissues; a decomposition product of nuclein.

adenitis, inflammation of lymph nodes or a gland.

adenocarcinoma, malignant tumor cells occurring in glandular tissue.

adenofibroma, benign tumor cells arising from connective tissue frequently found in the uterus.

adenoids, lymph glands in the upper pharynx which function to trap germs which can enlarge to the point of hindering nasal breathing.

adenoidectomy, the removal of the adenoids by excision.

adenoiditis, inflammation of the adenoids.

adenoma, a benign epithelial tumor in a gland.

adenomatosis, the development of multiple grandular growths.

adenomyofibroma, a fibroma containing muscular and glandular elements.

adenopathy, enlargement and morbid change of glands and lymph nodes.

adenosarcoma, a malignant tumor composed of both glandular and sarcomatous elements.

adenosine, derived from nucleic acid consisting of adenine and the pentose sugar D--ribose.

adenosis, abnormal development of a gland; gland disease.

adenovirus, virus causing disease of the upper respiratory tract.

adermia, absence of skin, congenital or acquired.

adhesion, the abnormal joining of structures or organs which have been separated by incision.

adhesive, adhering; sticky.

adipose, pertaining to fat accumulations in cells.

adiposis, an increase of fat in the body; obesity.

adjuvant, an additive to a drug which enhances the action of a principal prescription.

adnerval, near or toward a nerve.

adnexa, accessory parts of a structure or organ.

adnexopexy, attaching the fallopian tube and ovary to the abdominal wall.

adolescence, beginning of puberty until maturity.

adrenal, pertaining to the kidney or its function.

adrenal gland, an endocrine gland attached to the kidney.

adrenalectomy, excision of the adrenal glands.

adrenalin, epinephrine, a drug used as a heart and circulatory stimulant.

adrenaline, the hormone epinephrine.

adrenergic, activated by epinephrine.

adrenocortical, pertaining to the cortex of the adrenal gland./

adrenocorticotropic hormone, ACTH, an anterior pituitary hormone that stimulates the adrenal cortex of the adrenal glands.

adsorb, to attract and retain other substances.

adsorption, the action of a substance in attracting and retaining other materials to its surface.

adult, having reached full maturity.

adventitia, the outer coat of a structure or organ.

aeration, an exchange of carbon dioxide for oxygen by the blood in the lungs.

aerobe, a microorganism that lives and thrives only in the presence of free oxygen.

aeroembolism, an obstruction within the blood vessel by air or gas.

aeroneurosis, a nervous disorder occurring to aviators.

aerophagia, habitual air-swallowing.

aerosol, a drug or suspension that is dispensed in a fine spray.

afebrile, without fever.

affect, cognitive display of emotion reflecting a mental state.

affective, pertaining to the emotions.

afferent, transporting impulses toward a center.

affinity, a tendency to unite with another object or substance.

afflux, a sudden rush of blood to a part of the body.

afterbirth, after childbirth, the placenta and membranes that are expelled from the uterus.

afterhearing, sensations of sound heard after the stimulus has ceased.

afterimage, the persistence of images after the cessation of stimulus.

afterpains, cramplike pains after expulsion of placenta in the uterus.

aftertaste, a persistent taste after cessation of stimulus.

agar, a colloidal substance from red algae used in solid culture media for microorganisms; also used as a treatment for constipation.

agensia, an imperfect development; sterility.

agglutination, the clumping together of bacteria when exposed to immune serum; a process in wound healing.

agglutinogen, a substance that stimulates the production of agglutinin.

aggregation, a clumped mass of material such as platelets induced by agents.

aglaucopsia, inability to distinguish bluish-green and green tints.

aglossia, the absence of a tongue at birth.

aglossostomia, the absence of the tongue and mouth opening at birth.

agnosia, inability to comprehend sensory impressions.

agonad, an individual without sex glands.

agoraphobia, an extreme fear of open spaces.

agranulocytosis, a marked decrease in the number of granulocytes in the white blood cell count characterized by high fever and prostration.

agraphia, a loss of ability to express thoughts in writing.

agromania, morbid desire to live in solitude.

ague, intermittent malerial fever, characterized by fever, sweating, and chills.

ahypnia, insomnia; sleeplessness.

ailurophobia, unusual fear of cats.

air embolism, an obstruction of a blood vessel brought about by a bubble of air.

akatamathesia, inability to comprehend.

akathisia, motor restlessness due to anxiety.

akinesia, lacking muscular movement.

ala, resembling a wing; winglike appendage.

alalia, unable to speak because of vocal organs paralysis or defect.

alanine, a natural amino acid.

albinism, congenital absence of normal pigmentation; albino.

albumin, a water-soluble protein found in blood, milk, and the white of an egg.

albuminuria, albumin found in urine indicating a kidney disorder.

alcohol, organic compound which can be used as an astringent or antiseptic. Also a common name for ethyl alcohol found in alcoholic beverages.

alcoholism, an addictive disease characterized by a craving for alcohol which interferes with an individual's health, relationships, and economic functioning.

aldehyde, a colorless, flammable liquid resulting from the oxidation of a primary alcohol.

aldosterone, a hormone secreted by the adrenal cortex which regulates the electrolyte and water balance of the organism.

aleukemia, absence of white blood cells.

aleukocytosis, deficiency of white blood cell production.

alexia, inability to read; form of aphisia.

algae, various water plants, including the seaweeds.

algesia, increased sensitivity to pain.

algogenic, producing pain; lowering body temperature.

algophobia, unusual fear of pain.

alienation, a mental disorder; insanity.

alimentary, pertaining to nutrition and digestion.

alkalemia, abnormal alkalinity of the blood.

alkali, a caustic base such as sodium or potassium hydroxide that can neutralize acids to form salts.

alkalinuria, alkali found in urine.

alkaosis, an accumulation of high concentrations of alkali in blood and tissues.

allele, one of two alternative forms of a gene, dominant or recessive, which occupy the same locus on a designated pair of chromosomes that determine heredity.

allergen, any substance inducing hypersensitivity or allergy.

allergist, a specialist in allergies.

allergy, sensitivity to an allergen.

allopathy, a treatment based on producing a condition antagonistic to the condition being treated.

allorhythmia, an irregular heart beat or pulse that recurs regularly.

allotropism, possessing different forms of the same element with unlike properties.

aloe, a plant whose juices are used in pharmaceutical preparations.

alopecia, baldness; an absence of normal body hair.

alum, a crystaline substance used as an astringent and stypic.

aluminosis, chronic inflammation of the lungs due to aluminum-bearing dust.

alveolar, the cavities or sockets found in the jaw for the teeth.

alveolus, a small hollow; socket of a tooth; an air cell of the lungs.

Alzheimer's Disease, a mental disease causing deterioration similar to senility.

A.M.A., American Medical Association.

amalgam, an alloy containing mercury; mixture; blend.

amara, bitters.

amarthritis, inflammation of more than one joint.

amaurosis, loss of vision in which there is no evidence of pathology within the eye itself.

ambidextrous, one who is able to use either hand with equal proficiency.

ambivalence, simultaneous conflicting feelings or emotions toward a goal, person, or object.

Amblyomma, hard-bodied ticks.

amblyopia, dullness of vision without a detectable cause sometimes called ''lazy eye''.

ambulatory, able to move about and not confined to bed.

ameba, a single celled protozoan which moves about and absorbs food by completely surrounding it. Some amebae cause amebic dysentery in man. Also known as amoeba.

amebiasis, ulceration and infection of mucous membranes of the intestinal walls with Entameoba histolytica, the causative agent of amebic dysentery.

amelioration, the improvement of a condition.

amelodential, pertaining to dentin or dental enamel.

amenorrhea, the absence or suppression of menstruation which is normal before puberty, after menopause, and during pregnancy or lactation.

amentia, feeble-mindedness or mental deficiency marked by mental confusion and subnormal intelligence.

ametropia, an abnormal condition of the eye in which vision is affected due to imperfect focus of images on the retina as in astigmatism, hyperopia, and myopia.

amino acid, one of a group of organic compounds containing both an amino and a carboxyl radical which are the building blocks of protein.

aminopyrine, an antipyretic and analgesic which has longer lasting effects in smaller doses than an antipyrine.

aminuria, accumulations of nitrogen-containing compounds found in the urine.

amitosis, cell division without changes in the nucleus or formation of chromosomes.

amitriptyline, an antidepressant drug.

amniocentesis, a surgical procedure which penetrates the uterus for aspiration of amniotic fluid to determine genetic defects.

amnion, the inner membrane which surrounds the fetus and holds the amniotic fluid.

amniotic fluid, the albuminous fluid within the amniotic sac which is colorless and functions to protect the floating fetus.

amnionitis, inflammation of the amnion.

amoeba, see: ameba.

amorphous, shapeless and having no specific form.

amphetamine, a drug used to stimulate the central nervous system. Misuse may lead to drug dependence.

amphoteric, showing or having opposite characteristics and capable of neutralizing both acids and bases.

ampule, a small container for hypodermic solutions.

ampulla, a dilatated end of a tubular structure such as a canal or duct.

amputation, the act of cutting off a limb or appendage by a surgical procedure.

amusia, loss of ability to produce or recognize musical sounds.

A.M.W.A., American Medical Women's Association.

amyelia, absence of the spinal cord at birth.

amygdaline, shaped like an almond; pertaining to a tonsil.

amylaceous, resembling starch.

amylase, pancreatic and salivary juices with enzymes that convert starch into sugar.

amyloid, starchlike, translucent material formed in a variety of diseases and deposited intercellularly.

amylolysis, the conversion of starch into sugar in the process of digestion.

amylopsin, an enzyme in pancreatic juice which converts starch into sugar maltose.

amylum, corn starch used as dusting powder.

amyocardia, weakness of the heart muscle.

amyosthenia, muscular weakness and lacking muscle tone.

amyotrophy, muscular wasting that is painful.

amyxorrhea, an absence of mucous secretion.

ana, used in medical ingredients meaning in equal proportions or of each.

anabiosis, restoration of life after an apparent cessation of vital processes.

anabolism, opposed to catabolism in the metabolic process by which the body substance is built up.

anabolite, a complex substance of anabolism.

anadipsia, intense thirst.

anaerobe, a microorganism that thrives without oxygen.

anakusis, total deafness.

anal, a ring, pertaining to the rectal opening; near the anus.

analeptic, drug that gives strength and is restorative.

analgesic, drug that relieves pain without loss of consciousness.

anallergic, not allergic or hypersensitive.

analysis, separation and or act of determining the compound parts of a substance; separation into compound parts; psychoanalysis involving diagnosis and treatment.

analyst, one who analyzes.

anamnesis, recollection; past history of a patient and his family.

anaphase, third stage in mitosis between metaphase in which longitudinal halves of chromosomes separate and move toward opposite poles.

anaphia, diminished sense of touch.

anaphoresis, insufficient activity of the sweat glands.

anaphrodisia, loss of sexual desire.

anaphrodisiac, a substance that represses sexual desire.

anaphylaxis, an increased sensitivity to a drug, so that a second dose brings about a severe reaction, severe enough to cause serious shock.

anaplasia, an alteration in cells which is believed to produce characteristics of tumor tissue.

anaplastic, restoring of an absent part.

anarthria, speechlessness resulting from the loss of the ability to articulate words.

anasarca, severe generalized edema.

anastaltic, very astringent.

anastomosis, the surgical formation of a passage between two normally distinct organs or spaces; the joining together of parts such as nerves or connective tissue fibers; the union of arteries or veins.

anatomist, one skilled in anatomy.

anatomy, the scientific study of structures of organisms.

anconal, pertaining to the elbow.

ancylostomiasis, infestation with hookworms which gain entrance into the body through the skin of the bare foot of a person causing inflammation, itching, allergic reactions, pneumonia-like symptoms, nausea, and diarrhea. Excessive blood loss leads to anemia.

androgen, a substance producing male characteristics, as testosterone.

androgynous, resembling an androgynoid and without definite sexual characteristics.

androsterone, a male hormone found in urine.

anemia, a reduction in hemoglobin, or in the volume of packed red blood cells. It occurs when hemoglobin is less than 13--14 gm. per 100 ml. for males or 11--12 gm. per 100 ml. for women.

anemic, having anemia.

anencephaly, an absence of brain and spinal cord, a congenital defect.

anesthesia, a lost sense of feeling due to disease or induced to permit the performance of surgery and other painful procedures.

anesthesiology, a branch of medicine which studies the administration of anesthetics.

anesthetist, a person trained to administer anesthetics.

anesthetize, to place under an anesthetic agent.

aneurin, thiamine, or Vitamin B1.

aneurysm, a widening of a blood vessel due to pressure on weakened tissues causing the formation of a sac of blood that may become clotted.

angiasthenia, a loss of tone in the vascular system.

angiitis, inflammation of the coats of either blood or lymph vessels.

angina, a choking, spasmodic, or suffocating pain that characterizes any disease.

angina pectoria, severe pain about the heart that radiates to the shoulder and down the left arm, usually caused by interference with the oxygen supply to the heart muscle.

angiocardiogram, a film produced by an X-ray of the heart and the great vessels after intravenous injection of a radiopaque solution.

angiocarditis, inflammation of the heart and the great blood vessels.

angiography, an examination of blood vessels and lymphatics by roentgen rays which are made visible by injection of a diagnostic solution.

angiology, the scientific study of blood vessels and lymphatics.

angioma, a tumor which is usually benign believed to be misplaced fetal tissue consisting of blood vessels and lymphatics.

angiomyosarcoma, a tumor consisting of a mass of blood vessels or lymphatics resembling elements of angioma, myoma, and sarcoma.

angioneurectomy, excision of blood vessels and nerves.

angioplasty, reconstruction of blood vessels by surgery.

angiospasm, excessive contractions of blood vessels.

angiostaxis, trickling of blood; oozing of blood as in Hemophilia.

angiostenosis, narrowing of a blood vessel.

angulation, angular loops which form in the intestine.

anhidrosis, deficiency of secretion of sweat.

anhydremia, deficiency of the normal fluid content in the blood.

anhydrous, without water.

anhypnia, insomnia.

animation, the quality of being alive, or active. (**suspended, a.** temporary suspension of vital activities).

aniridia, absence of the iris at birth.

anisocoria, inequality in size of the pupils, a normal condition or congenital.

anisocytosis, excessive variations in size of red blood cells indicating an abnormal condition.

ankle, the joint between leg and foot.

ankylo-, combining word form meaning bent or crooked.

ankylocolpos, pathological closure of the vagina.

ankylosis, partial or complete rigidity of a joint as a result of disease, injury, or surgical procedure.

ankyroid, hook-shaped.

anlage, the beginning of cell formation in an embryo which will develop specific tissue, organ, or part.

annular, ring-shaped.

annulus, a ring-shaped structure.

anococcygeal, refering to the anus and coccyx.

anodyne, a medication that relieves pain.

anomalous, irregular or abnormal.

anomaly, deviation from normal resulting from congenital or hereditary defects; a malformation.

anoia, idiocy.

anomia, inability to name objects or to recognize names of persons.

anonychia, without nails.

anopheles, widely distributed mosquitoes, many of which are vectors of malaria.

anopsia, defective vision resulting from strabismus, cataract, or refractive errors.

anorexia, loss of appetite for food.

anorexia nervosa, a lack or complete loss of appetite usually seen in girls and young women; sometimes the disease is accompanied by induced vomiting, emaciation, and amenorrhea. The psychophysiologic condition may also occur in males.

anosmia, absence of the sense of smell.

anostosis, defective development of bone.

anovarism, absence of the ovaries.

anoxemia, reduced oxygen level in the blood.

anoxia, absence of oxygen to body tissues despite adequate blood supply.

ant-, anti-, prefix meaning opposed to or counteracting.

Antabuse, trademark for disulfiram used in treatment of alcoholism.

antacid, an alkali that neutralizes acids in the stomach.

antagonism, opposition between similar muscles, medicines, or organisms.

antagonist, counteracting the action of anything.

antalkaline, neutralizing alkalinity.

ante-, prefix meaning before.

antefebrile, before a fever.

anteflexion, the forward bending of an organ; the normal forward bending of the uterus.

antemortem, occurring before death.

antenatal, before birth.

antepartum, before labor commences.

anterior, directed toward the front.

anterolateral, in front and situated to one side.

anteversion, tipping forward of an organ.

anthelmintic, an agent which is destructive to parasitic intestinal worms.

anthemorrhagic, medication for preventing hemorrhage.

anthracosis, a pneumoconiosis due to the inhalation of coal dust.

anthrax, a disease man contracts from animal hair or waste; a carbuncle; the disease may be of two forms, one on the skin and the other in the lungs. If untreated, anthrax may often be fatal.

anthropo-, prefix denoting relation to man.

anthropogeny, origin of man.

anthropoid, resembling man; tailless apes such as the gorilla, orangutan, and chimpanzee.

anthropology, the science of man in relation to origin, classification, race, physical and mental constitution, environmental and social relations, and culture.

anthropometry, the science of measuring the size, weight, and proportions of the human body.

anthropophobia, a morbid fear of a particular person, or of society. May be the onset of mental illness.

anthypnotic, hindering sleep.

anti-, prefix meaning against.

antianaphylaxis, desensitization to antigens.

antiarrhythmic, an agent alleviating cardiac arrhythmias.

antibacterial, destroying or hindering the growth of bacteria.

antibiotic, a substance produced by a microorganism which has the capacity to inhibit or destroy other microorganisms. Antibiotics are produced by bacteria and fungi and can be made synthetically.

antiblennorrhagic, a substance used to prevent or cure gonorrhea or catarrh.

antibody, a protein produced by the body in response to the presence of an antigen.

anticholineric, an agent that blocks the passage of impulses through the parasympathetic nerves; parasympatholytic.

anticoagulant, acting to prevent clotting of blood; any substance which prevents or delays the coagulation of blood.

anticonvulsive, inhibiting or relieving convulsions.

antidepressant, acting to relieve or prevent depression.

antidiuretic, a substance that acts to suppress excretion of urine by the kidneys.

antidotal, acting as an antidote.

antidote, an agent which neutralizes poison or its effects.

antiemetic, an agent that prevents or alleviates nausea and vomiting.

antienzyme, an agent which inhibits enzymatic action; an enzyme produced by the body retarding the activity of another enzyme.

antiepileptic, an agent that combats epilepsy.

antifebrile, relieving fever.

antigalactic, an agent that suppresses the secretion of milk.

antigen, any substance which induces the formation of antibodies when bacteria or foreign blood cells are introduced into the body.

antihistamine, a substance which counteracts the effects of histamine such as used in treatment of allergies.

antihypertensive, reducing high blood pressure.

antimalarial, acting to relieve or prevent malaria, such as quinine.

antimicrobial, preventing or destroying the development of microbes.

antimony, a metallic element with a crystalline structure used in medicine.

antimycotic, preventing the growth of fungi.

antiparkinsonian, an agent used in treatment of parkinsonism.

antipathy, aversion or disgust; a chemical incompatibility.

antiperistalsis, the peristaltic contractions moving toward the oral end of the gastrointestinal tract.

antiphlogistic, relieving inflammation.

antiprothrombin, anticoagulant.

antipyretic, an agent effective against fever.

antipyrine, an odorless, white crystalline powder used to reduce pain and fever.

antiscabious, relieving or preventing scabies.

antiscorbutic, effective against scurvy such as Vitamin C.

antisepsis, pertaining to sepsis, preventing the growth of germs.

antiserum, a serum containing antibodies specific for the antigen.

antispasmodic, relieving or preventing spasms.

antitoxin, a substance produced by the body capable of neutralizing a specific poison or toxin.

antitussive, an agent which relieves or prevents coughing.

antivenin, a substance used in treatment of animal venom poisoning.

antiviral, an effective agent inhibiting a virus.

antivitamin, an antagonistic substance which inhibits certain vitamins.

antrum, any nearly closed chamber or cavity in bones.

anuresis, a condition in which the kidneys fail to secrete urine.

anuria, failure to produce urine.

anus, outlet of the rectum leading from the bowel.

anvil, one of the three small bones of the middle ear between the stirrup and the hammer.

anxiety, an emotional feeling indicating uneasiness and apprehension; a psychological term.

aorta, the main artery arising from the left ventricle of the heart.

aortic stenosis, a narrowing of the aorta due to lesions of the wall with scar tissue from infection often seen resulting from rheumatic fever or embryonic anomalities.

aortitis, inflammation of the aorta.

apandria, an aversion to men.

apaneuria, impossibility of cloitus.

apathetic, indifferent; lacking interest.

apathy, sluggish; without feeling or emotion.

aperient, a mild laxative usually given at night on an empty stomach.

aperitive, an appetizer; a gentle purgative.

aperture, an opening.

apex, the extremity of anything; used to indicate the uppermost part of a body organ.

aphagia, inability to swallow.

aphakia, absence of crystalline lens behind the pupil of the eye.

aphasia, inability to express oneself through speech; a loss of verbal comprehension.

aphemia, loss of speech due to a central lesion.

aphonia, lack of voice with intact inner speech due to chronic laryngitis, hysteria, psychological problems, or diseases of the vocal cords.

aphrasia, inability in using connected phrases in speaking.

aphrodisia, extreme or morbid sexual passion.

aphrodisiac, a substance that excites sexual desire.

aphtha, a white spot or small ulcer occurring in the mouth.

aphthous stomatitis, recurring blister-like ulcers inside the mouth and on the lips; canker sores.

aphylaxis, absence of immunity.

aplasia, defective development of an organ or tissue.

apnea, temporary cessation of breathing due to reduction of stimuli to respiratory center; may occur during Cheyne-Stokes respiration.

apocrine, cells which lose part of their cytoplasm while functioning, especially mammary gland and certain sweat gland cells.

apodal, having no feet.

apomorphine, a morphine derivative used as an emetic and expectorant.

aponeurosis, a fibrous sheet of connective tissue which attaches muscle to bone or other tissues at insertion.

apophysis, a projection from a bone; an outward growth without a center of ossification.

apoplectic, pertaining to apoplexy.

apoplexy, sudden loss of consciousness followed by paralysis resulting from rupture of a blood vessel of the brain; a stroke.

appendage, anything attached to a larger part.

appendectomy, surgical removal of the vermiform appendix.

appendicitis, inflammation of the vermiform appendix.

appendix, an appendage; the vermiform appendix attached to the cecum.

appestat, a section of the brain, centrally located, controlling the appetite.

appetite, chiefly a desire for food, not necessarily hunger.

apraxia, loss of ability to carry out familiar purposeful movements without motor or sensory impairment.

apyrexia, absence of fever; nonfebrile period of an intermittent fever.

aqua, water; solution.

aquaphobia, unusual fear of water.

aqueous, containing water.

aqueous humor, watery transparent liquid produced by the iris, ciliary bodies, and cornea which circulates through the anterior and posterior chambers of the eye.

arachnoid, resembling a web.

arachnoid membrane, the thin, transparent center membrane that covers the brain and spinal cord.

Aran-Duchenne disease, muscular atrophy beginning in the extremities and progressing to other parts of the body; a progressive muscular atrophy.

archiform, bow-shaped.

arcus, an arc or arch.

arcus senilis, the opaque white ring which appears around the periphery of the cornea, seen in aged persons due to lipoid degeneration.

areola, a small area in a tissue; a small space between tissues that surrounds a skin lesion such as a boil; the colored circle surrounding the nipple; the part of the iris that surrounds the pupil.

areolar, containing small cavities in a tissue such as the glands lying beneath the breasts with ducts opening on its surface; connective tissue within the innerspaces of the body.

ariboflavinosis, a condition caused by a deficiency of riboflavin (Vitamin B2 or G).

arnica, a substance derived from plants used as an application to wounds.

aromatic, a drug or medicine having a fragrant odor.

arrectores pilorum, involuntary muscle fibers contracting under the influence of cold or fright and raising the hair follicles resulting in "goose-flesh".

arrhythmia, a disturbance of rhythm in the heartbeat.

arrhythmic, without regularity; abnormal rhythm of the heartbeat.

arsenic, a poisonous chemical element used in medicine and industry.

ateria, an artery.

arterial, pertaining to an artery or arteries.

arterial bleeding, bright-red blood pumped out of an artery, may be arrested by pressure on the proimal side of the blood vessel nearest the heart.

arterialization, changing venous blood to arterial by aeration.

arteriogram, a radiograph of arterial pulse.

arteriography, radiography of an artery or arterial system after injection with a contrast medium into the blood stream.

arteriola, arteriole, a minute artery, especially one which leads into a capillary at its distal end.

arterioplasty, surgical reconstruction of an artery.

arteriosclerosis, a thickening or hardening and loss of elasticity of the blood vessels and arteries.

arteriospasm, pain in an artery caused by spasms.

arteriostenosis, constriction of an artery.

arteriovenous, pertaining to both arteries and veins.

arteritis, inflammation of an artery.

artery, one of the many vessels carrying blood from the heart to the tissues of the body.

arthralgia, pain in a joint.

arthritic, pertaining to a joint; pertaining to arthritis; a person afflicted with arthritis.

arthritis, inflammation of the joints.

arthrography, an x-ray of a joint after injection with an opaque solution.

arthropathy, any joint disease.

arthroplasty, a surgical procedure upon a joint to make it function.

arthrosclerosis, stiffening of the joints, occurring especially in the aged.

arthrosis, a joint; degeneration of a joint.

arthrosynovitis, inflammation of the synovial membrane of a joint.

articular, pertaining to the joint.

articulation, connection of bones or joints; clearly enunciated speech; in dentistry, the contact relationship of the surfaces of the teeth.

artifact, artificially produced; a structure produced in a tissue or cell by staining.

artificial, not natural; formed in imitation.

artificial insemination, mechanical injection of seminal fluid within the vagina or cervix.

artificial respiration, maintaining respiratory movements by mouth-to-mouth breathing or by mechanical means.

artus, a joint or limb.

arytenoid, resembling a ladle, usually referring to the larynx and relating to cartilage or ligaments.

arytenoiditis, inflammation of arytenoid cartilage.

asaphia, inability to articulate normally due to a cleft palate.

asbestosis, lung disease caused by the inhalation of asbestos particles.

ascaris, infestation of an intestinal parasite.

ascites, excessive fluid accumulation in the peritoneal cavity or abdominal cavity.

ascorbic acid, Vitamin C which occurs naturally or may be produced synthetically.

asepsis, absence of germs; sterile, free from microorganisms.

aseptic, free from germs.

asexual, not sexual.

Asiatic cholera, an acute infectious disease of epidemic proportion.

aspergillosis, a condition produced by Aspergillus fungi producing mycotic nodules in the lungs, liver, kidneys, or on any mucous surface.

aspermia, lack of semen, or failure to ejaculate sperm.

asperous, minute, uneven elevations; roughness.

asphyxia, an interruption of effective gaseous exchange, oxygen and carbon dioxide, resulting in respiratory interference or suffocation.

asphyxiate, to cause asphyxia.

aspirate, to remove by suction; to inhale.

aspiration, to draw foreign bodies in or out by suction through the nose, throat, or lungs; withdrawal of fluid from a body cavity with an instrument called an aspirator.

aspirin, a derivative of acetylsalicylic acid used as an analgesic, antipyretic, and antirheumatic.

astasia, motor incoordination resulting in the inability to sit, stand, or walk normally.

asteatosis, an absence of sebaceous secretion.

asternal, not connected to the sternum.

asthenia, loss of strength; weakness originating in muscular or cerebellar disease.

asthenic, pertaining to asthenia.

asthenopia, tiring or weakness of eye muscles due to fatigue: painful vision.

asthma, a chronic condition characterized by difficulty in breathing and wheezing due to spasmodic bronchial contractions.

asthmatic, pertaining to asthma: one who suffers from asthma.

astigmatic, pertaining to astigmatism.

astigmatism, an imperfection of the eye caused by differences in curvature of the lens and refractive surfaces of the eye so that light rays are not focused properly on the retina.

astragalus, the talus, or anklebone of the foot.

astraphobia, unusual fear of lightening and thunderstorms.

astringent, styptic or contracting: an agent that has an astringent effect; a constricting or binding effect which checks hemorrhages and secretions.

astrocyte, a neuroglial cell resembling a star-shape, collectively named astroglia.

astrocytoma, a malignant tumor composed of astrocytes.

asynergia, incoordination between muscle groups.

asynovia, insufficient secretion of synovial fluid of a joint.

asystole, abnormal contractions of ventricles of the heart.

atactilia, inability to distinguish tactile impressions.

ataractic, a drug that produces ataraxia.

atavism, reappearance of a disease or abnormality experienced by an ancestor.

ataxia, muscular incoordination affecting voluntary muscular movements.

atelectasis, partial or total collapse of the lung; a condition in which lungs of a fetus remain unexpanded at birth.

atelencephalia, congenital anomaly, an imperfect development of the brain.

atelocardia, congenital anomaly, an incomplete development of the heart.

atelocephalus, having an incomplete head.

atelocheilia, incomplete development of the lip; harelip.

atheroma, a sebaceous cyst: a thickening of the wall of larger arteries.

atherosclerosis, localized accumulations of deposits of lipids within the inner surfaces of blood vessels, one of the causes of arterial occlusion.

athetosis, repeated involuntry, purposeless, muscular distortion involving the entire body, especially hands, fingers, feet, and toes.

athlete's foot, a fungus infection of the foot which is contagious: ringworm of the foot.

athrombia, defective blood clotting.

athymia, without emotion or feeling.

atlas, the first cervical vertebra which supports the head.

atom, the smallest particle of an element.

atomizer, a device for dispensing liquid into a fine spray.

atonic, lack of normal tone.

atony, flaccidy and lack of strength; lack of muscular tone.

atopy, a group of diseases of an allergic nature; an acquired or inherited hypersensitivity of the skin to an agent.

atresia, closure of a normal body opening or congenital absence of a body orifice such as anus or vagina.

atrioventricular, pertaining to an atrium and ventricle of the heart.

atrium, the auricles; receiving chambers of the heart.

atrophic, pertaining to or characterized by atrophy.

atrophy, degeneration of the body or of an organ or part.

atropine, an anticholinergic alkaloid which acts to block stimulation of muscles and glands and used as a smooth muscle relaxant; used to dilate the pupil of the eye.

attenuation, the act of thinning or weakening.

attic, the upper part of the tympanic cavity of the ear.

audiogram, a drawing of the audiometer.

audiometer, an instrument for testing the acuity of hearing.

auditory nerve, a sensory nerve of hearing leading to the brain; the eighth cranial nerve.

aura, a subjective feeling that precedes the onset of an attack, such as experienced in epilepsy or hysteria.

aural, pertaining to the ear; pertaining to an aura.

aureomycin, a trademark for chlortetracycline, an antibiotic.

auricle, auricula, the external ear; pina or flap; the atrium of the heart.

auricular, pertaining to an auricle or to the ear.

auriscope, an instrument for making an aural examination.

aurotherapy, treatment of rheumatoid arthritis using gold salts.

auscultate, to examine by listening to the sounds of the viscera.

ascultation, process of listening for sounds produced in the body cavities such as the chest and abdomen to detect abnormalities with a stethoscope.

autism, a self-centered mental state in which thoughts and behavior are not subject to correction by external information.

autistic, self-centered; living in a phantasy of wish fulfillment.

autoclave, an airtight apparatus used to sterilize materials by steam pressure for a specified length of time.

autodigestion, digestion of tissue by their own secretion.

autogenous, self-produced; originating within the body.

autograft, a tissue graft taken from one part of a person's body and transferred to another part of the same body.

autohypnosis, self-induced hypnosis.

autoinfection, infection by microorganisms present within one's own body.

autoinoculation, inoculation of organisms obtained from another part of the body.

autointoxication, poisoning within the body by toxic substances produced within the body.

autolysis, digestion of tissue or cells by ferment in the cells themselves, even after death.

automatism, automatic actions and behavior without conscious volition; the activity of tissues or cells spontaneously such as the movement of cilia or the contractions of smooth muscles or organs removed from the body.

autonomic nervous system, spontaneous control of involuntary bodily functions as part of the nervous system which innervates glands, smooth muscle tissue, blood vessels, and the heart.

autophobia, abnormal fear of being alone.

autoplasty, a replacement of diseased or injured parts with a graft taken from the patient's own body.

autopsy, dissection of a body after death to determine the cause of death; a postmortem examination of a body.

autosome, any non-sex-determining chromosome of which there are 22 pairs in man.

autosuggestion, suggestion or thought originating within one's self.

autotoxemia, self-poisoning due to absorption of a poisonous substance generated within the body.

autotoxin, a toxin generated within the body upon which it acts.

avitaminosis, a condition caused by a lack of vitamins in the diet; a deficiency disease.

avivement, a procedure to hasten wound healing by refreshing the edges of the wound.

avulsion, a forcible pulling away of a part or structure.

axalein, a red dye.

axanthopia, yellow blindness.

axilla, armpit.

axion, pertaining to the brain and spinal cord.

axis, a line, real or imaginary, that runs through the center of the body; the second cervical vertebra of the neck on which the head turns.

axon, axone, a process of a nerve cell which conducts impulses away from the cell body.

azoospermia, absence of spermatozoa from the semen.

azotenesis, a condition caused by an excess of nitrogen in the body.

azoturia, an increased accumulation of nitrogenous compounds in urine.

azygous, singled, not in pairs.

azymia, lack of an enzyme.

B

Babes-Ernst bodies, metachromatic bodies seen in bacterial protoplasm.

Babinski reflex, backward flexion of the great toe when the sole of the foot is stroked, a normal reaction found in children up to one year of age. When the reflex is found in adults it indicates pyramidal tract involvement.

bacillary, relating to or being caused by bacilli, rod-like structures.

bacillemia, presence of bacilli in the blood.

bacilluria, bacilli in the urine.

bacitracin, an antibiotic effective against a wide range of infections.

back, posterior surface of the body; the region of the body from neck to pelvis.

backbone, vertebral or spinal column.

bacteria, bacterium, plant-like microorganisms without chlorophyll.

bacterial, pertaining to, or caused by bacteria.

bactericidal, being able to destroy bacteria.

bactericide, an agent capable of destroying bacteria.

bacteriology, the scientific study of bacteria.

bacteriolysis, destroying bacteria or dissolving them by a specific antibody.

bacteriophagia, destruction of bacteria by a virus capable of inducing lysis.

bacterioscopy, a microscopic examination of bacteria.

bacteriostasis, arresting bacterial growth.

bacterium, (singular of bacteria) single-celled microorganisms called Schizomycetes, having rod-shaped, round, or spiral bodies found in animal tissue, soil, and water.

bacteriuria, bacteria found in urine.

bag-of-waters, the amnion that surrounds the fetus.

baker's itch, eczema caused by yeast irritation.

baker's leg, knock-knee.

balanitis, inflammation of the glans penis.

balanus, the glans penis or glans clitoridis.

barbiturate, a salt used for its sedative effects; hypnotic.

basal metabolism, the process and measurement of cellular activity necessary to maintain life in the fasting and resting state based on oxygen requirements of the individual.

Basedow's disease, Graves's disease; exopthalmic goiter.

basiphobia, morbid fear of walking.

basocytopenia, a decrease of basophil leukocytes in the blood.

basocytosis, excess of basophil leukocytes in the blood.

basophil, applied to cells which are readily stained with basic dyes; a type of white blood cell.

bathophobia, extreme fear of looking downwards from high places.

bathycardia, a condition in which the heart is fixed in an abnormally low position.

battarism, stuttering.

B complex, see Vitamin B complex.

bedsore, see decubitus.

bedwetting, see enuresis.

behavior, conduct; the observable actions and activity of an individual.

behaviorism, a psychological theory based upon objective observation and measurable data, rather than subjective ideas and emotions.

belch, an involuntary escape of gas from the stomach through the mouth.

belladona, a poisonous plant from which a drug is manufactured to relieve spasmodic disorders; active principle of atropine.

Bell's palsy, paralysis of facial nerves and muscles; an acute inflammatory reaction causing distortion to facial muscles.

belly, stomach.

bends, a decompression illness caused by bubbles of nitrogen in the blood and tissues.

benign, not malignant.

Benzedrine, proprietary name for amphetamine; a central nervous system stimulant.

benzocaine, a nontoxic local anesthetic; found in an ointment.

beriberi, a deficiency caused by faulty nutrition and the lack of Vitamin B, uncommon in the United States.

bicarbonate, a salt containing two parts of carbonic acid and one part of a base.

biceps, a muscle with two heads; a major muscle in the upper arm and in the thigh.

bicuspid, premolar tooth; having two cusps; mitral valve between left atrium and left ventricle of the heart.

bifid, split into two parts; cleft or forked.

bifocal, having two foci as seen in eyeglasses that correct both near and far vision.

bifurcate, having two distinct branches; forked.

bifurcation, a division into two branches.

bilateral, relating to two sides of the body.

bile, a bitter secretion of the liver which aids digestion.

bile acids, complex acids which occur as salts and which are important to the digestion of fats in the intestines.

bile duct, a tube which conveys the liver secretion as it leaves the gall bladder.

biharzia, a term used for Schistosoma, the human blood fluke.

biliary, pertaining to the bile or gallbladder or to the passages conveying bile.

bilifulvin, bilirubin mixed with other substances, resulting in a tawny pigment.

bilious, an excess of bile due to a disorder of the liver.

bilirubin, a reddish-yellow pigment in bile, also found in blood and urine.

biliverdin, a greenish pigment found in bile formed in oxidation of bilirubin.

bilobate, having two lobes.

bilocular, divided into two cells or compartments.

bimaxillary, afflicting both jaws.

binocular, pertaining to two eyes.

binovular, derived from two ova.

bioassay, determining the strength of a drug by observing its effects on test animals and comparing these effects with a standard substance.

biocatalyst, a biochemical that dissolves; an enzyme.

biochemistry, the scientific study of living things and the chemical changes that occur during vital processes.

bioclimatology, pertaining to the relations or effect of climate on living things.

biodynamics, the science of energy; biophysiology.

biogenesis, the origin of living organisms.

biokinetics, the science of movement occurring in the developing of organisms.

biological, pertaining to biology; medical preparations used in the treatment or prevention of disease such as serums and vaccines.

biological block, pertaining to the internal mechanism in living organisms that direct the rhythmic cycles of varied involuntary processes.

biologist, a specialist who studies biology.

biology, the scientific study of life and living things; the study of plants and animals.

biometry, the study and computation of life expectancy.

bion, any living organism.

bionomy, the science pertaining to vital functions within the organism.

biophysics, the scientific study of living organisms using the principles of physics.

biopsy, tissue excised from a living organism for examination under the microscope.

biostatics, vital statistics.

biotics, pertaining to the law of living things.

biotin, a component of the vitamin B complex of which the therapeutic value has not been proven.

biotomy, vivisection on living animals for physiological and pathological study.

biotype, a genotype; the basic constitution of an organism.

biovular twins, twins from two separate ova.

biparous, giving birth to twins.

biramous, having two branches.

birth, the act of being born.

birth control, the prevention of pregnancy; any method used to prevent conception such as artificial devices or drugs.

birthmark, a permanent mark from birth injury found on the skin of an infant; nevus.

birth trauma, the emotional stress experienced by an infant at birth which may be a source of neurosis as an adult according to psychoanalytic theory.

bisexual, having both sexes in one individual; hermaphroditic; possessing genital and sexual characteristics of both man and woman.

bisferious, having a double pulse; dicrotic.

bismuth, a silvery white metallic element; it is used in its salt form as an antiseptic, astringent, sedative, and in treatment of diarrhea.

bistoury, a small surgical knife, used for minor surgery.

bitemporal, referring to both temporal bones in the skull.

bituminosis, pneumoconiosis originating from inhalation of dust or soft coal.

black death, a contagious and malignant disease known as bubonic plague.

blackhead, a fatty deposit of dried sebum in a sebaceous gland.

blackout, a sudden temporary loss of consciousness and vision.

blackwater fever, a form of malaria characterized by a sudden rise in body temperature, enlarged liver and spleen, epigastric pain, vomiting, jaundice, dark bloody urine, and shock.

bladder, collecting sac for urine; a reservoir.

bland, mild or soothing; pertaining to diet in which irritating food is avoided.

Blandin's glands, glands near tip of tongue.

blastocyst, a group of undifferentiated cells, the bastula, which develop into an embryo; a stage in the development of an embryo which follows the morula.

blastogenesis, the transmission of characteristics from parents to offspring by genes.

blastoma, a granular tumor.

blastomere, one of the cells into which fertilized ovum separate into segments.

blastomyces, pathogenic yeastlike organisms producing disease.

blastula, an early stage in the development of an ovum that develops into an embryo.

bleb, a blister or pustule.

bleeder, one who bleeds an abnormal amount; see hemophilia.

bleeding time, a natural stoppage of bleeding from a wound or cut, usually about three minutes or less.

blennorrhagia, an accumulative amount of discharge from mucous membranes, esp. gonorrheal discharge from the genital or urinary tract; gonorrhea.

blepharitis, inflammation of the eyelids involving hair follicles and glands causing swelling, redness and crusting.

blepharon, the eyelid.

blindness, inability to see partially or totally; visual impairment as a result of disease, irritation, or accident.

blind spot, a region on the retina where the optic nerve enters the eye and that is in-sensitive to light.

blister, a collection of fluid under the skin due to pressure or injury.

bloated, an abnormal swelling beyond normal size.

blood, the fluid which circulates throughout the body carrying nourishment and oxygen to the cells and tissue, and, at the same time, takes away waste matter and carbon dioxide.

blood bank, a storing place and processing center for reserve blood kept for emergency transfusions.

blood cell, a minute chamber; a corpuscle in the blood; red or white corpuscle.

blood clot, a coagulated mass of blood cells which forms when blood vessels are injured.

blood corpuscle, a circulating cell in the blood; a red cell, erythrocyte, or a white cell, leukocyte.

blood count, determination of the number and type of red and white blood cells per cubic millimeter of blood.

blood group, a classification into which human blood can be based or grouped; blood groups are designated as O, A, B, and AB.

bloodletting, an old method for treating disease by opening a vein and allowing a person to bleed for the specific purpose to reduce blood volume and hence the amount of work required by the heart; phlebotomy.

blood plasma, the colorless fluid of the blood separated by centrifuging.

blood poisoning, a diseased condition caused by the entrance of toxins or microorganisms into the blood stream; toxemia; pyremia; septicemia.

blood pressure, the pressure existing against the inner walls of the large arteries at the height of the pulse when the heart contracts, systolic pressure, and when the heart relaxes, diastolic pressure.

blood serum, the clear liquid that separates from the blood when it is allowed to clot; blood plasma from which fibrogen has been removed.

bloodshot, excessive congestion of capillaries causing inflammation and redness of the eyes.

blood smear, a drop of blood spread on a slide for microscopic examination.

blood sugar, glucose circulating in the blood, normally 60--90 mg. per 100 ml. of blood.

blood test, test of blood sample to determine blood type or the contents (such as sugar) of the blood.

blood transfusion, a technique for transferring the blood from one individual to another directly without being exposed to air.

blood type, determining classification of blood according to blood groups such as O, A, B, or AB.

blood vessel, vessels of the body that transport blood; three major types of bloodvessel: artery, capillary, and vein.

blotch, usually a red or pink spot on the skin.

blue baby, an infant born with a bluish color due to a mixture of venous and arterial blood caused by a defect in the heart.

boil, a microbic infection of the skin; a furuncle.

bolus, a pill-shaped mass.

bone, the hard, dense connective tissue consisting of bone cells that form the skeleton.

bone reflex, a reflex action resulting from a tapping; actually a tendon or muscle response or reflex.

borborygmus, a rumbling sound in the bowels; intestinal flatus.

boric acid, an odorless, white, crystalline powder used as a mild antiseptic, especially for the eyes, mouth, and bladder. In large amounts taken by children it may be poisonous.

botulinic acid, a toxic substance found in putrid meat.

botulism, severe food poisoning containing the toxin produced by Clostridium botulinum.

bougie, an instrument for dilating canals and passages of the body.

boulimia, abnormal hunger sensation after a meal.

bowels, see intestines.

bowleg, an outward bending of the leg.

brachialgia, extreme pain in the arm.

brachium, pertaining to the upper arm from shoulder to elbow.

brachycardia, slowness of heartbeat.

brachycephalic, short headed.

brachydactylia, shortness of fingers.

brachymetropia, nearsightedness; myopia.

bradycardia, unusually slow heart action.

bradykinesia, extremely slow movements.

bradyphagia, slowness in eating.

bradypnea, abnormally slow breathing.

bradyrhythmia, slow pulse rate.

bradyuria, slowness in passing urine.

brain, a large mass of nerve tissue which fills the cranium of man and other vertebrates.

brain fever, meningitis.

brain storm, a temporary outburst of mental excitement often seen in paranoia.

breakbone fever, a sudden febrile disease of epidemic proportion.

breast, the upper anterior aspect of the chest; mammary gland.

breath, inhaled and exhaled air in act of respiration.

breathing, respiration; taking in air and exhaling carbon dioxide.

breech, the buttocks.

breech presentation, the appearance of the buttocks or feet first instead of the head in childbirth occurring in about 3% of all labors.

bregma, the junction of the coronal and sagittal sutures on the surface of the skull.

Bright's disease, a disease of the kidneys usually associated with faulty uric acid elimination and high blood pressure.

broad-spectrum, any antibiotic that is effective against a wide variety of bacteria.

Brocca's area, the speech center in the left hemisphere of the brain which controls the movements of the tongue, lips, vocal cords, or motor speech.

bromides, the salts of bromine used in medication as a sedative and a hypnotic.

bromism, brominism, state of poisoning due to prolonged use of bromides.

bromomania, psychosis induced by use of bromides.

bromopnea, an offensive breath.

bronchadenitis, inflammation of the bronchial glands.

bronchi, plural of bronchus; primary divisions of the thrachea.

bronchial, pertaining to the bronchi or bronchioles.

bronchial tubes, the bronchi that lead from the trachea or windpipe.

bronchiectasis, a condition arising from inflammed bronchial tubes, usually secreting large amounts of offensive, infectious pus.

bronchiole, the smallest branch of the bronchi within the lungs.

bronchitis, an inflammation of the membranes lining the bronchi.

bronchopneumonia, inflammation of the bronchi and lungs caused by various types of pneumococci, pathogenic bacteria as well as viruses, rickettsias, and fungi.

bronchoscope, an instrument for examination of the interior of the bronchi.

bronchospasm, contractions of the smooth muscles of the bronchi which occurs in asthma.

bronzed skin, characteristic of Addison's disease due to adrenal cortical insufficiency.

brow, the forehead; the prominence over the eyes.

brucellosis, an infectious disease which primarily affects cattle, swine, and goats but sometimes affects man; caused by bacteria Brucella.

bruise, a contusion; an injury produced by impact without skin breakage but causing blood vessels to rupture and discolor surrounding tissues.

bruit, a murmur or sound heard in auscultation by means of a stethoscope.

bruxism, the grinding of teeth while sleeping.

bubo, an inflammed or enlarged lymph node, especially in the groin or axilla.

bubonic plague, an acute, infectious disease, frequently fatal, caused by infected rats and ground squirrels who carry the rat-flea which ultimately infects man through its bite; the black death of the Middle Ages.

buccal, pertaining to the cheek or mouth.

Buerger's disease, a recurring inflammatory disease affecting the veins and arteries of the limbs, seen mostly in males between the ages of 15 and 50 years.

bulbous, bulb-shaped; swollen or enlarged.

bulimia, unusual hunger experienced a short time after eating a meal.

bulla, a large blister; a skin vesicle or bubble filled with a watery fluid; the dilated portion of the bony external meatus of the ear.

bundle, group of fibers; a bundle of fibers of the impulse-conducting system of the heart.

bundle branch block, formation of a heart block in which the two ventricles contract independently of each other.

bunion, inflammation and thickening of the bursa of the joint of the great toe resulting from chronic inflammation.

burn, injury to the tissues of the skin as a result of excessive high heat, chemical, or radio-active exposure; burns are classified according to the extent of damage to the layers of skin.

bursa, a sac lined with synovial membrane containing synovial fluid which acts as a lubricant and reduces friction between joints and surrounding structures.

bursectomy, surgical removal of the bursa.

bursitis, inflammation of a bursa.

butacaine, used as a local anesthetic.

butalbital, a sedative.

buttocks, the fleshy prominence formed by the gluteal muscles of the lower back which joins the thighs.

bypass, a shunt performed by surgery creating an alternate pathway for the blood to bypass an obstructed main artery.

bysma, a plug.

byssinosis, a pulmonary disease from inhalation of cotton dust.

byssus, growth of pubic hair.

C

cachet, a wafer in which medicine is placed; capsule.

cachexia, a condition of malnutrition and wasting occurring in chronic illness in the later stages.

cachinnation, hysterical laughter.

cadaver, corpse; dead body.

cadaverous, resembling the appearance or color of a corpse.

caduceus, a symbol of the medical profession.

caesarean, see cesarean.

caffeine, an alkaloid found in coffee and tea which is used as a stimulant, diuretic, and as a treatment for headache.

caffeinism, chronic effects from excessive use of coffee causing heart palpitations, trembling, general depression, anxiety, insomnia, and agitated states.

caisson disease, a painful condition occurring in divers when air pressure is reduced too rapidly after coming to the surface causing nitrogen in the blood and tissues to be released as bubbles; the bends.

calamine, a pink, watery substance composed of zinc and iron oxides used externally as a protective astringent, skin lotion or ointment.

calcaneus, heel bone.

calcar, a spurlike process or projection.

calcareous, containing calcium carbonate; chalky.

calcemia, an excess of calcium in the blood.

calcic, pertaining to calcium or lime.

calcicosis, a pulmonary condition caused by inhaling dust from limestone, especially by marblecutters.

calciferol, vitamin D2 derived from ergosterol; used in treatment of rickets and hypocalcemic tetany.

calcification, the deposit of calcium in the tissues and bone.

calcinosis, an abnormal condition caused by deposits of calcium in tissues.

calcipenia, a calcium deficiency in the body.

calcium, a silvery white metallic element; the basic element of lime, necessary to skeletal structure and body function.

calcium carbonate, a white tasteless powder used as an antacid.

calculus, resembling a stone composed of mineral salts, found in kidneys, bladder, urethra, or other organs and ducts in the body under abnormal conditions.

calf, the fleshy part on the back of the leg below the knee.

calibrator, an instrument for measuring openings.

calisthenics, a systematic exercise routine for improving health, strength, and flexibility in movement.

callus, a thickening or horny layer of skin; the osseous material at the ends of a fractured bone and eventually replaced by new bone growth.

caloric, relating to heat or calories.

calorie, calory, a unit of heat; a measure of energy intake and output of the body; the amount of heat necessary to raise the temperature of one gram of water one degree centigrade.

calorimeter, an apparatus for determining the heat of the body.

calosity, callositas, the formation of thick skin due to pressure, friction, or irritation.

calvaria, human skull cap; cranium skull.

calvities, alopecia, baldness.

calyx, a cup-shaped organ or cavity such as the cup-like structure of the kidney pelvis.

camphor, a gum derived from an Asian evergreen tree used as a topical antipruitic.

camphorated, containing camphor.

canal, a passage or duct.

canaliculus, a tubular small channel or passage.

cancellate, latticelike or porous.

cancer, a malignant tumor; neoplasm; sarcoma or carcinoma characterized by abnormal growth of cells which spread to other tissues.

cancerous, pertaining to malignant growth.

cancroid, appearance of a cancer; skin cancer.

cancrum, a rapidly spreading cancer or ulcer.

canine, pertaining to upper and lower teeth between the incisors and molars of which there are four in number.

canker, a mouth ulcer; thrush; gangrenous inflammation of the mouth.

canker sore, an ulceration of the lips or mouth.

cannabis, the dried tops of hemp plants which produces euphoric states when used as a narcotic; hashish and marijuana.

cannula, a tube used for insertion into a duct or cavity for the purpose of withdrawing fluid or injecting medication into the body.

cannular, a hollow needle.

cantharis, a strong substance derived from crushed blister beetles used in medicine as a diuretic stimulant to reproductive or urinary organs; Spanish fly.

canthectomy, excision of a canthus.

canthitis, inflammation of the canthus.

canthus, the junction or angle of the upper and lower corner of both sides of the eyelids.

capiat, an instrument for removing foreign materials from body cavities, especially the uterus.

capillaritis, inflammation of the capillaries.

capillarity, action by which the liquid's surface is elevated or depressed at the point of contact with a solid.

capillary, minute blood vessel which connects the smallest arteries with the smallest veins.

capital, pertaining to the head.

capitate, head-shaped; having a rounded end.

capitatum, small capitate bone in the hand.

capitellum, the rounded projection or knob of the humerus articulating with the radial head.

capsitis, crystalline lens.

capsula, resembling a capsule; internal capsule of the brain.

capsular, referring to a capsule.

capsulation, enclosed within a capsule.

capsule, a covering usually of gelatin which envelops medication; a small membranous sac.

caput, head; upper part of an organ.

carbohydrase, an enzyme such as amylase and lactase that aids in the digestion of carbohydrates.

carbohydrates, a group of compounds including starches, sugars, celluloses, and gums; organic compounds composed of carbon, oxygen, and water, and classified as monosaccharides, disaccharides, and polysaccharides; carbohydrates provide 47% of calories in the diet and are one of the major sources of nourishment.

carbolic acid, used as an antiseptic and disinfectant derived from coal tar.

carbon, a nonmetallic element found in all living matter in various forms; coal is a common form, a diamond is a crystallized form, and in food it is a fuel which creates heat in animal life.

carbon 14, used in cancer research and archaeological studies.

carbon dioxide, an acid-tasting gas which is heavier than air and exhaled by all living animals; found in the atmosphere as a colorless, odorless non-combustible gas necessary to all plant life.

carbon monoxide, a colorless, odorless, tasteless, poisonous gas which is formed as a result of incomplete combustion and oxidation.

carbon monoxide poisoning, poisoning produced as a result of breathing in carbon monoxide gas and mixing with the hemoglobin of the blood which prevents oxygen from being carried to the tissues of the body causing difficult breathing, dizziness, pounding of the heart, headache, reddish color to face and chest, faintness, and nausea. If the victim can inhale fresh air, he will recover, but if not found in time convulsions, paralysis, and death may occur.

carbuncle, large boil.

carcinogenic, causing cancer.

carcinoid, a benign epithelial growth resembling a cancer.

carcinoma, a cancer; a malignant tumor which infiltrates connective tissues and spreads.

carcinomatophobia, extreme fear of carcinoma.

carcinomatosis, having a widespread dissemination of carcinoma throughout the body.

carcinosarcoma, pertaining to a mixed tumor of both carcinoma and sarcoma.

cardia, the region of the heart; the part of the stomach surrounding the esophagus.

cardiac, heart failure; having heart disease; referring to cardiac orifices surrounding the stomach; a heart medication.

cardiac failure, inability of the heart to pump blood in sufficient volume to meet body needs.

cardiac hypertrophy, enlargement of the heart.

cardiasthenia, weakness of the heart muscles with cardiac symptoms.

cardiataxia, very irregular heart contractions.

cardiectomy, a surgical procedure which involves the excision of the cardiac portion of the stomach.

cardiogram, record of electrical energy changes of the heart cycle.

cardiograph, apparatus for recording the heart cycle on a graph.

cardiologist, a specialist in the treatment and diagnosis of the heart.

cardiology, scientific study of the heart and its functions.

cardioneurosis, functional neurosis with cardiac symptoms such as rapid heart beat.

cardiopathy, any disorder or disease of the heart.

cardiophobia, extreme fear of heart disease.

cardiopulmonary, pertaining to the lungs and heart.

cardiopyloric, referring to both the cardiac and pyloric ends of the stomach.

cardiosclerosis, thickening and hardening of the cardiac tissues and arteries.

cardiospasm, spasm or contraction of the cardiac sphincter of the stomach when the esophagus fails to function properly.

cardiosphygmograph, an apparatus for recording movements of the heart and pulse.

cardiotomy, incision of the heart.

cardiovalvulitis, inflammation of the valves of the heart.

cardiovascular, pertaining to the heart and blood vessels.

carditis, inflammation of the heart muscles.

caries, decay and disintegration of bone or teeth.

carminative, a drug that will remove flatus from the gastrointestinal tract.

carnal, relating to the flesh.

carnophobia, abnormal fear to eat meat.

carotene, a yellow, orange, or red pigment found in some plants and animal tissues; stored in the liver and kidney and converted into Vitamin A in the body.

carotid, the main artery of the neck which divides into the left and right branch that transports the blood from the aorta to the head.

carpal, relating to the joint of the wrist.

carpophalangeal, pertaining to the carpus and the finger bones.

carpus, eight bones of the wrist.

carrier, an individual carrying disease germs without being infected himself; one who transmits a disease without suffering from it himself.

car sickness, motion sickness.

cartilage, dense connective tissue consisting of cells embedded in compact matrix but without blood vessels; gristle; the cartilage or elastic connective tissue composing the skeletal structures of the embryo is converted into bone after birth.

cartilaginous, pertaining to cartilage.

caruncle, an abnormal fleshy growth.

cascara, a laxative.

caseation, conversion of necrotic tissue into a cheese-like granular mass in some diseases; formation of casein during coagulation of milk.

case history, information about a patient's personal or family's history recorded during interview, used especially in social work, medicine, or psychiatry.

casein, the principle protein in milk occurring in milk curds.

caseous, resembling cheese.

cassia, used as a laxative derived from a plant in the form of senna.

cast, a mold made of plaster of Paris to hold a bone rigid and straight as in fractures, dislocations, and other serious injuries.

castor oil, a sticky oil used as a purgative derived from the castor bean.

castrate, to remove the testicles or ovaries.

castration, destruction or excision of the testicles or ovaries.

castration complex, morbid fear of castration.

catabasis, decline of a disease or illness.

catabolic, pertaining to catabolism.

catabolism, the breaking-down phase of metabolism in which complex substances are converted to simpler substances; the opposite of anabolism.

catalepsy, a neurosis characterized by a temporary loss of the senses and the power to move the muscles; trance-like.

catalyst, an agent that causes a chemical reaction or change.

catamenia, menses; periodic menstrual discharge from the uterus.

catamnesis, the medical history of a patient documented by the physician after the first examination including subsequent visits.

cataphasia, a speech disorder causing involuntary or constant repetition of the same phrase or word.

cataphora, lethargy with intermittent periods of waking.

cataphoria, a condition in which a downward turning of the visual axis of each eye continues after the visual stimuli have been removed.

cataplasia, degeneration change in which cells and tissues revert to earlier, more primitive conditions.

cataplasm, a poultice, usually with a medication.

cataplexy, cataplexia, resembling a stroke; sudden shock with a temporary loss of muscular weakness and muscle tone; often a result of emotional shock, sudden onset of an illness, or associated with narcolepsy.

cataract, a condition of the eye caused by a clouding of the crystalline lens or its capsule or both which prevents normal vision.

catarrh, inflammation of the mucous membranes with a discharge of mucus secretions, particularly from the upper respiratory tract.

catatonia, type of schizophrenia characterized by immobility and unresponsiveness; stupor; exhibiting fixed posturing and refusal to communicate.

catatonic, pertaining to catatonia.

catatropia, the downward turning of both eyes.

catgut, a cord or surgical thread that is sterile and absorbable used for tying or binding blood vessels, usually made of twisted sheep's intestine or silk.

catharsis, a purging of the bowels; in psychoanalysis, experiencing emotional release by recalling an event that precipitated a psychoneurosis; abreaction.

cathartic, pertaining to catharsis.

catheter, a tube of elastic, elastic web, rubber, glass, or metal used for evacuating or injecting fluids.

catheterization, inserting a catheter into a body channel or cavity.

cathexis, the attachment of emotional or mental energy to an idea or object.

cauda, taillike structure.

caudad, toward the tail or posterior direction of the body.

caudal, pertaining to any tail-like structure; inferior in position.

caudate, having a taillike projection.

caul, the great omentum; membranous amnion covering the head of the fetus at birth.

causalgia, burning pain.

caustic, corroding and burning; an agent capable of destroying tissue.

cauterization, burning or cauterizing a part.

cauterize, to burn or sear with a cautery.

cautery, destroying tissue by application of electricity, heat, or corrosive chemicals.

caval, pertaining to the vena cava.

cavernous, containing hollow spaces.

cavity, hollow space; a hollow place within the body or one of the organs; hole in a tooth or a dental cavity.

cecectomy, surgical removal of part of the cecum or incision of the cecum.

cecitis, inflammation of the cecum.

cecoileostomy, an opening or stoma into the ileum.

cecoptosis, displacement of the cecum.

cecostomy, surgical creation of an artificial opening into the cecum.

cecum, a pouchlike formation at the beginning of the large intestine and bears at its lower end the vermiform appendix; any blind sac.

celiac, pertaining to the abdominal cavity.

celiac disease, a chronic intestinal disorder occurring in infants and children due to a dietary deficiency.

cell, a small enclosed chamber containing a nucleus within a mass of protoplasm which is the basic structure of all living things.

cellular, pertaining to, or composed of cells.

cellulase, an enzyme produced by snails or molluscs used in medicine to convert cellulose to celloboise; used as a digestive aid.

cellulitis, inflammation of connective tissues.

celluloneuritis, inflammation of nerve cells.

cellulose, a carbohydrate forming the framework of plants; plant fiber.

cell wall, boundary lying outside the cell membrane.

cementum, thin layer of bony tissue deposited by cementoblasts which form the dentine or outer surface of the root of a tooth.

cenogenesis, appearance of characteristics in a person which are absent in ancestors and which do not have a phylogenetic importance.

cenotype, common or original type.

centigrade, pertaining to a thermometer in which the boiling point is 100° and the freezing point is 0°.

central nervous system, abbr. CNS, brain and spinal cord, including nerves and end organs which control voluntary action; voluntary nervous system.

centrifuge, an apparatus used in testing corpuscles in the blood, and solids in urine by employing centrifuging force which hastens sedimentation.

cephalad, toward the head.

cephalagia, pain in the head; headache.

cephalhematoma, a swelling of the subcutaneous tissues containing blood, frequently found on the head of a newborn infant a few days after delivery.

cephalic, pertaining to the head.

cephalitis, encephalitis; inflammation of the brain.

cephalometer, an instrument for measuring the head.

cephalonia, enlarged head marked by idiocy.

cera, wax.

cerebellar, pertaining to the cerebellum.

cerebellitis, inflammation of the cerebellum.

cerebellospinal, relating to the cerebellum and spinal cord.

cerebellum, posterior portion of the brain which controls voluntary muscular movements, equilibrium, and posture.

cerebral, pertaining to the cerebrum or brain.

cerebral hemorrhage, resulting from a ruptured blood vessel in the brain associated with disease, accident, or high blood pressure.

cerebral palsy, brain damage, usually occurring at birth, characterized by incoordination of muscular activity, spasms, and abnormal speech.

cerebritis, inflammation of the brain.

cerebromalacia, softening of the brain.

cerebromeningitis, inflammation of the brain and its membranes.

cerebrosclerosis, hardening of the brain, esp. of the cerebrum.

cerebrospinal, pertaining to the brain and spinal cord.

cerebrospinal fluid, a watery substance produced by the choroid plexuses in the lateral ventricles situated at the base of the brain which acts as a cushion protecting the brain.

cerebrum, the largest part of the brain consisting of the left and right hemisphere being united by the corpus callosum and the anterior and posterior commissures.

cerumen, earwax.

cervical, pertaining to the neck of the womb.

cervicitis, inflammation of the cervix.

cervitamic acid, crystalline ascorbic acid; Vitamin C.

cervix, narrow part of the uterus; part of an organ resembling a neck.

cervix vesicae, the neck of the bladder.

cesarean, abdominal operation to remove an infant from the womb; cesarean section.

cestode, belonging to the subclass Cestoda; a parasitic tapeworm found in the alimentary tract.

cestoid, resembling a tapeworm.

cetrimonium bromide, a quaternary ammonium compound used as an antiseptic and detergent; applied topically to the skin as a disinfectant.

chafe, injury by friction or rubbing.

chalazion, a sty; small, hard sebaceous cyst developing on the eyelids.

chancre, a syphilitic ulcer usually occurring two or three weeks after infection.

chancroid, a nonsyphilitic soft veneral ulcer, highly contagious.

change of life, menopause; climacteric.

chapped skin, skin which becomes dry, split, and cracked due to overexposure to a harsh environment and decreased activity of glands in the surrounding area.

charting, recording the progress of an illness or disease which also gives information about the patient and his treatment; a clinical chart or record.

chauffage, treatment with a cautery at low heat that is applied close to the tissue.

cheek, fleshy portion of either side of the face below the eyes; pertaining to the mucous membranes within the inner surface of the mouth.

cheekbone, zygomatic bone.

cheilitis, inflammation of the lip.

cheilosis, a condition of the lips characterized by dry scaling, fissures, and reddened appearance at the angles of the mouth, resulting from Vitamin B deficiency.

cheirospasm, writer's cramp; spasms of the muscles of the hand.

chemical, pertaining to chemistry.

chemocautery, application of a caustic substance in cauterization.

chemoprophylaxis, prevention of a disease by drugs or chemical agents.

chemosis, edema of the conjunctiva of the eye.

chemosurgery, destruction of diseased tissue by chemical agents for therapeutic purposes.

chemotaxis, movement of living cells in response to a chemical stimulus.

chemotherapy, treatment of disease by chemical agents.

cherophobia, extreme fear of and aversion to gaiety.

chest, the thorax which encloses the ribs.

Cheyne-Stokes respiration, irregular type of arrhythmic breathing occurring in acute illness or in certain acute diseases of the central nervous system, heart, lungs, and occasionally involving intoxication.

chiasm, a crossing of tendons or nerves; a structure in the forebrain formed by fibers of the optic nerves.

chickenpox, varicela; a highly contagious disease characterized by vesicular eruptions on the skin and mucous membranes.

chiggers, a six-legged reddish mite larva which burrows beneath the skin producing wheals, intense itching and sever dermatitis.

chilblain, inflammation, swelling, and itching of the ears, fingers, and toes produced by frostbite.

childbed, puerperal period in childbearing.

childbirth, process of giving birth; parturition.

chill, shaking of the body when affected by cold temperatures or occurring with certain diseases such as malaria; shivering.

chiropodist, podiatrist; one who treats foot irregularities.

chiropractic, manipulative treatment based on the theory that all diseases are caused by interference with spinal nerves and can be treated by adjusting the spinal column.

chiropractor, one who practices chiropractic manipulation.

chirospasm, see cheirospasm.

chloasma, discoloration of pigment in skin occurring in yellowish brown patches or spots.

chloral, an oily, bitter tasting substance derived from chlorine and alcohol.

chloral hydrate, colorless crystalline substance used as a sedative and hypnotic.

chloramphenicol, a broad-spectrum antibiotic made synthetically used especially to treat typhoid fever.

chloride, a salt of hydrochloric acid.

chlorinated, treat with chlorine.

chlorinated lime, used in solution as a bleach and as an antiseptic derived from calcium hypochlorite.

chlorine, a yellowish-green irritating gas used in compounds as a bleaching agent and germicide; a poisonous gas which can cause severe damage to the mucous membranes of the respiratory passages and cause death if inhaled in excessive amounts.

chloroform, colorless, heavy liquid with a sweet taste and ethereal odor used as a solvent, general anesthetic, locally in liniments, and internally as a carminative or a sedative.

chloroma, green cancer of the cranial bones; a greenish colored malignant tumor found in myeloid tissue.

Chloromycetin, trademark for chloramphenicol, an antibiotic.

chloromyeloma, multiple growths in bone marrow.

chlorophyll, green coloring matter found in plants and which acts in the manufacture of simple carbohydrates.

chloropsia, vision in which all things appear green.

chlorosis, iron deficiency anemia.

chlorpromazine, a major tranquilizer used in treatment of psychotic states; trademark name is Thorazine; used as an antiemetic.

chlorpropamide, an oral hypoglycemic used to treat mild diabetes.

chlortetracycline, a broad-spectrum antibiotic which destroys strains of streptococci, staphylococci, pneumococci, rickettsiae, and some viruses; trademark name is Aureomycin.

choke, to interrupt respiration by obstruction or by constriction about or by the neck; strangle; spasm of the larynx; suffocate.

cholangitis, inflammation of the bile ducts.

cholecystectomy, surgical removal of the gallbladder.

cholecystitis, acute or chronic inflammation of the gallbladder.

cholesystography, examination of the gallbladder by x-ray.

cholecystolithiasis, cholelithiasis, the formation of gallstones in the gallbladder.

cholecystopathy, any gallbladder disease.

cholecystotomy, incision of gallbladder to remove gallstones.

choledochitis, inflammation of the common bile duct.

choleic, pertaining to the bile.

cholelithotomy, surgical removal of gallstones.

cholemia, presence of bile pigments in the blood causing jaundice.

cholera, an acute, infectious disease caused by Vibrio cholerae, characterized by diarrhea, severe cramps of muscles, vomiting, and exhaustion.

choleretic, an agent that increases bile production.

choleric, quick-tempered; easily irritated.

cholesteatoma, a small, pearl-like tumor occurring in the brain.

cholesterol, fatty, steroid alcohol found in animal tissues, occurring in egg yolk, oils, fats, and organ tissues; constitutes the largest portion of gallstones; most of the cholesterol is synthesized in the liver, and it is important to bodily metabolism.

choline, an amine found in plant and animal tissues which is important to normal fat and carbohydrate metabolism.

cholinergic, pertaining to nerve endings which produce acetylcholine which is important in the transmission of nerve impulses.

chondral, pertaining to cartilage.

chondroma, a slow growing cartilaginous tumor.

chondromalacia, abnormal softening of cartilage.

chondropathy, any disease of the cartilage.

chorda, referring to a chord, string, or tendon.

chorditis, inflammation of the vocal cord.

chorea, muscular twitching of the limbs; known as St. Vitus' dance or Sydenham's chorea, a disease of the central nervous system; Huntington's chorea is a hereditary form marked by mental deterioration.

chorion, the outermost embryonic membrane from which chornionic villi develop and connect with the endometrium from which the fetal part of the placenta forms.

chorionic, pertaining to the chorion.

chorioretinitis, inflammation of the choroid and retina.

choroid, the vascular coat of the eye between the sclera and retina.

choroiditis, inflammation of the choroid membrane.

chromatelopsia, color blindness.

chromatid, either of the two chromosomal bodies resulting from cell division, each drawn to a different pole.

chromatin, the specific portion in the nucleus of a cell that stains readily with basic dyes, and is considered to carry hereditary characteristics in the genes.

chromatosis, pathological skin pigmentation.

chromaturia, abnormal color of the urine.

chromocystoscopy, examination of kidney functions by use of dyes.

chromoscopy, examination of renal function by color of urine after dyes have been administered; testing for color vision.

chromosomal, pertaining to chromosomes.

chromosome, found in all plant and animal cells; a structure in the nucleus containing threads of DNA responsible for transmitting genetic information; there are 23 pairs of chromosomes in man.

chronic, recurring or occurring over a long period of time; in reference to a disease that is not acute.

chyle, a milklike substance found in the intestinal lymphatic vessels, produced during digestion, especially fats.

chylopoiesis, the formation of chyle.

chylothorax, chyle in the pleural cavity or chest.

chylous, pertaining to chyle.

chyme, the liquid mixture of partially digested food and gastric juices during digestion found in the stomach and small intestine after a meal.

chymotrypsin, an enzyme found in the intestine combined with trypsin which hydrolyzes protein to peptones.

cicatrix, healed wound; scar.

cilia, hairlike projections that arise from epithelial cells as found in bronchi, which transport mucus and dust particles upward; eyelashes.

ciliary, pertaining to eyelashes and to eye structures such as ciliary body.

ciliary body, consists of ciliary processes and ciliary muscle that extends from the iris base to the choroid.

cillosis, spasmodic twitching of the eyelid.

cinchona, a tree or shrub whose bark is the source of quinine.

cinchonism, poisoning resulting from overdoses of cinchona or quinine, characterized by headache, deafness, dizziness, and ringing of the ears.

circulation, movement of blood through the blood vessels of the body maintained by the pumping action of the heart.

circulatory, pertaining to circulation.

circumcision, the cutting around or removal of the foreskin of the penis.

cirrhosis, inflammation of an organ characterized by degenerative changes, particularly the liver.

cirrhotic, affected with or pertaining to cirrhosis.

cirsectomy, surgical removal of a part of a varicose vein.

cirsotomy, treatment for varicose veins with multiple incisions.

citric acid, an acid derived from citrus fruits used to flavor pharmaceuticals; important to metabolism.

citric acid cycle, Kreb's cycle, involved and complicated reactions pertaining to the oxidation of pyruvic acid in metabolism and converting it into energy for the body.

clamp, used for surgical procedures to compress a part or structure such as a blood vessel.

clap, see gonorrhea.

claudication, lameness; limping due to severe pain in the muscles of the calf resulting from decreased blood flow.

claustrophobia, an obsessive, intense fear of closed spaces.

clavicle, collarbone; a curved bone which joins the sternum and the scapula.

clavicular, pertaining to the clavicle.

clavus, a corn.

cleft palate, a congenital malformation in the roof of the mouth which forms a communicating opening between the mouth and the nasal cavities.

cleidorrhexis, bending or fracturing the clavicles of the fetus to ease delivery.

cleptomania, the impulsive act of stealing.

climacteric, menopause; cessation of a woman's reproductive period; corresponding period in a male characterized by decreased sexual activity.

clinic, a medical center for examination, diagnosis, and treatment for non-hospitalized patients.

clinical, pertaining to a clinic; pertaining to actual observation and treatment of patients.

clinician, a specialist in clinical procedures such as a clinical physician, teacher, or nurse; practicing physician.

Clinistix, trademark for glucose oxidase reagent strips to test urine for glucose.

clitoris, an organ of the female genitalia; an erectile structure located beneath the anterior part of the vulva.

clonic, alternate contraction and relaxation of muscle groups in rapid succession.

clonicity, condition of being clonic.

clonus, opposite of tonus.

Clostridium, a genus of spore-bearing anaerobic, rod-shaped bacteria commonly found in soil and in the intestinal tract of animals and man; frequently found in wound infections and the primary cause of gangrene and tetanus.

clot, coagulated blood or lymph; a thrombus.

clotting time, see coagulation time.

clouding of consciousness, state of mental confusion characterized by disorientation of time and place, amnesia, and decreased reaction time due to illness.

cloudy swelling, degeneration of tissues which become swollen and turbid.

clubbed fingers, broadening and rounding of the fingertips due to swelling, often seen in children with congenital heart disease and adults with pulmonary disease of long duration.

club-foot, congenital foot deformity.

clumping, see agglutination.

clunes, buttocks.

clysis, injection of a cleansing fluid for washing out blood in a cavity.

C.N.S., see central nervous system.

coagulability, being capable of forming clots.

coagulant, an agent responsible for coagulation.

coagulate, cause a clot or to become clotted.

coagulation, process of clotting.

coagulation time, period of time required for blood to clot or coagulate which is indicated when fibrin appears in tiny threads; normal clotting time is between 3 to 7 minutes.

coagulum, clump of clotting blood.

coarctate, pressed together; to tighten.

coarctation, compression of vessel walls; narrowing or tightening.

coarctotomy, division of a stricture by incision.

coat, a layer in the wall of an artery.

cobalt, a chemical element; cobalt 60 is a radioisotope of cobalt used in radiation therapy.

cocaine, a bitter alkaloid obtained from coca plants used in medicine as a local anesthetic and as a narcotic.

cocarcinogenesis, the development of cancer in preconditioned cells.

coccidia, sporozoa which are commonly found in epithelial tissue of the intestinal tract, the liver, and other organs in the body.

coccygeal, pertaining to the coccyx.

coccygectomy, removal of the coccyx by surgery.

coccygodynia, pain in the coccyx and the surrounding area.

coccyx, usually referring to the last four bones of the spine which attach to the sacrum.

cochlea, a cone-shaped, winding structure in the inner ear containing the organ of corti which is the receptor for hearing.

cochleitis, inflammation of the cochlea.

cocoid, resembling a cocus.

coconscious, coconsciousness, a conscious objective state in which subconscious impressions may rise to the surface and influence the stream of consciousness.

cocoa butter, a fat obtained from cocoa seed used as a lubricant in pharmaceuticals.

cocus, a spherical bacterium; organisms of the genus staphylococcus, and micrococcus.

codeine, an alkaloid from opium or synthetically produced, used as an analgesic and hypnotic sedative.

cod liver oil, a fixed oil obtained from cod fish livers used for its Vitamin A and D.

cohabitation, sexual intercourse; living together.

coherent, sticking together; being logically consistent.

cohesion, the process of sticking together; adhering; causing particles to unite.

coitus, sexual intercourse; copulation.

colchicum, a drug derived from the Colchicum seed used to relieve symptoms of gout.

cold, common viral infection of the respiratory mucous membranes causing symptoms of nasal congestion, headache, coughing, body aches, fatigue, fever, and chills.

cold sore, a fever blister particularly around the mouth caused by herpes simplex virus.

colectomy, excision of part of the large intestine or colon.

colic, spasms accompanied by abdominal pain; pertaining to the colon; occurring in infants, especially in the first few months of life.

colicstitis, cystitis caused by Eschericia coli.

colitis, inflammation of the colon.

collagen, a substance composed of white fibers of connective tissue found in the skin, tendons, cartilage, and bone; a body protein composed of connective tissue fibers.

collapse, a sudden caving in of the walls of an organ; an extreme loss of vital functioning of organ systems producing shock or breakdown.

collarbone, the clavicle.

collecting tubules, small ducts which receive urine from the renal tubules.

Colles' fracture, fracture of the distal end of the radius (just above the wrist bone).

colliculus, small anatomical mound.

collodion, a substance applied to the skin which forms a very thin protective layer.

colloid, a gelatinous protein found normally in thyroid secretion.

colloma, colloid degeneration found in cancerous tissue.

collutory, used as a gargle or mouth wash.

collyrium, a neutral solution used as an eyewash.

coloboma, an eye defect, usually due to an abnormal closure of the fetal fissure which may affect any part of the eye.

colon, the section of the large intestine between the cecum to the rectum.

color blindness, a hereditary condition in which a person is totally or partially unable to distinguish between certain primary colors; chromatolepsia:

colostomy, a surgical procedure that provides an opening between the colon and the abdominal wall creating a stoma.

colostrum, the first secretion of the breasts after childbirth before lactation commences, within a two to three day period, containing high protein and immunity factors for the newborn.

colotomy, incision of the colon.

colpalgia, vaginal pain.

colpitis, vaginitis.

colpocystitis, inflammation of both the bladder and vagina.

copocystocele, prolapse of the bladder into the vagina.

colpohysterectomy, excision of the uterus through the vagina.

coloplasty, plastic repair involving the vagina.

colpoptosis, prolapse of the vagina.

colporrhapy, suturing the vaginal wall for the purpose of narrowing it.

colposcope, an instrument for examining the cervix and vagina.

coma, a state of abnormal unconsciousness from which a person cannot respond to external stimuli due to illness or an injury; stupor.

comatose, pertaining to coma.

comedo, a blackhead caused by dried sebum blocking a duct in the skin.

comminute, breaking into pieces such as a shattered bone.

comminution, comminuting or reducing to fine particles.

commissure, joining together of corresponding structures such as lips or eyelids; a band of nerve fibers coming together.

communicable disease, transmission of a disease from one person to another either directly or indirectly.

compensation, making up for some abnormality.

complemental, adding something that is deficient.

complex, a group of associated ideas which are usually unconscious, believed to be influencing factors of abnormal attitudes and mental states.

complication, a complex state in which disease or accident is added to an existing illness without being related specifically.

compos mentis, sane; of sound mind.

compound, a substance composed of two or more parts.

compound fracture, bone which is broken and pierces the skin.

compress, a soft pad, moist or dry, applied to a part of the body with pressure to prevent hemorrhage, or to apply medication, heat or cold.

compression, being pressed together.

compulsion, an insistent, repetitive, and unwanted urge to perform an irrational act; state of being compelled.

compulsive, exhibiting repetitive patterns of behavior.

concave, a rounded, hollowed out surface, or cavity.

concavity, a concave surface.

concavoconvex, being concave on one side and convex on the other side; pertaining to the lens of the eyes.

conceive, to become pregnant; to form a mental image or an idea.

concentration, increasing in strength of a substance by evaporation.

concept, a mental image of an idea.

conception, the beginning of pregnancy when the ovum is fertilized by a sperm forming a zygote.

concha, a structure resembling a shell; the pinna or outer ear; one of the three bones on the nasal cavity.

conchitis, inflammation of a concha.

concretion, a calculus; an inorganic mass found in a body cavity or tissues.

concubitus, sexual intercourse, copulation, coition.

concussion, an injury resulting from a collision or impaction with an object; partial or complete loss of bodily functions resulting from a violent shock or a blow to the head.

conditioned reflex, acquired response through repetition and training.

condom, a thin rubber sheath to be worm over the penis during sexual intercourse to prevent impregnation or veneral disease.

condyle, a rounded projection at the end of a bone which articulates with another bone.

condylectomy, excision or removal of a condyle.

condyloma, a wartlike lesion on the skin occurring on the mucous membranes or external genitals or near the anus.

confabulation, an unconscious replacing of imaginary experiences due to memory loss, seen principally in organic mental disorders.

confinement, period of childbirth or puerperal state.

confusion, disturbance in orientation to time, place, or person; a psychological evaluation pertaining to a disordered consciousness.

congenital, present at birth, including conditions arising from fetal development or the birth process that are not hereditary.

congest, to cause an abnormal amount of blood to accumulate in an organ.

congestion, the presence of an excess amount of fluid in an organ or in tissue.

congestive, pertaining to congestion.

conization, excision of a cone of tissue pertaining to the cervix.

conjugate, paired; working together; an important measurement in the diameter of the pelvis.

conjugation, a coupling.

conjunctiva, mucous membranes lining the eyelids and covering the anterior surface of the eyeball.

conjunctivitis, inflammation of the conjunctiva.

connective tissue, primarily functions to support or bind together bodily tissues, organs, and parts; other functions include food storage, blood formation, and defensive mechanisms.

consanguinity, kinship; blood relationship.

conscience, associated with superego; a person's set of moral values which controls his behavior and performance.

conscious, being aware of one's existence and having the ability to respond subjectively to stimuli; awake.

consciousness, awareness; being conscious.

consolidation, the process of becoming solid, referring to a condition in the lungs due to an accumulation of fluid in acute pneumonia.

constipation, irregular, difficult, or sluggish defecation.

constitution, the functional habits and physical properties of the body; a disposition, temperament, or condition of the mind.

constitutional, pertaining to the whole body.

constriction, a narrowing of a part or opening.

consultant, acting in an advisory capacity.

consultation, two or more specialists who deliberate about diagnosis and treatment of a client.

consumption, pertaining to tuberculosis; wasting away of the body.

consumptive, one afflicted with tuberculosis.

contact, one who has been exposed to a contagious disease; touching of two bodies.

contact lens, a thin concave disk which fits on the convex surface of the eyeball and floats on the fluid of the eye, helpful in correcting impaired vision.

contagion, the process of spreading a disease from one person to another by direct or indirect contact.

contagious, a readily transmitted disease either directly or indirectly from one person to another; communicable.

contaminate, the act of soiling or exposing to infectious germs into normally sterile objects; render impure by contact or mixture.

continence, the practice of self-restraint in sexual indulgence.

contortion, a spasmodic twisting or writhing of the body; distortion.

contraception, the prevention of conception.

contraceptive, an agent or device to prevent conception or impregnation.

contraction, a shortening or drawing up of a muscle; a shrinking.

contracture, a permanent contraction or shortening of a muscle due to spasm, fibrosis of tissues, or paralysis.

contraindication, a condition or circumstance that indicates that a form of treatment of medication is inappropriate in a specific case.

contralateral, affecting the opposite side of the body.

contuse, to injure or wound by bruising.

contusion, an injuring to the skin without breaking the flesh; a severe bruise.

convalescence, a recovery period after an illness, operation, or injury.

convalescent, pertaining to convalescence; a patient who is recovering from an illness, operation, or injury.

convergence, coordinating the movements of both eyes toward a common point.

convex, having an elevated or rounded surface.

convexoconcave, having one convex and one concave surface, especially the lens.

convolute, rolled or coiled up, as a scroll.

convolution, a folding or coiling of anything which is convoluted; the many folds on the surface of the brain or the intestines.

convulsant, medication or a drug which causes convulsions.

convulsion, severe involuntary muscle contractions with a temporary loss of consciousness due to many causes.

convulsive, pertaining to, characterized by convulsions.

Coombs' test, used in the diagnosis of several forms of hemolytic anemias.

coprolalia, abnormal desire to use obscene words in ordinary conversion.

coprophagy, ingesting of feces.

coprophilia, abnormal attraction to feces and defecation.

coprophobia, an abnormal disgust of filth and feces.

coprostasis, fecal impaction.

copulation, sexual coitus, or the act of copulating.

coracoid process, pertaining to the upper anterior surface of the scapula.

Coramine, trademark for nikethamide used as a respiratory stimulant.

cord, the umbilical cord; stringlike structures such as vocal cords, the spinal cord, or the spermatic cord.

cordate, heart-shaped.

corectomy, surgical removal of the iris.

corium, the dermis; the layer of skin immediately beneath the epidermis which contains vascular connective tissue, nerve endings, hair follicles, sebaceous glands, sweat glands, and smooth muscle fibers.

corn, a horny and thickened area of the skin which may be either soft or hard depending on its location on the foot due to pressure or friction.

cornea, the transparent membrane covering the iris and pupil of the eye.

corneal, pertaining to the cornea.

corneitis, inflammation of the cornea.

corneous, horn-shaped.

cornification, conversion of stratified squamous epithelium cells into keratin, or horn.

corona, resembling a crown.

coronal, pertaining to corona; referring to the suture which joins the parietal and frontal bones in the skull.

coronary, pertaining to a circle or crown.

coronary arteries, two arteries which supply blood to the heart muscles.

coronary occlusion, closure or blockage of one of the coronary arteries.

coronary thrombosis, clotting of blood in the blood vessels which supply the heart; a common cause of myocardial infarction.

coroner, a county officer who investigates any death from unknown causes or violent crimes.

corpulence, obesity.

corpulent, being stout, fat, obese.

corpus, principle part of an organ; any mass or body.

corpuscle, any minute rounded body; a blood cell.

corpusculum, corpuscle.

corpus luteum, a yellowish endocrine substance secreted by the ovary after the rupture of a Graafian follicle and the release of ovum; during pregnancy the corpus luteum persists in secreting the hormone progesterone.

corrode, to wear away by chemical action.

corrosion, disintegrating; the process of corroding.

corrosive, an agent that is destructive to the tissues.

cortex, outer portion of an organ, the brain, and the adrenal glands.

cortical, pertaining to the cortex.

corticosteroids, hormones produced by the adrenal glands.

cortin, a hormone secreted by the adrenal cortex.

cortisone, a hormone extracted from the adrenal cortex of the adrenal gland and also prepared synthetically, important to fat metabolism.

coryza, nasal catarrh resulting from inflammation of the mucous membranes; common head cold.

costa, rib.

costae, the rib cage composed of twelve ribs on each side.

costal, pertaining to the ribs.

costalgia, pain in a rib, or intercostal spaces.

costive, constipated.

costoclavicular, pertaining to the ribs and clavicle.

costovertebral, the joining of a rib to a vertebrae.

cough, a more or less violent expulsion of air from the lungs in an attempt to expel an irritant from the respiratory tract.

counterirritant, the application of an agent to reduce or relieve another irritation.

courses, menses.

cowperitis, inflammation of the Cowper's glands.

Cowper's glands, two composed tubular glands the size of a pea beneath the bulb of the urethra in males.

cowpox, pustular eruptions of milk cows on areas of udder and teats resembling smallpox in man; when virus is contained in vaccine and given to humans against smallpox, it offers some degree of immunity against the disease.

coxa, the joint in the hip or hip bone.

coxalgia, pain in the hip.

cramp, a spasmodic, involuntary contraction of a muscle or group of muscles with pain.

cranial, pertaining to the cranium or skull.

cranial nerves, originating in the brain; there are twelve pairs of cranial nerves.

craniectomy, excision of part of the skull.

craniometry, the science of skull measurement.

cranioplasty, plastic repair on the skull.

craniopuncture, an exploratory procedure in which the skull is punctured.

cranium, including all of the bones of the head that enclose the brain.

crapulent, crapulous, excessive drinking of alcohol; intoxication.

creatine, a nitrogenous compound synthesized in the body which serves as a source of high energy phosphate.

Crede's method, a procedure used in obstetrics whereby the placenta is expelled by employing a downward pressure on the uterus through the abdominal wall; treatment of the eyes of the newborn with 1% silver nitrate solution immediately after birth for prevention of infection.

cremaster, one of the fascialike muscles suspending the testicles and spermatic cord.

cremation, burning of dead bodies by heat.

crepitant, a crackling sound; making a grating sound.

cresol, a substance used as a disinfectant derived from coal tar.

crest, a ridgelike formation on a bone.

cretin, one afflicted with cretinism.

cretinism, a congenital affliction caused by abnormal thyroid secretion, characterized by stunted physical and mental development.

crevice, a small fissure or crack.

cribbing, swallowing air.

cribriform, sievelike; having many small openings.

cribriform plate, a thin, perforated bone in the skull through which many nerve filaments pass.

cricoid cartilage, the lowermost, ringlike cartilage of the larynx.

crinogenic, stimulating secretions in a gland.

crisis, the turning point of a disease marked by a sudden decrease in high temperature to normal; a turning point in illness for better or worse.

cross-eye, esotropia.

cross-matching, testing before transfusion to determine blood compatibility.

croup, a disease occurring in children characterized by inflammation of the respiratory passages causing difficult breathing, laryngeal spasm, coughing, and sometimes exudation due to the formation of a membrane.

crowning, stage in delivery when the fetal head appears at the opening of the birth canal.

crural, pertaining to the leg or thigh.

crus, the leg.

crush syndrome, renal failure following the severe crushing of the lower extremities.

crust, crusta, a scab; an outer covering.

crutch, used to support the body weight in walking. A staff which extends from the armpit to the ground.

cryanesthesia, the inability to perceive cold.

cryesthesia, having an abnormal sensitivity to cold.

cryocautery, cold cautery; a device used for application of solid carbon dioxide.

cryogenic, pertaining to low temperatures.

cryosurgery, the application of extreme low temperatures to destroy or remove diseased tissue.

cryotherapy, crymotherapy, the therapeutic use of cold.

crypt, a small sac or cavity which extends into epithelial or glandular surfaces.

cryptogenetic, of unknown origin.

cryptorchidism, a condition in which the testicles fail to descend into the scrotum.

crystalline, resembling a crystal; clear.

crystalline lens, the lens of the eye behind the pupil.

crystaluria, the appearance of crystal formations in the urine.

crystalluridrosis, urinary elements appearing on the skin as crystallized sweat.

cubital, pertaining to the forearm.

cubitus, elbow; forearm; ulna.

cuboid, referring to the outermost bone of the tatsal or instep bones which connect with the 4th and 5th metatarsus.

cul-de-sac, a blind cavity or pouch.

culdoscopy, a visual examination of the female viscera of the pelvic cavity through an endoscope introduced into the vagina.

Culex, a genus of mosquitoes found throughout the world which are vectors of malaria producing organisms.

culture, a mass of microorganisms growing in a culture medium in the laboratory.

cumulative, increasing in effect or amount; an accumulation of drugs by successive additions or dosages.

cupula, an inverted cup-shaped cap or dome over a structure.

curare, curari, an extract obtained from tropical plants used as an arrow poison by South American Indians; used in anesthesia to control convulsions, spasms, and for skeletal muscle relaxation.

curet, curette, a spoon-shaped instrument used in scraping a cavity to remove foreign matter or a diseased surface.

curettage, scraping of a cavity with a curette.

curie, a standard unit of radioactivity.

curietherapy, radium therapy.

cusp, a point of a crown of a tooth.

cuspid, a canine tooth, of which there are four; a cuspidate tooth.

cuspidate, having cusps.

cutaneous, pertaining to the skin.

cuticle, a layer of solid or semisolid nonliving skin that surrounds fingernails and toenails.

cutis, the skin.

cyanemia, dark blue-colored blood.

cyanide, a fast-acting poison.

cyanocobalamin, Vitamin B12.

cyanopsia, objects appear tinged with blue due to a defect in vision.

cyanosis, a bluish, slatelike, or dark purple skin color due to excessive concentration of reduced hemoglobin in the blood.

cyanotic, pertaining to cyanosis.

cycle, a series of events or a sequence of movements.

cyclic, pertaining to cycles.

cyclitis, inflammation of the ciliary body or ciliary region of the upper eyelid.

cyclomate, an artificial sweetener with no nutritional value.

cycloplegia, paralysis of the ciliary muscles.

cyclothyme, one afflicted with cyclothymia.

cyclothymia, a cyclic disorder of the mind characterized by recurring and alternating periods of sadness and elation.

cyesis, pregnancy.

cyst, a pouch or closed sac under the skin or in the body which contains fluid, semifluid, or solid matter.

cystadenoma, a tumor containing cysts.

cystalgia, a painful urinary bladder.

cystectomy, removal of a cyst; removal of the gallbladder; excision of the urinary bladder or part of it.

cystic, pertaining to a cyst; pertaining to the urinary bladder, or to the gallbladder.

cystic fibrosis, a disease occurring in childhood involving the exocrine glands resulting in pancreatic insufficiency and chronic respiratory disease; believed to be hereditary.

cystitis, inflammation of the bladder.

cystocele, a protrusion of the urinary bladder into the vagina.

cystocolostomy, a surgical procedure that creates a permanent communication between the gallbladder and the colon.

cystoid, resembling a cyst; bladderlike.

cystolith, having a calculus or stone in the urinary bladder.

cystolithectomy, excision of calculus from the bladder.

cystoma, a cystic tumor.

cystoplasty, plastic repair upon the bladder.

cystoscope, an instrument for examining the bladder.

cystoscopy, examination of the bladder with a cystoscope.

cystospasm, a spasmodic contraction of the urinary bladder.

cystostomy, surgical procedure of the urinary bladder to make an opening.

cytobiology, biology of the cells.

cytoblast, a cell nucleus.

cytochemistry, the scientific study of the structure and chemistry of living cells.

cytochromes, iron-containing compounds found in animal and human tissue which play an important role in cellular respiration.

cytogenesis, the origin and development of cells.

cytokalipenia, a deficiency of potassium in the body.

cytokinesis, the movement of cytoplasm into two parts during cell division.

cytology, the study of the structures and functions of cells.

cytolysis, the destruction or degeneration of cells.

cytoplasm, the protoplasm of a cell not including the nucleus.

cytosine, a component of nucleic acid common to both DNA and RNA.

cytoscopy, a diagnostic microscopic examination of cells.

cytotropism, the movement of cells in response to external stimuli.

cytula, the impregnated ovum.

cyturia, the presence of various cells in the urine.

D

dacrocystitis, dacryocystitis, inflammation of the lacrimal or tear sac.

dacryadenitis, dacroadenitis, inflammation of a lacrimal (tear) gland.

dacryocele, protrusion of a lacrimal (tear) sac.

dacryocystotomy, surgical operation of the lacrimal sac.

dacryolith, a calculus or stone in the tear duct.

dacryorrhea, excessive flow of tears.

dactyl, a finger or toe.

dactylitis, inflammation of a finger or toe.

dactylography, the study of fingerprints.

dactylology, communicating by sign language made with the hands and fingers.

dactylolysis, loss or amputation of a finger or toe.

dactylomegaly, abnormally large fingers or toes.

dactylus, referring to a finger or toe; a digit.

daltonism, color blindness, especially in differentiating between red and green.

D and C, pertaining to dilatation of the cervix and curettage of the uterus.

dandruff, dry scales of epidermis forming on the scalp which shed, sometimes due to seborrheic dermatitis.

dandy fever, an acute febrile disease which occurs in the tropics; dengue.

dartos, a fibrous layer beneath the skin of the scrotum.

darwinian ear, a congenital deformity of the helix of the ear.

deaf, lacking the sense of hearing.

deaf-mute, unable to hear or speak.

deafness, complete or partial loss of hearing.

deamination, the removal of the amino group from a compound.

dearterialization, changing arterial to venous blood by deoxygenation.

death rattle, a rattling sound heard in the throat of the dying.

debilitant, drug to reduce excitement.

debilitate, producing weakness or debility.

debility, weakened condition of the body and loss of bodily function; feebleness.

debridement, the removal of foreign matter or dead tissue from a wound.

decalcification, the removal of lime salts from bones; loss of bone calcium.

decalcify, softening of bone by removal or loss of calcium or its salts.

decannulation, to remove a cannula or tube.

decant, to pour off liquid with sediment remaining in the bottom of the flask or container.

decapitation, beheading; to remove the head from the body.

dechloridation, dechlorination, decrease sodium chloride in the body by the removal of salt from the diet.

decibel, a unit of sound measuring intensity and volume.

decidua, the endometrium when conception occurs which divides itself into three layers enveloping the impregnated ovum.

decidual, pertaining to the decidua.

deciduoma, a uterine tumor containing decidual tissue.

deciduous, shedding at a particular stage of growth, especially of temporary teeth.

decimeter, one-tenth of a meter.

declinator, an instrument used in surgery to retract or hold apart the dura matter.

decline, a declining period of a disease or illness.

decoloration, bleaching or the removal of color.

decompensation, the ability of the heart or other organs in the body to maintain adequate functioning; a term used in psychiatry which implies the failure of defense mechanisms resulting in disintegration of personality.

decomposition, decaying process.

decompression, removal of pressure, or removing of air pressure from a chamber; a normal bodily adjustment to atmospheric pressure.

decongestant, a substance or drug that reduces congestion and swelling, especially in nasal passages.

decontamination, rendering free of contamination as in an object or person contaminated by poisonous gas or radioactive substances.

decortication, removal of the surface layer from structures or organs.

decrepit, wasted or worn down by the infirmities caused by the aging process.

decrepitude, senile breaking down.

decubation, recovery stage of an infectious disease.

decubitus, a bedsore; a pressure wound.

decussate, crossing of parts.

decussation, crossing of structures or nerves which form an X; chiasma.

defecation, evacuation of the bowels, or the expulsion of fecal matter.

defective, imperfect; physically or mentally deficient.

defeminization, loss or absence of female sexual characteristics.

deferens, to carry away, as in ductus deferens, excretory duct of the testicles.

deferent, to carry downward.

deferentitis, inflammation of the ductus deferens.

defervescence, subsidence of fever to normal body temperature.

defibrillation, terminating atrial or ventricular fibrillation or irregular heart muscle contractions.

deficiency disease, any disease caused by a dietary insufficiency.

defluvium, sudden loss of air.

defluxion, a flowing down of a copious discharge of any kind.

deformation, disfiguration or malformation.

deformity, a malformation or misshapen part of the body or organ; a distortion of the body or part of the body which may be acquired or congenital.

degenerate, a sexual pervert; to deteriorate.

degeneration, impairment or deterioration of an organ or its parts.

deglutition, act of swallowing.

degradation, act of degrading; conversion of a chemical compound to one less complex.

degustation, act of tasting.

dehiscence, bursting open; separation of the layers of a surgical wound.

dehydrate, to lose moisture or water.

dehydration, excessive loss of body fluids or water; the process of dehydrating.

déjà vu, a sensation that what one is seeing is a repetition of a previous experience.

dejecta, feces.

dejection, dejecture, feeling of being downcast; a state of mental depression; excrement.

delacrimination, a constant overflow of tears.

delactation, cessation of lactation; weaning.

deleterious, injurious or harmful to health or well-being.

delinquent, antisocial, criminal, or illegal behavior, especially significant in a minor exhibiting such behavior.

deliquescence, liquefaction of salts by absorption of water from the air.

delirious, pertaining to delirium.

delirium, a temporary disorientation, usually accompanied by illusions and hallucinations due to various causes such as fever, intoxication, or trauma.

delirium tremens, an acute mental disorder characterized by delirium, trembling, great anxiety, mental distress, sweating, and gastrointestinal symptoms, caused by excessive alcohol consumption.

delivery, giving birth; parturition.

delomorphous, having a definite form or shape.

deltoid, referring to a large triangular muscle which covers the shoulder prominence.

delusion, a false belief which is firmly maintained despite obvious evidence to the contrary.

delusional, pertaining to delusions.

demented, out of one's mind; insane.

dementia, mental deterioration; organic loss of intellectual functioning.

dementia praecox, schizophrenia; an obsolete descriptive term for schizophrenia.

demineralization, abnormal loss of mineral salts from the body by excessive secretion and excretion.

demonomania, obsolete term for an irrational belief that one is possessed by demons or evil spirits.

demulcent, a substance that will soothe and soften the skin.

demyelinate, to remove the myelin sheath from a nerve or nerves.

denatured, to change the nature of a substance; to render unfit for human consumption without impairing usefulness for other purposes, as alcohol.

dengue, an infectious tropical disease carried by mosquitoes characterized by fever and severe pain in the joints and muscles.

dental, pertaining to the teeth.

dental caries, decay of the teeth.

dentalgia, toothache.

dental hygienist, one trained to clean teeth, provide instruction on general tooth care, and assist a dentist.

dentate, notched, or toothed.

denticle, a small tooth; projecting toothlike point.

dentifrice, a substance for cleaning teeth.

dentin, dentine, the main hard tissues of a tooth enclosing the pulp which is covered by enamel on the crown and cementum on the roots.

dentist, a practioner who cares for and treats the gums and teeth.

dentistry, the branch of medicine which is concerned with the care of teeth, and with the prevention, diagnosis, and treatment of diseases of the teeth and gums.

dentition, the teeth in situ or in the dental arch.

dentures, false teeth; artificial teeth.

denudation, act of denuding; removal of a protective covering.

denutrition, malnutrition.

deodorant, an agent that masks offensive odors.

deodorize, to remove offensive and foul odors.

deossification, loss of mineral elements from bone.

deoxidation, process of depriving or reducing oxygen.

deoxycholic acid, a crystalline acid found in bile.

deoxyribonuclease, an enzyme produced by some streptococci.

deoxyribonucleic acid, see DNA.

depersonalization, a neurosis characterized by feelings of unreality and lost sense of personal identity; a lessened sense of one's perception of self, may occur in a mild form in a normal person.

depilate, to remove or pluck out hair.

depilation, the process of removing hair.

depilatory, a substance used for hair removal.

deplete, to empty or relieve, as in blood letting or purging.

deplumation, loss of eyelashes due to illness or disease.

deposit, collecting of matter in an organ part, or in an organism; sediment.

depraved, one perverted or abnormal; deteriorated.

depressant, a substance that depresses any functional body activity; an agent that depresses; sedative.

depressed, pertaining to depression.

depression, a depressed region or hallow; lowering of a body part or vital function; a morbid sadness, melancholy, or lack of hope.

depressomotor, an agent which retards muscular movements.

depressor, a device for depressing the tongue or a body part.

depurate, an agent that purifies.

deradentis, inflammation of a lymph gland in the neck.

derangement, a mental disorder.

dereistic, day dreaming.

derm, derma, true skin, beneath the epidermis.

dermal, pertaining to the true skin.

dermatitis, inflammation of the derma.

dermatoautoplasty, grafting of skin taken from the patient's own body.

dermatogen, an antigen produced from a skin disease.

dermatoid, resembling skin.

dermatologist, a skin specialist.

dermatology, the branch of medicine concerned with the skin and its diseases.

dermatomycosis, a skin infection caused by fungi; athlete's foot.

dermatomyositis, inflammation of the skin and muscles.

dermatone, an instrument used for cutting thin sections of skin for transplants.

dermatoneurosis, skin disease caused by a nervous disorder.

dermatophobia, morbid fear of contracting a skin disease.

dermatophyte, a plant parasite which infects the skin of animals and man causing diseases such as eczema and ringworm; a parasitic plant fungus.

dermatoplastic, pertaining to the grafting of skin.

dermatorrhea, excessive secretion from sebaceous glands.

dermatosis, any skin disease.

dermis, see derm, derma.

desensitization, to lessen hypersensitivity reactions by giving subsequent injections of an antogen; in treatment of phobias, a patient is intentionally exposed to emotionally distressing stimuli.

desiccant, a medication which causes drying.

desiccate, to dry up.

desmalgia, pain in a ligament.

desmectasis, stretching of a tendon.

desmitis, inflammation of a ligament.

desmoid, resembling a ligament; a very tough and fibrous tumor.

desmology, science of ligaments and tendons.

desmotomy, incision of a ligament.

desquamate, shedding of the epithelium.

desquamation, shedding of skin or cuticle.

detelectasis, collapse of an organ.

deteriorate, to become worse, to degenerate.

determinism, the theory that nothing in a person's emotional or mental life results by chance alone but rather from specific causes known or unknown.

detoxify, to decrease the toxic properties of a substance; to remove the effects of a toxic drug.

detritus, any degenerative or broken down tissue.

detrusor urinae, the longitudinal muscular layer of the bladder that helps to excrete urine.

detumescence, the subsidence of a swelling or of erectile tissue.

deutencephalon, the interbrain.

deuteranopia, defective color vision, especially an inability to distinguish between green and red.

deviant, varying from a normal standard or condition.

deviated septum, a congenital or acquired cartilaginous partition between the nostrils or septum.

devitalize, to weaken; to deprive of life or vitality.

devolution, degeneration as in catabolism.

dexter, pertaining to the right side.

dextral, pertaining to the right side.

dextrocardia, the heart positioned on the right side of the chest.

dextrose, a simple form of sugar, also known as glucose or grape sugar; a constituent of corn syrup and honey.

dextrosuria, the presence of dextrose in the urine.

diabetes, any one of various diseases which indicate the body's inability to handle glucose.

diabetes insipidus, a disease characterized by the excretion of excessive amounts of pale urine with no sugar or albumin, and extreme thirst, weakness, and dry skin.

diabetes mellitus, a disorder of carbohydrate metabolism characterized by an elevated blood sugar and the presence of sugar in the urine, resulting from decreased insulin production or utilization.

diabetic, pertaining to one afflicted with diabetes.

Diabinese, trademark for chlorpropamide which is used in selected patients for management of diabetes mellitus.

diagnosis, recognition of diseases based on examination, and microscopic and chemical results of laboratory findings.

diagnostic, pertaining to diagnosis.

diagnostics, the science concerned with diagnosis of diseases.

dialysis, the passage of small molecules or solute through a membrane; a procedure used to purify colloidal substances enclosed in a thin membraneous sac, and exposing to water or solvent which continually circulates outside the sac.

dialyze, to loosen or separate by a dialyzer.

dialyzer, a membrane used in performing dialysis such as a coiled cellophane tube.

diameter, measured by a straight line passing through the center of a circle or body surface and connecting opposite points on its circumference.

diapason, a tuning fork used in diagnosing diseases of the ear.

diapedesis, the passage of blood cells outward through unruptured capillary walls.

diaphane, translucent membrane of a cell.

diaphoresis, excessive or profuse perspiration or sweating.

diaphoretic, pertaining to profuse perspiration; an agent which increases perspiration.

diaphragm, a membraneous partition separating the abdominal and thoracic cavity which serves in inspiration and expiration; any separating membrane; female contraceptive placed over the cervix.

diarrhea, an abnormal evacuation of the intestines characterized by watery and frequent stools.

diarthric, pertaining to two or more joints.

diarthrosis, an articulation in which the bones move freely; a synovial or hinged joint.

diarticular, pertaining to two joints.

diastalsis, a forward movement due to a wave of inhibition before a downward contraction of the intestines.

diastase, an enzyme or ferment found in plant cells of grains and malt, and in the digestive juice which converts starch into sugar.

diastasis, an injury to a bone occurring during surgery in which an epiphysis is separated; pertaining to the rest period of the cardiac cycle between the diastole and the systole.

diastole, the normal period of dilatation of the heart, especially the ventricles.

diastolic, pertaining to the diastole of the heart; referring to diastolic pressure; it is the point of the greatest cardiac relaxation.

diathermia, diathermy.

diathermic, being permeable by heat waves.

diathermic surgery, the application of high frequency heat to remove tissue as in cauterization.

diathermy, therapeutic use of heat within the body in treatment of disease or injury.

diathesis, a constitutional perdisposition to certain diseases.

dichotomy, dichotomization, dividing into two parts, or dividing into pairs.

dichromasy, partial colorblindness.

diachromatic, perceiving only two colors.

dicliditis, inflammation of a cardiac valve.

dicoria, double pupil in each eye.

dicrotic, having one heartbeat for two arterial pulsations; a double pulse.

dicrotism, the state of having a double pulse.

Dicumarol, trademark for bishydroxycoumarin, an anticoagulant used in treatment of intravascular clotting.

didactylism, having only two digits on a hand or foot.

didelphic, having a double uterus.

didymitis, inflammation of the testicle.

diencephalon, second portion of the brain which includes the epithalamus, thalamus, metathalamus, and hypothalamus.

diet, one's nutritional intake; a prescribed food exchange adapted for a particular health problem; to eat sparingly according to prescribed rules to reduce body weight.

dietetic, pertaining to diet.

dietetics, science of nutrition and diet.

dietitian, one trained in dietetics and nutritional needs and who is part of the treatment team in hospitals and institutions in charge of diets.

dietotherapy, the regulation of diet in the treatment of disease.

differential blood count, microscopic determination of the number and variety of white and red blood cells in a cubic millimeter of a blood specimen.

differential diagnosis, a diagnosis of symptoms of two or more diseases by comparison.

differentiation, pertaining to distinct differences between individuals, groups or objects.

diffuse, irregular spreading or scattering of a substance; to pass through a tissue or substance.

diffusion, the process of becoming diffused; widely spread.

digest, to undergo digestion.

digestion, the process of converting food by enzymatic action into chemical substances and assimilation into the body.

digestive tract, the system responsible for the conversion of food in the body which includes the mouth, pharynx, esophagus, stomach, small intestine, large intestine, and accessory glands.

digit, a finger or toe.

digital, pertaining to digits.

digitalis, a drug obtained from common foxglove, or Eurasian herbs used in powdered form as tablets or capsules which acts as a heart stimulant and indirectly as a diuretic.

digitalism, a condition caused by the poisonous effects produced by digitalis.

digitalization, the administration of the drug digitalis in scheduled dosages designed to produce and maintain optimal therapeutic results.

digitate, having digitlike appendages.

digitoxin, a cardiotoxic, bitter-tasting glycoside obtained from Digitalis purpurea used as a heart stimulant and in treatment of congestive heart failure.

Dilantin, trademark for phenytoin used as an anticonvulsant in the treatment of epilepsy.

dilatation, enlargement or expansion of an organ or vessel; expansion of an opening with a dilator.

dilation, see dilatation.

dilator, an instrument used to dilate or stretch muscles, cavities, or openings.

dilute, rendering less potent by mixing with water.

dilution, process of diluting a substance; weakening the strength of a substance.

dimercaprol, a metal antagonist used as an antidote in heavy metal poisoning which is effective against arsenic, gold, and mercury poisoning.

diminution, act of reducing.

dimpling, a retracting of the subcutaneous tissue in the formation of a dimple which occurs in certain carcinomas.

dinical, vertigo.

Diodoquin, trademark for diodohydroxyquin used as an antiamebic drug.

diopsimeter, an apparatus for exploring the visual field.

diopter, something that can be seen through such as a lens with refractive power with focal distance of 1 meter; one diopter is used as a unit of measurement in refraction.

dioptometer, an instrument for measuring ocular refraction and accommodation.

dioptric, pertaining to refraction of light.

dioxide, a compound consisting of two atoms of oxygen and another element such as carbon dioxide.

dipeptidase, an enzyme that converts dipeptids into amino acids by hydrolysis.

dipeptide, a derived protein by hydrolysis.

diphasic, having two phases.

diphtheria, an acute infectious disease affecting the mucous membranes of the nose, throat, or larynx with symptoms of fever, pain, and respiratory obstruction; toxins produced by the causative organism Corynebacterium diphtheriae may also cause myocarditis and neuritis.

diphtheritic, pertaining to diphtheria.

diphyodont, having two sets of teeth, as in man.

diplegia, a paralysis of similar parts occuring on both sides of the body.

diplococcus, gram positive bacteria occurring in pairs.

diploe, cancelled tissue between the inner and outer walls of the skull bones.

diploetic, diploic, pertaining to the diploe.

diploid, having two sets of chromosomes, as in somatic cells.

diplophonia, diphonia, producing two different voice tones at the same time in speaking.

diplopia, having double vision.

dipsomania, having an uncontrollable craving for alcoholic beverages.

dipsophobia, abnormal fear of drinking alcohol.

dipsosis, abnormal thirst.

disaccharide, any of the group of sugars in carbohydrates yielding two monosaccharides in hydrolysis.

disarticulation, separation or amputation through a joint.

disc, disk, a round, platelike structure or organ such as the fibro-cartilaginous disc between two vertebrae in the spinal column.

disease, any interruption of the normal function of any body organ, part, or system that presents an abnormal or pathological body state.

disinfect, to free from infection or destroy bacteria by physical or chemical means.

disinfectant, a chemical agent which kills bacteria; germicide.

disjoint, to separate bones from their natural positions in a joint.

dislocate, to move out of position or joint.

dislocation, the act of dislocating.

dismemberment, amputation.

disorganization, state of being disorganized or confused.

disorientation, being disoriented; inability to perceive one's self in relation to time, place, or person; a state of confusion.

dispensary, clinic for free dispensation of medicines or medical treatment; a place in which medicines are dispensed.

displacement, a defense mechanism in which an emotion is transferred unconsciously from its original object to one more acceptable; removal from the normal or usual position such as a body part.

disposition, a natural tendency or aptitude within a person; having susceptibility to disease.

dissect, to divide or cut apart tissues for the purpose of anatomical study; to separate tissues of a cadaver.

dissection, referring to the cutting of parts or tissues and studying of same.

dissector, one who dissects such as an anatomist.

disseminated, to scatter or spread over a wide area.

dissociation, a state of being separated; a defense mechanism through which emotional attachment is separated from an object, idea, or situation, usually an unconscious process.

dissolution, the process of dissolving of one substance into another; liquefaction; death.

dissolve, to cause a solid substance to pass into solution.

distal, farthest from the medial line or center of the body.

distemper, an infectious disease of animals.

distend, to swell up, stretch out, or to become inflated.

distill, to purify by vaporization of heat, condensing a volatile substance.

distillation, the process of purifying a liquid by vaporizing it and then condensing the substance.

districhasis, the growing of two hairs from the same follicle.

distrix, the splitting of ends of the hairs.

disulfiram, a drug used in treatment of alcoholism to deter ingestion of alcohol by producing an unpleasant reaction, nausea, and vomiting.

diuresis, abnormal secretion of urine.

diuretic, an agent which increases urinary output.

divagation, incoherent speech.

divergent, radiating or separating in different directions.

diver's paralysis, an occupational disease occurring after working under high air pressures and returning too suddenly to normal atmospheric pressure; the bends.

diverticula, pertaining to diverticulum; a pouch or sac in the walls of a canal or cavity.

diverticulitis, inflammation of the diverticulum.

diverticulosis, the presence of diverticula without inflammation.

divulsion, the act of pulling apart.

divulsor, an apparatus for dilation of a part.

diztgotic twins, fraternal twins, who are the product of two ova.

dizziness, state of being dizzy; foolish; vertigo.

DNA, deoxyribonucleic acid, a complex protein found in all cells, considered the chemical basis of heredity; a nucleic acid found in chromosomes consisting of a long chain molecule of repeated combinations of four basis (two purines, adenine and guanine, and two pyrimadines, thymine and cystosine).

doctor, one licensed to practice medicine and graduated from a college of medicine, dentistry, or veterinary medicine.

dolichocephalic, a long head; having a skull with a long front to back diameter.

dolichoderus, having a long neck.

dolichomorphic, having a thin, long body type.

dolor, pain, sorrow.

dolorific, producing pain.

dolorus, expressing pain, or grief.

domatophobia, morbid fear of being in the mouse; pertaining to a form of claustrophobia.

dominant, exerting control or influence; in genetics, the expression of a trait or characteristic which is inherited from one parent and excluding a contrasting trait from the opposite parent; a dominant allele or trait.

donor, a person who furnishes blood for transfusion or an organ for transplant.

dorophobia, morbid aversion to touching animal fur.

dorsad, toward the back.

dorsal, pertaining to the back; thoracic.

dorsalgia, pain in the back.

dorsiflect, bending backward.

dorsiflexion, backward flexion, as in bending backward either a hand or foot.

dorsolateral, pertaining to the back and the side.

dorsosacral, pertaining to the lower back.

dorsum, pertaining to the back or posterior surface of a body part.

dosage, the determination and regulation of the amount of medicine to be given at one time.

dose, a prescribed amount of medication to be taken at one time.

dosimeter, a device for measuring doses of radiation or X-rays.

dosimetry, a scientific determination of radiation; measurement of doses.

dotage, feeblemindedness or senility of old age.

double vision, seeing two images of an object at the same time.

double-blind, in reference to a study in which neither the administrator nor the subject knows which treatment the subject is getting.

douche, a stream of hot or cold water directed against a body part or cavity used for hygenic or medicinal purposes, especially the vagina.

DPT, diptheria-pertussis-tetanus vaccine.

Down's Syndrome, a common form of mental retardation caused by a chromosomal abnormality; mongolism.

drainage, the withdrawal of fluids and discharges from a cavity or wound.

dram, drachm, dr., a unit of liquid measure of the apothecaries system, containing 60 minims; a unit of weight equal to 60 grains, 1/8 ounce of the apothecaries' system.

Dramamine, trademark for dimenhydrinate, effective in the prevention and treatment of nausea, vomiting, and vertigo associated with surgery, motion sickness, and radiation sickness.

dreams, images that occur during sleep.

dressing, a protective covering for treatment of a wound caused by disease or injury to aid the healing process.

drip, to fall in drops; a slow injection of glucose or saline a drop at a time; intravenously.

drive, the urge or force that activates and motivates animals and man.

drop foot, inability to raise the foot upwards due to paralysis, of dorsal flexor muscles.

dropsy, a condition characterized by generalized accumulation of fluids in the tissues and cavities; see edema.

drug, a medicinal substance used internally or externally in treatment of disease or for diagnostic purposes.

drug addiction, a physical dependence on a drug caused by excessive or continued use of habit-forming drugs.

druggist, pharmacist.

drum, the middle ear; the tympanic membrane which serves to separate the tympanic cavity from the exterior acoustic meatus.

duct, a narrow tube or channel which serves to convey secretions from a gland.

ductless, having no duct, or secreting internally; see endocrine glands.

ductule, a small duct.

ductus arteriosus, the fetal blood vessel which communicates between the pulmonary artery and the aorta.

dumb, unable to speak; mute.

duodenal, pertaining to the duodenum.

duodenectomy, an operation excising all or part of the duodenum.

duodenitis, inflammation of the duodenum.

duodenostomy, a surgical procedure of making a permanent opening into the duodenum through the abdominal wall.

duodenum, the first segment of the small intestines connecting with the pylorus of the stomach and extending to the jejunum.

dural, pertaining to the dura mater, the outermost covering of the brain and spinal cord.

durematoma, an accumulation of blood between the arachnoid and dura membranes.

dwarf, an undersized human being.

dwarfism, being abnormally small in size.

dynamia, having vital energy or an ability to combat disease.

dynamometer, an apparatus for measuring muscular strength.

dynamoscopy, to examine the muscles by auscultation.

dysacousia, dysacousma, discomfort caused by loud noises, or having a hypersensitivity to sounds.

dysarthrosis, disease or deformity of a joint.

dyscrasia, a disordered condition of the body; an abnormal condition of the blood.

dysenteric, pertaining to dysentery.

dysentery, any of a group of intestinal disorders characterized by inflammation and irritation of the colon, with diarrhea, abdominal pain, and the passage of mucous or blood.

dysergia, incoordination in voluntary muscular movements.

dysfunction, impairment or absence of total function of the body or an organ.

dysgenesis, defective development, or malformation.

dysgenics, research study into causative factors in degeneration or deterioration in offspring.

dysgerminoma, a slow-growing, malignant tumor of the ovary; the seminoma is the counterpart in testicular neoplasm.

dysgraphia, inability to write due to a brain lesion; writer's cramp.

dyskinesia, any of a number of diseases which produce defective voluntary movements; impairment of normal movement.

dyslexia, difficulty in reading and visual confusion resulting from a brain lesion; inability to comprehend written language due to a central lesion.

dysmenorrhea, painful menstruation.

dyspepsia, indigestion due to any one of many causes.

dysphagia, difficulty in swallowing.

dysphemia, stuttering; a speech disorder.

dysphonia, any voice impairment causing difficulty in speaking; hoarseness.

dysphoria, restlessness; having a feeling of unrest and depression without cause.

dysplasia, abnormal growth of tissue, as in pathology; irregular growth in size, shape, and structure of cells.

dyspnea, difficult and labored breathing; shortness of breath, which may be accompanied by pain.

dystonia, impairment of muscle tone or tonicity.

dystrophy, defective nutrition; any disorder due to poor nutrition marked by degeneration of the muscles.

dysuria, painful urination.

E

ear, the organ of hearing and equilibrium composed of three different sections: the external, middle, and internal ear.

earache, pain in the ear usually caused by inflammation.

eardrum, the tympanic membrane.

earwax, cerumen.

eburnation, changes in bone structure causing a hardening of bone into an ivory-like mass.

ecbolic, an agent which hastens labor or abortion by causing the uterine muscles to contract.

eccentric, deviating from a center; peripheral; peculiar or abnormal behavior.

ecchondroma, a cartilaginous tumor of slow growth.

ecchymosis, a hemorrhagic, non-elevated, irregularly-formed discolored area of the skin caused by the seepage of blood beneath the epidermis.

eccrinology, the study of glandular secretions.

eccyesis, extrauterine pregnancy.

ecderon, pertaining to the epidermis or outer portion of the skin.

ecdysis, the sloughing off or shedding of skin; desquamation.

echidin, the venom of poisonous snakes.

Echinococcus, a genus of tapeworms whose larvae may develop in mammals and form cysts, especially in the liver.

echinosis, a change in the appearance of blood corpuscles such as losing their smooth outlines; crenation of red blood cells.

echolalia, uncontrollable senseless repetition of words spoken by others.

eclampsia, a major toxemia occurring in pregnancy or childbirth characterized by high blood pressure, albuminuria, decreased urine formation, edema, convulsions, and coma.

eclectic, choosing from a wide variety of sources what appears to be the best.

ecmnesia, forgetfulness of recent events, as seen in senility.

ecologist, a specialist in ecology.

ecology, the study of the physiology of organisms as affected by environmental factors.

ecomania, extreme humbleness in the presence of those in authority but having a dominating and irritable attitude toward family members; manifested in chronic alcoholism.

ecphoria, reestablishment of a memory trace.

ecthyma, an infection of the skin as a result of neglected treatment of impetigo.

ectiris, the external part of the iris.

ectoblast, ectoderm, the outer layer of cells in a developing embryo; from this outer layer, the epidermis, nails, hair, skin glands, nervous system, external sense organs, and the mucous membrane of the mouth and anus are derived.

ectodermosis, ectodermatosis, a disorder or illness resulting from congenital maldevelopment of organs.

ectogenous, developing from outside a body structure, as infection from pathogenic bacteria.

ectomere, any of the cells forming the ectoderm.

ectomorphic, having body structures that are slightly developed characterized by linearity and leanness; referring to body tissues derived predominantly from the ectoderm.

ectoparasite, pertaining to a parasite living outside the host's body.

ectopia, displacement of an organ or structure.

ectopic pregnancy, a pregnancy occurring in the abdominal cavity of a fallopian tube.

ectoplasm, the outer portion of the cell protoplasm.

ectopotomy, surgical removal of the fetus in ectopic pregnancy.

ectopy, displacement or malposition.

ectoretina, outer portion of the retina.

ectotoxemia, introduction of a toxin into the blood.

ectromelia, congenital absence of a limb or limbs.

ectropic, pertaining to complete or partial turning outward of a part such as eversion of the eyelid.

ectropion, eversion of a part or edge, especially of an eyelid.

eczema, an inflammatory condition of the skin which may be acute or chronic, characterized by itching or burning, tiny papules and vesicles, oozing, crusting, and scaling; dermatitis.

eczematous, resembling eczema.

edema, swelling of body tissues due to an excessive accumulation of fluid in connective tissue or a serous cavity.

edematous, pertaining to edema.

edentia, without teeth.

edulcorant, sweetening.

edulcorate, to sweeten; to wash out acids, or salts.

EEG, electroencephalogram.

effect, a result or consequence of an action.

effector, a motor nerve ending having the efferent process terminate in a muscle or gland cell.

effemination, having feminine qualities in a man.

efferent, conducting impulses from the brain or spinal cord to muscles, glands, and organs.

effervescence, the formation of bubbles of gas rising to the surface of a liquid; to show exhilaration or excitement.

efflorescence, a rash, eruption, or redness of the skin.

effluvium, a noxious or foul exhalation.

effusion, the escape of fluid into a cavity, as the pleural space.

egersis, extremely alert; abnormal wakefulness.

egest, excrete or discharge from the body.

egesta, excrement or waste matter eliminated from the body.

egestion, eliminating undigested matter.

egg, a female gamete or egg; a female reproductive cell before fertilization.

ego, the conscious part of the psyche that maintains its identity and tests reality; in psychoanalysis, the ego mediates between the id and the superego.

egocentric, self-centered and withdrawing from the external world; having most of one's thoughts and ideas centering on self.

ego ideal, an unconscious perfection or desired standard of character usually identified with significant others or esteemed and admired persons.

egoism, an overevaluation of self; self-seeking personal advantage at the expense of other people.

egomania, egotism developed to a pathological degree.

egotism, an overevaluation of self.

egotist, a boastful and self-centered person.

eidoptometry, measuring visual acuteness.

eighth cranial nerve, the acoustic nerve.

eikonometry, determining distance of an object by measuring the image produced by a lens with an instrument.

ejaculation, the sudden ejection of seminal fluids from the male reproductive organs.

ejaculatio precox, premature ejaculation.

EKG, electrocardiogram.

elastin, an albuminoid material forming the main constituent of yellow elastic tissue found in tendons and cartilage.

elation, emotional excitement, or joyous emotion; euphoria.

elbow, the joint of the arm and forearm.

Electra complex, the suppressed, unresolved libidinal feelings a daughter has for her father, accompanied by strong feelings of jealousy toward her mother.

electroanesthesia, a local anesthesia injected into tissues by electricity.

electrocardiogram, a record of heart action by an electrocardiograph.

electrocardiograph, an apparatus used for recording variations in heart muscle activity.

electrocardiography, the study and recording of electrocardiograms produced by an electrocardiograph of the heartbeat.

electrocatalysis, chemical decomposition using electricity.

electrocautery, cauterization by means of an instrument containing a platinum wire heated by a current of electricity.

electrocoagulation, coagulation of tissue using a high frequency electric current.

electroconvulsive, using electric current to induce convulsions in treatment of mental illness.

electroencephalogram, a record of electrical activity in various areas of the brain.

electroencephalograph, an instrument for recording electrical activity of the brain.

electroencephalography, the study of changes in electrical fluctuations of the brain made by an electroencephalograph.

electrohemostasis, stopping of hemorrhage by electrocautery.

electrolysis, the destruction of a chemical compound by an electric current passing through it; the removal of body hair by electric current.

electrolyte, a solution which is capable of conducting electricity.

electrolytic, pertaining to electrolysis, or to an electrolyte.

electromassage, application of electrization in massage.

electromyogram, a graphic record of muscle contraction resulting from electrical stimulation.

electromyography, the preparation, study, and interpretation of an electromyogram.

electronarcosis, inducing narcosis or anesthesia by the application of electricity which is used in treatment of mental illness.

electropathology, the study of electrical reaction of muscles and nerves as a means of determining a diagnosis.

electroretinograph, an apparatus for measuring the electrical responses of the retina using light stimulation.

electroshock, shock induced by an electric current used in treatment of mental illness.

electrosurgery, surgery performed by electricity.

electrotherapy, treatment of disease by use of low-intensity electricity.

electuary, a medicinal substance mixed with a powdered drug and honey or syrup to form a paste.

elephantiasis, a chronic disease due to a tropical infection characterized by inflammation and obstruction of the lymphatics, and hypertrophy of the skin and subcutaneous tissues, affecting the lower extremities and the scrotum most frequently.

elinguation, surgical removal of the tongue.

elixir, a sweetened, aromatic alcoholic liquid used in oral preparations.

elytrocleisis, surgical closure of the vagina.

elytrotomy, surgical incision into the vaginal wall.

emaciate, to become extremely thin or lean; wasting.

emaciation, wasting of flesh; the state of growing extremely thin.

emaculation, removal of spots from the skin.

emasculation, removal of the testicles; castration.

embalming, a procedure to retard decomposition in treatment of the dead.

embedding, a process by which a piece of tissue is fixated in a medium such as paraffin to keep it intact during cutting into thin sections for microscopic examination.

embolic, pertaining to or caused by embolism.

embolism, an obstruction of a blood vessel by a clot of blood or foreign substance.

embololalia, including meaningless words or phrases in a spoken sentence.

embolus, a plug or clot of blood present in a blood or lymphatic vessel having been brought from another vessel and obstructing the circulation within the smaller vessel.

emboly, invagination of one part into another such as the formation of the gastrula by the bastula.

embradure, to widen an opening.

embrocation, fomentation, such as the application of heat and moisture to a diseased or bruised part of the body; a drug rubbed into the skin.

embryectomy, the removal of an extrauterine embryo by excision.

embryo, the offspring of any organism in the process of development from the fertilized ovum; prenatal development of a mammal between the ovum and the fetus; in humans, the stage of development between the second week to the eighth week after conception.

embryogeny, study of the origin or development of the embryo.

embryology, the science of the development of the individual organism during the embryonic stage.

embryoma, a dermoid cyst; a tumor consisting of embryonic germ tissue but devoid of organization.

embryonic membrane, derived from the zygote but outside the embryo, an additional embryonic structure in vertebrates providing additional nutritive and protective value.

emesis, vomiting.

emetic, an agent or substance to induce vomiting.

emetine, a white powdered alkaloid derived from ipecac with emetic properties used as an antiamebic.

eminence, a projection or bony prominence.

emissary, providing an outlet.

emissary veins, small veins which penetrate the skull carrying blood from the sinuses.

emission, an involuntary discharge of semen by the male, particularly during sleep.

emmenagogue, a medicine that stimulates menstrual functioning.

emmenia, the menstrual flow.

emmenic, pertaining to the menses.

emmeniopathy, any menstrual dysfunction.

emmetropic, normal vision.

emollient, an agent that softens and soothes the skin.

emotion, a mental state or strong feeling accompanied by physical bodily changes; any intense state of mind such as hate, love, anger, joy, or grief which precipitates physiological changes.

empathy, an attempt to identify one's feelings with those of another; having understanding and recognition of another's feelings.

emphysema, a distention caused by accumulated air in tissues or organs; pulmonary emphysema, a disease of the lungs due to overdistention of lung tissues and atrophic changes such as loss of elasticity and thinning of lung tissues.

emphysematous, pertaining to emphysema.

empiric, based on experience and observation.

empirical, pertaining to empiric, or based on experience.

Empirin, trademark for acetylsalicylic acid, phenacetin, and caffeine combined in a tablet used as an analgesic and antipyretic compound.

empyema, accumulation of pus in certain cavities of the body such as the chest cavity.

emulsify, to make into an emulsion.

emulsion, a mixture of two liquids not mutually soluble, one being divided into droplets and dispersed throughout the other.

enamel, the hardest substance in the body forming a white, dense covering for the crown of the teeth.

enanthesis, a skin eruption or rash originating from internal disorders or diseases.

enarthritis, inflammation of a ball-and-socket joint.

enarthrosis, any ball-and-socket joint.

encanthis, a new growth at the inner angle of the eye.

encelialgia, abdominal pain; belly-ache.

endoderm, inner layer of cells of an embryo.

endosteitis, inflammation of the medullary cavity of a bone.

endosteum, the membrane lining the medullary cavity of the bone which contains the marrow.

endothelial, pertaining to the endothelium.

endothelioma, a malignant growth of the endothelial lining of blood vessels.

endothelium, a lining formed of epithelial cells which line the blood and lymphatic vessels, heart, and the serous body cavities.

endothermy, surgical diathermy.

endotoscope, an instrument to examine the ear; and ear speculum.

endotoxin, bacterial toxin present within the body of a bacterium, liberated only when the bacterium disintegrates.

end plate, the terminal mass of a motor nerve ending which joins a skeletal muscle fiber.

enema, introduction of water or solution into the rectum and colon to evacuate the contents of the lower intestines, or as a means of introducing nutrients or medicine for therapeutic purposes.

energy, having the ability to work or take part in any activity.

enervation, weakness; lack of energy or strength.

engorged, distended with blood.

engorgement, the state of being engorged or distended; vascular congestion.

engram, the lasting impression of a physical experience upon nerve cells.

enomania, a craving for alcohol; delirium tremens.

enophthalmus, -mos, recession of the eyeball into its orbit.

ensiform, sword-like structure of the lower part of the sternum.

enstrophe, turning inward, especially of the eyelids.

enteral, pertaining to the small intestine.

enteralgia, pain in the intestines; colic or intestinal cramps.

enterectomy, surgical excision of part of the intestines.

enteric, pertaining to the intestines.

enteric fever, typhoid fever.

enteritis, inflammation of the intestines, usually of the small intestines.

enterocele, intestinal hernia; posterior vaginal hernia.

enterocinesia, movement of the intestines; peristalsis.

enterococcus, any streptococcus found in the intestines of man.

enterocolitis, inflammation of the intestines and colon.

enterocolostomy, surgical joining of the small intestine to the colon.

enteroenterostomy, surgical joining between two segments of the intestine after a diseased portion has been excised.

enterogastritis, inflammation of the intestines and of the stomach.

enterogenous, originating in the intestines.

enterohepatitis, inflammation of both large and small intestines and the liver.

enterlith, an intestinal calculus.

enterology, the study of the large and small intestines.

enteromegalia, enteromegaly, abnormal enlargement of the intestines.

enteron, the alimentary canal with specific reference to the small intestine.

enteropathy, referring to intestinal diseases.

enteroplasty, surgical plastic repair of the intestine.

enteroplegia, paralysis occurring in the intestines.

enterospasm, painful peristaltic movement in the intestines; resembling colic.

enterostenosis, narrowing of the intestine; a stricture.

enterostomy, creating a permanent opening into the intestine through the abdominal wall by a surgical procedure.

entoderm, see endoderm.

entopic, pertaining to the eyeball.

entoptoscopy, examining the interior of the eye.

entropion, turning inward of the edges of the lower eyelid.

enucleate, to remove the entire tumor or structure without rupturing; to remove the nucleus of a cell.

enuresis, being incontinent, involuntary complete or partial discharge of urine.

environment, external surroundings which influence an organism.

enzygotic, developing from the same ovum.

enzyme, a complex colloidal substance produced by living cells which induces chemical changes in another substance without being changed; a catalyst in the metabolism of organisms.

enzymology, the science that studies enzymes and enzymatic activity.

eonism, sexual perversion, as in transvestism of the male.

eosin, an acid dye used for diagnostic purposes and microscopic examination.

eosinophil, a cellular structure that stains readily with eosin dye.

epencephalon, the anterior portion of the embryonic hindbrain which develops into the pons and cerebellum.

ependyma, membrous lining of cerebral ventricles and the spinal cord's central canal.

ephedrine, an alkaloid, usually produced synthetically, known for its therapeutic properties as a bronchodilator in treatment of asthma, and for its constricting effects on the nasal passages in colds.

epicardia, the abdominal part of the esophagus which extends from the diaphragm to the stomach.

epicardiac, pertaining to the epicardium.

epicardium, the visceral layer of the pericardium which forms a serous membrane surrounding the outer layer of the heart wall.

epicranium, soft section covering the cranium.

epicritic, extreme sensitivity of the skin in discriminating between varying degrees of sensation produced by touch or temperature.

epidemic, infectious disease affecting many people at the same time and in the same region; a contagious disease widely diffused and quickly spreading and of high morbidity.

epidemiology, the study of epidemic diseases.

epidermal, pertaining to the epidermis.

epidermatoplasty, grafting with pieces of skin.

epidermis, outer layer of skin.

epidermitis, inflammation of the epidermis.

epididymis, a small, oblong structure resting upon and beside the posterior section of the testes.

epididymitis, inflammation of the epididymis.

epidural space, outside of the dura matter of the brain or spinal cord.

epigastric, the upper region of the abdomen, pertaining to the epigastrium.

epigastrium, region over the pit of the stomach or belly.

epiglottis, the thin, lid-like structure behind the posterior section of the tongue which covers the entrance of the larynx when swallowing.

epilation, removal of hair by the roots.

epilepsy, an episodic disturbance of the brain function characterized by a loss of consciousness, sensory disturbance, and generalized convulsions; three major types of epilepsy are: grand mal, petit mal, and focal seizures.

epileptic, one who is afflicted with epilepsy.

epileptoid, resembling or similar to epilepsy.

epimysium, a fibrous sheath of connective tissue surrounding the skeletal muscle.

epinephrine, a hormone produced by the adrenal medulla which is a powerful stimulant of the sympathetic nervous system, and a potent vasopressor which acts on the cardiovascular system and stimulates the myocardium to increase cardiac output; other medicinal uses include increasing metabolic activity, relaxing bronchioles in treatment of asthma, and inducing uterine contractions.

epinephritis, inflammation of the adrenal gland.

epineurium, the connective tissue sheath around the trunk of a nerve.

epiphora, abnormal excessive flow of tears.

epiphylaxis, to increase defensive powers within the body.

epiphyseal, pertaining to an epiphysis.

epiphysis, the end part of a juvenile long bone separated by cartilage from the main shaft but which later becomes a part of the larger bone through ossification.

epiphysitis, inflammation of an epiphysis, mostly of the hip, knee, and shoulder in infants.

epiploic, pertaining to the omentum.

episiotomy, surgical cutting of the vaginal opening to avoid the tearing of tissues in childbirth.

epistasis, a substance which rises to the surface like scum instead of sinking; the checking of a discharge; in heredity, a presence of a determining gene which prevents another gene not allelomorphic to it from expressing itself.

epistaxis, hemorrhage from the nose.

episternum, upper part of the sternum.

epithelial, pertaining to the epithelium.

epithelioma, malignant tumor consisting of epithelial cells; a carcinoma.

epithelium, the cellular layer forming the epidermis of the skin and internal and external covering of mucous and serous membranes.

equilibrium, a balance between opposing forces.

equivalent, equal in force or value.

erection, a distended state of an organ or part, especially in erectile tissue when filled with blood; becoming rigid.

erector, muscle that raises another part.

eremophobia, morbid fear of being alone.

erepsin, an enzyme found in intestinal juice which causes a peptide-splitting action.

erethism, excessive irritability or excitement.

ereuthrophobia, morbid fear of blushing.

ergograph, a device for recording muscle contractions and measuring the amount of work done.

ergonovine, an alkaloid derived from ergot, also produced synthetically; used to prevent hemorrhage after childbirth and to relieve migraine.

ergophobia, abnormal dread of working.

ergosterol, found in animal and plant tissues, and also derived from yeast, ergot, and other fungi; resembles cholesterol, and may be converted into Vitamin D by ultraviolet radiation.

ergot, a drug derived from fungi used to cause contractions of the uterus and control hemorrhage after childbirth.

ergotamine, a crystalline substance derived from ergot, used to treat migraine and to stimulate uterine contractions.

ergotism, poisoning resulting from excessive use of ergot, or from infected rye or wheat by fungus Claviceps purpurea, producing symptoms marked by spasms, cramps, or dry gangrene.

erogenous, sexual excitability; producing sexual desire.

eroticism, excessive libido; a condition of intense but normal sexual desire.

erotomania, abnormal, unrestrained libido.

erotopathia, any perverted sexual impulse.

erotophobia, an aversion to sexual love.

erubescence, a reddening of the skin, as in blushing.

eructation, bringing up of gas from the stomach; belching.

eruption, the appearance of a skin rash which accompanies a disease such as measles; the breaking through of a tooth through the gum.

erysipelas, an infectious disease of the skin due to infection with Streptococcus pyogenes characterized by fever and vesicular and bulbous lesions.

erysipeloid, a contagious dermatitis resembling erysipelas.

erythema, unusual redness of the skin caused by capillary congestion, resulting from inflammation, as in heat or sunburn.

erythrism, unusual redness of hair with a ruddy-colored skin.

erythroblast, a nucleated cell which possesses hemoglobin; the precursor of the erythrocyte.

erythrocyte, a mature red blood corpuscle, or cell.

erythrocythemia, an increase in the number of erythrocytes in the blood.

erythrocytosis, an abnormal increase in the number of red blood corpuscles.

erythrodermia, erythroderma, abnormal redness of the skin over a large area.

erythromycin, an antibiotic effective against many gram-positive organisms, used in treating amoebic and other diseases.

erythropoiesis, producing red blood corpuscles.

eschar, a sloughing or crusting which forms on the skin after cauterization or a burn.

esophagismus, spasms of the esophagus.

esophagitis, inflammation of the esophagus.

esophagoscope, a device used to examine the esophagus.

esophagus, the muscular canal extending from the pharynx to the stomach, approximately 9 inches in length.

esophoria, a tendency for the visual lines to converge.

esophoric, pertaining to esophoria.

esotropia, a marked turning inward of one eye toward that of the other causing crossed eyes.

ester, the combination of an organic acid with an alcohol; esters usually have fruity or flowery odors in liquid form.

esterase, an enzyme that catalyzes the hydrolysis of esters.

esthesioneurosis, loss of feeling in a body part without any apparent organic lesion.

estradiol, a hormone found in the ovary with estrogenic properties used in treatment of estrogen deficiency.

estriol, a hormone found in the urine of pregnant women.

estrogen, an estrogenic hormone produced by the ovarian follicle and other structures, responsible for the development of secondary female characteristics and changes in the epithelium of the vagina and the endothelium of the uterus; the natural estrogens include estradiol, estrone, and estriol.

estrone, a female sex hormone found in urine of pregnant women, used in the treatment of estrogen deficiencies.

estrum, estrus, the recurrent period of sexual receptivity in mammals called "heat."

ether anesthetic, a thin, colorless, highly volatile, and highly inflammable liquid widely used for general anesthesia and having a great margin of safety.

ethmoid, sievelike, cribriform plate which forms the nasal fossae and part of the floor of the skull.

ethmoidal, pertaining to the ethmoid bone.

ethmoidectomy, surgical removal of ethmoid cells.

ethmoiditis, inflammation of the ethmoidal cells causing headache, pain between the eyes, and nasal discharge.

ethmoid sinus, air spaces inside the ethmoid bone.

etiology, the study of any of the causes of diseases or abnormal body states.

eucalyptus, an oily substance derived from fresh plant leaves used as an expectorant and antiseptic.

eugenics, the scientific study of inheritance and the improvement of the human offspring.

eunuch, one with testicles removed; castrated male.

euphoria, feeling of mild elation and a sense of well-being.

euplastic, healing quickly and organizing well, as in tissue repair.

eupnea, normal respiration.

eupraxic, normal functioning.

eustachian tube, the auditory tube that connects the middle ear with the pharynx.

eustachitis, inflammation of the eustachian tube.

euthanasia, known as mercy killing; the ending of life for those who have an incurable disease or condition.

evacuant, an agent which promotes evacuation; cathartic.

evacuate, to discharge or expel, especially from the bowels.

evacuation, the process of evacuating.

evagination, the protrusion of an organ or part of an organ from its natural place.

eversion, a turning inside out, or turning outward.

evert, to turn outward; to turn inside out.

evisceration, the removal of viscera, contents of a cavity, or internal organs.

evolution, a developmental process from a rudimentary to a more complex state.

evulsion, a forcible extraction, or the act of tearing away of a part.

exacerbation, an increase in the severity of symptoms in a disease.

exaltation, a state of mind characterized by excessive or abnormal feelings of joy, optimism, elation, self-importance, or personal well-being.

examination, the process of inspecting the body and its products as a means of diagnosing a disease or as to physical fitness.

exanthema, any eruptive disease accompanied by inflammation of the skin, fever, or rash, as in measles or smallpox.

exanthrope, any cause of a disease originating externally.

exarteritis, inflammation of the outer coat of an artery.

exarticulation, amputation of a limb, or partial removal of a joint.

excipient, a substance such as jelly or sugar which is added to a drug to give it more consistency.

excise, to cut off or remove.

excision, the act of cutting out or removing, as in removing an organ or part of an organ.

excitability, susceptible to being stimulated.

excitant, an agent producing excitation of vital functions of the brain.

excitation, the condition of being excited, stimulated, or irritated.

excitor, a nerve which stimulates to greater activity.

excoriate, to abrade or wear off the surface of the skin or cuticle.

excoriation, the abrasion of the skin or the coating of an organ caused by disease or injury.

excrement, excreta, feces, or dejecta.

excreta, waste material expelled from the body.

excretion, the elimination of waste materials from the body.

excretory, pertaining to excretion.

exenteration, the surgical removal of the internal organs; evisceration.

exercise, physical exertion for health improvement; voluntary muscle activity.

exfoliation, the falling off of dead tissue in scales.

exhalation, breathing outward; the opposite of inhalation.

exhaustion, state of being extremely fatigued; weariness; the using up of a supply of something.

exhibit, to administer, as a drug or medicine; to show.

exhibitionism, an abnormal compulsion to expose the genitals to the opposite sex; a psychoneurosis.

exhibitionist, one with an abnormal impulse to exhibit the genitals to attract attention.

exhumation, disinterment of a body, or corpse.

exocrine, external secretion of a gland; excretion which reaches epithelial tissue or a duct.

exodontia, dentistry concerned with tooth extraction.

exodontist, one who practices exodontics.

exoenzyme, an enzyme that functions outside the cell which secretes it.

exogastritis, inflammation of the peritoneal coat of the stomach.

exogenous, originating outside an organ.

exometritis, inflammation of the peritoneal coat of the uterus.

exophoria, visual axes diverging outward.

exophthalmia, an abnormal protrusion of the eyeballs.

exormia, any skin rash.

exoserosis, an oozing or discharge of exudate.

exostosis, a bony growth projecting from the surface of a bone capped by cartilage.

exoteric, developing outside the body.

exotoxin, a toxin excreted by a microorganism into its surrounding medium.

expectorant, an agent having the quality of liquefying sputum or phlegm.

expectoration, ejecting or expelling mucus or phlegm from the lungs and throat; spitting.

expiration, the process of breathing out air from the lungs.

expire, to exhale; to die.

exploration, examining of an organ, part of an organ, or a wound by various means.

exploratory, pertaining to exploration.

expulsion, the act of expelling.

exsanguinate, to deplete of blood; bloodless;

exsanguination, the process of draining blood from a part.

exsanguine, anemic.

exsection, to cut out; excision.

exsiccation, the process of drying by heat.

extima, the outermost layer of blood vessels.

extirpation, to cut out totally; removal by the roots.

extraction, pulling out a tooth; the process of removing the active part of a drug.

extrasystole, an abnormal or premature contraction of part of the heart.

extrauterine, occurring outside the uterus.

extravasate, to escape into the tissues from a blood vessel.

extravasation, an escape of blood into the surrounding tissues; process of being extravasated.

extravascular, occurring outside a vessel.

extremity, a limb of the body; a terminal part of a structure.

extrinsic, originating externally.

extroversion, the direction of one's energy or attention turned outward from the self and toward objects.

extrude, to push out of a normal position.

extrusion, the process of being extruded, as in a tooth being pushed out of alignment.

extubation, removal of a tube.

exudate, the accumulation of fluid or pus in a cavity.

exudation, abnormal oozing of fluids, as in inflammatory conditions.

eye, the organ of vision; a globular structure consisting of three coats: the retina, uvea, and sclera with the cornea; the three layers enclose two cavities. The anterior cavity is divided by the iris into an anterior chamber and a posterior chamber which are filled with a watery aqueous humor. The cavity behind the lens is much larger in proportion and is filled with a jelly-like substance vitreous humor.

eyebrow, the ridge containing hair above the eye.

eyedrops, ophthalmic solutions for the treatment of eye disorders.

eyeglass, a lens for aiding impaired sight.

eyelash, a cilium or stiff hair on the edge of the eyelid.

eyelid, a movable protective fold of skin which covers the eyeball.

eyesight, having the ability to see.

eyestrain, fatigue of the eye due to excessive use or to an uncorrected visual defect.

eyetooth, a cuspid or upper canine tooth.

F

fabella, small fibrocartilages which develop in the head of the large muscle of the leg, or gastrocnemius.

face, the anterior or front part of the head from the forehead to the chin.

facet, facette, a small smooth surface on a bone.

facial, pertaining to the face.

facies, a specific surface of an organ or body structure; face.

faciocephalalgia, a neuralgia affecting the face and head.

facioplasty, plastic surgery of the face.

facioplegia, facial paralysis resulting from a stroke, or injury.

factitious, artificial or not natural; contrived.

faculty, having the ability to function.

faint, syncope; to feel weak and about to lose consciousness; temporary loss of consciousness.

fainting, the loss of consciousness.

falcate, sickleshaped; hooked.

fallectomy, excision of part of the fallopian tube.

fallopian tube, one of two tubes or ducts which extend laterally from the uterus to the ovary, and that function to convey the ova from the ovary to the uterus.

fallostomy, a surgical procedure to create an opening of the fallopian tube.

Fallot, tetralogy of, stenosis of the pulmonary artery which is a congenital defect occurring in newborns.

fallotomy, surgical division of the fallopian tubes.

false ribs, the lower five ribs which are not directly attached to the sternum.

falx, a sickle-shaped structure.

familial, common to the same family.

family, members of a group descended from a common progenitor.

fantasy, mental images which satisfy unconscious wishes or desires.

faradism, an interrupted current of electricity used to stimulate muscles and nerves.

farcy, a form of glanders which is a contagious infection in animals that may be communicated to man.

farsighted, clarity of vision at a distance.

fascia, a fibrous membrane of connective tissue supporting, and separating muscles and body organs.

fascicle, fasciculus, a small bundle of muscle fibers or nerves; a synonym for tract.

fasciectomy, surgical removal of strips of fascia.

fasciola, a small group of nerve or muscle fibers.

fascioplasty, plastic repair on a fascia.

fasciotomy, surgical incision and separation of a fascia.

fascitis, inflammation of a fascia.

fastidium, aversion to eating.

fastigium, the highest point of the 4th ventricle of the brain; the period of maximum temperature during the development of acute, infectious diseases.

fasting, going without nourishment.

fat, obese; corpulent; oily consistency; a group of organic compounds composed of carbon, oxygen, and hydrogen.

fatigue, a feeling of weariness resulting from excessive mental or physical exertion; temporary loss of capacity to respond to stimulation.

fauces, a passage leading from the mouth to the pharynx or throat cavity.

faucial, pertaining to the fauces.

faucitis, inflammation of the fauces.

faveolus, a depression on the skin.

favus, a contagious skin disease which may spread all over the body and scalp which is characterized by yellowish crusts resembling honeycomb.

febricula, a mild fever of short duration.

febrifacient, fever producing.

febrifuge, an agent which lessens fever such as an antipyretic.

febrile, pertaining to a fever.

fecal, pertaining to feces.

feces, excreta, dejecta, stools; waste products of the body discharged through the anus.

feculent, containing feces; having sediment.

fecundation, fertilization; impregnation.

fecundity, having the ability to produce offspring.

feeblemindedness, mental deficiency.

fellatio, oral stimulation of the penis.

felon, a purulent infection of the deeper tissues of the distal phalanx of a finger.

feminism, having female characteristics by the male.

feminization, adopting female characteristics.

femoral, pertaining to the femur or the thigh bone.

femur, the thigh bone which extends from the hip to the knee.

fenestra, a window-like open area in the inner wall of the middle ear covered by a membrane.

fenestration, surgical operation creating an artificial opening into the labyrinth of the ear.

fermentation, decomposition of complex substances by the action of anaerobic microorganisms' enzymatic conversion.

ferric, pertaining to iron; containing iron.

ferrotherapy, therapeutic use of iron compounds.

ferrous, pertaining to iron.

ferruginous, containing the color of iron rust; pertaining to iron.

fertile, capable of reproduction.

fertility, the ability to produce offspring.

fertilization, fecundation; impregnation of a sperm cell and an ovum.

fester, to become suppurate.

fetal, pertaining to a fetus.

fetalism, the retention of fetal structures after delivery.

fetation, pregnancy.

feticide, intentional destruction of a fetus.

fetid, having an offensive or foul odor.

fetish, an object or body part which excites the libido or sexual interest.

fetishism, belief that an object has certain power, or it is symbolically endowed with special meaning, especially that of a beloved person; the attraction of an object is associated with libido gratification and sexual desire.

fetor, an offensive odor such as halitosis; stench.

fetus, the developing young in utero of humans from the eighth week after fertilization.

fever, an elevation of body temperature above 98.6°F; pyrexia; characteristic of a disease such as typhoid fever or yellow fever in which the body temperature is abnormally elevated.

fiber, a threadlike structure as in a nerve fiber; the axonal part of a neuron; in nutrition, pertaining to constituents found in a diet.

fibra, pertaining to a fiber.

fibralbumin, globulin.

fibremia, fibrin formation which causes embolism or thrombosis in the blood.

fibril, an extremely fine filament or fiber.

fibrillar, pertaining to fibrils.

fibrillation, elements composed of fibrils; a quivering of muscle fibers which are uncoordinated; rapid and tremulous action of the heart.

fibrillolytic, dissolution of fibrils.

fibrin, a whitish, elastic protein formed by the action of thrombin on fibrinogen which forms a network of red and white blood cells and platelets, causing a clot.

fibrinogen, a soluble protein in the blood which through the action of thrombin and calcium ions is converted into fibrin, responsible for the clotting of the blood.

fibrinogenic, fibrogenous, producing fibrin.

fibrinolytic, pertaining to the dissolution of fibrin.

fibrinopenia, a deficiency of fibrin and fibrinogen in the blood.

fibroadenoma, fibrous tissue adenoma, a benign tumor occurring in the breasts of young women.

fibroangioma, a fibrous tissue angioma, usually benign.

fibroblast, a cell from which connective tissue is developed.

fibrocyst, a fibrous tumor with cystic degeneration.

fibrocystic, consisting of fibrocysts.

fibroid, a fibroid tumor.

fibroma, a fibrous benign tumor, slow in growth.

fibromatosis, having multiple fibromas developing simultaneously.

fibrosarcoma, a malignant tumor consisting of connective tissue, primarily.

fibrosis, an abnormal fibrous tissue formation.

fibrositis, inflammation of white fibrous connective tissue anywhere in the body.

fibrous, resembling fibers.

fibula, the outer and smaller bone of the leg, or calf bone, connecting the ankle to the knee.

fibulocaneal, pertaining to the fibula and calcaneus.

filaria, a threadlike worm.

filariasis, a disease caused by a long filiform worm which may be found in the lymphatic ducts, circulatory system, and connective tissues of man, causing inflammation, fibrosis, or blockage of the lymph flow that results in edema.

filtration, passage of a liquid through a semipermeable membrane such as a filter.

filum, a threadlike structure.

fimbria, resembling fringe.

finger, a digit of the hand.

first aid, emergency treatment given to persons who have been injured in an accident or have an acute illness prior to regular medical care.

first cranial nerve, olfactory nerve.

fissure, a natural division, cleft, or furrow in body organs such as the brain; an ulcer; a crack or break in tooth enamel.

fistula, an abnormal passage or duct between two internal organs, or between an internal organ to the body surface.

fistulous, pertaining to a fistula.

fit, a sudden attack or convulsion.

fixation, holding in a fixed position; arresting psychosexual development at an early stage, often resulting from childhood trauma.

flaccid, absence of muscular tone; relaxed; flabby.

flagellum, hairlike processes on the extremities of protozoa and bacteria.

flatfoot, an abnormal flatness of the arch of the foot causing the sole to rest upon the ground.

flatulence, excessive gas in the stomach and the alimentary canal.

flautus, gas formed in the digestive tract and expelled through the anus.

flavedo, yellowish pigment of the skin; jaundice.

fleam, an instrument used in venesection.

flection, flexion, to bend, as in bending a limb.

fletcherism, excessive chewing of small amounts of food.

flexibility, being capable of being bent without breaking; adaptability.

flexor, a muscle that bends a joint.

flexure, a bend, or curvature to a structure.

flight of ideas, skipping from one idea to another in a continuous stream of talk.

floaters, visual spots caused by deposits in the vitreous of the eye, occurring as benign degenerative changes.

floating kidney, a kidney displaced from its normal position in the body.

floating ribs, the 11th and 12th ribs which do not directly connect with the sternum.

flora, normal bacteria living in the intestines or the skin of humans; plant life.

fluid, liquid; gaseous substance.

fluid ounce, eight fluidrams.

fluidram, measure of liquid capacity equal to one-eight part of a fluid ounce.

fluke, any of several parasitic worms in man.

fluor albus, a whitish discharge from the uterus or vagina; leukorrhea.

fluorescein, a red crystalline substance used in diagnostic examination of the eye to detect corneal lesions or foreign bodies.

fluoridation, addition of fluorides to drinking water as a means of preventing tooth decay.

fluoride, any binary compound of fluorine, especially with a radical.

fluorine, a gaseous, nonmetallic element found in the soil in combination with calcium which is important to plant and animal life.

fluoroscope, an apparatus that permits visual observation of the deep structures of the body on a fluorescent screen.

fluoroscopy, the use of a fluoroscope for medical examination and diagnosis.

fluorosis, chronic fluorine poisoning often caused by an excess of fluoride in drinking water.

flush, sudden reddening to the skin; blushing; flushing a body cavity or part with water.

flutter, a rapid pulsation or regular movement, especially of the heart.

flux, an excessive evacuation or discharge of fluid matter from the body or a cavity; diarrhea.

focal, pertaining to a focus.

focus, foci, point at which convergent light rays or sound waves intersect; that part of the body or organ in which a disease is localized.

folic acid, a B- vitamin important in the diet of humans used in treatment of pernicious and macrocytic anemia, and gastrointestinal disorders.

follicle, a small secretory cavity, sac, or gland.

follicle-stimulating hormone, a pituitary hormone that stimulates estrogen secretions and the production of Graafian follicles in the female; the follicle-stimulating hormone (FSH) in males stimulates the seminiferous tubules to produce sperm more rapidly.

follicular, pertaining to a follicle.

folliculin, the oophorin hormone produced by the ovarian follicles.

folliculitis, inflammation of a follicle.

fomentation, the application of heat and moisture to relieve pain or inflammation.

fomes, any material or substance on which infectious disease-producing agents may be transmitted.

fontanel, fontenelle, the soft spot of an infant's head lying between the cranial bones of the skull.

food, any nutritive taken into the body which provides a source of energy for physical activity, growth support, and maintenance of body tissue repair.

food allergies, allergic reactions to certain foods in one's diet caused by a sensitivity to one or more foods ingested; the most common foods that cause sensitivity are: eggs, lettuce, milk, spinach, strawberries, and tomatoes.

food poisoning, an acute digestive disorder due to ingesting foods which contain poisonous substances.

foot, the terminal part of a leg.

foot-and-mouth disease, Aphthous fever, a disease of cattle characterized by ulcers in the mouth, the hooves, teats, and udder, which can be transmitted to man.

footdrop, a condition in which the foot falls in a planter-flexed position caused by paralysis of flexor leg muscles.

foramen, an opening or communication between two cavities of an organ, or a perforation in a bone through which vessels or nerves pass.

foramen magnum, a perforation in the occipital bone through which the spinal cord unites with the medulla oblongata.

foramen ovale, an opening between the left and right cardiac atria that normally closes after birth.

forceps, a two-pronged instrument resembling a pair of tongs used for holding or extracting.

forearm, the section of the arm between elbow and wrist.

forebrain, the part of the brain which develops from the anterior portion of the embryonic brain, comprising the diencephalon and telencephalon.

forehead, the brow above the eyes.

forensic medicine, legal aspects of medicine.

foreskin, the fold of skin or prepuce which covers the glans of the penis.

formaldehyde, a pungent, colorless gas used in solution as a disinfectant, preservative, astringent, and fumigant.

formalin, an aqueous solution of formaldehyde with the addition of methanol.

formication, a creeping sensation as if ants were crawling upon the body; form of paresthesia.

formula, a prescription of ingredients with proportions in the preparation of medicine.

formulary, book of formulas.

fornication, voluntary sexual intercourse on the part of an unmarried person.

fornix, fornices, a vault-like band of a fibrous formation connecting the cerebral lobes; an arch-like space formed by such a structure.

fossa, a hollow or depressed area in the body.

fossette, a small, deep corneal ulcer; a small fossa.

fourchet, fourchette, a transverse fold of mucous membrane connecting the posterior ends of the labia minora which forms the margin of the vulva.

fovea, a small pit or depression, often indicating the central fovea of the retina.

Fowler's position, a semi-sitting position with the back rest elevated or the head of the patient placed on several pillows to relieve dyspnea.

fracture, a break or rupture, especially in a bone.

fragilitas, a brittleness or fragility.

fragility, state of being brittle or frail.

fragmentation, breaking into small pieces.

fraternal twin, derived from two separate fertilized ova.

freckle, a small, localized brownish spot on the skin, often due to exposure to the sun.

fremitus, palpation of vibratory tremors felt through the chest wall.

frenum, a membranous fold which connects two parts, one more or less restrained in movement, as in the underside of the tongue.

frenzy, state of violent mental agitation; wild excitement; delirium.

Freudian, pertaining to Sigmund Freud, founder of psychoanalysis, and to his theories regarding the causes and treatment of neurosis and psychosis.

friable, easily pulverized or broken down into crumbs.

friction, act of rubbing.

frigidity, usually applied to the inability to respond to sexual desire or sexual stimuli; coldness.

frontal, pertaining to the forehead or the bones forming the forehead.

frontal lobe, the anterior portion of the cerebral hemisphere, the cerebrum.

frostbite, damage occurring by the freezing of part of the body such as nose, fingers, or toes causing numbness.

frottage, rubbing; massage; sexual gratification by rubbing against a person of the opposite sex.

frotteur, one who practices frottage.

fructose, fruit sugar; levulose.

FSH, see follicle stimulating hormone.

fugue, physical flight from home on a hysterical impulse; a state of personality dissociation accompanied by amnesia.

fulguration, destruction of tissue by electricity.

fulminating, pain occurring with rapidity and severity.

fumigation, exposing to poisonous fumes or gases for the purpose of destroying living organisms such as vermin; disinfecting of rooms by gases.

functional, pertaining to function and not to structure.

functional disease, one not organic but in which there is a pathological alteration in the functioning of an organ.

fundus, referring to the base part or body of a hollow organ; the part most remote from its opening.

fungicide, a bacteriede which destroys fungi.

fungoid, resembling fungus.

fungus, fungi, any of a group of eukaryotic protists such as yeasts, molds, or mushrooms that subsist on organic matter.

funiculus, small structure resembling a cord; small bundle of nerve fibers; umbilical or spermatic cord.

funny bone, outer part of the elbow where part of the ulnar nerve passes by the internal codyle of the humerus.

furfur, dandruff.

furfuraceous, resembling dandruff; flaky or scaling.

furuncle, a boil.

furunculosis, a condition marked by the presence of boils on the skin.

fusiform, spindle-like structures.

Fusobacterium, a genus of gram-negative anaerobic bacteria normally found in the mouth and large intestines, and in necrotic lesions.

fusospirillosis, Vincent's angina caused by fusiform bacilli and spirochetes.

G

gag, a device to hold the mouth open; to retch or to cause to retch or vomit.

gait, a manner of moving on foot or walking.

galactacrasia, an abnormal condition occurring in the composition of milk from the breast.

galactan, a carbohydrate which forms galactose upon hydrolysis.

galactemia, an abnormal milky condition of the blood.

galactic, pertaining to flow of milk.

galactidrosis, sweat that appears milklike.

galactischia, suppression of the secreting ducts and the flow of milk.

galactophore, a milk duct.

galactophoritis, inflammation of a milk duct.

galactorrhea, excessive flow of milk after cessation of nursing.

galactstasis, cessation of breast milk secretion.

galeophobia, morbid aversion to cats.

gall, pertaining to the gall-bladder bile.

gallbladder, a pear-shaped organ containing bile produced in the liver, located beneath the right lobe of the liver.

gallstone, a stonelike mass formed in the gallbladder or bile ducts.

galvanism, the use of direct electric current to the body for therapeutic purposes.

galvanometer, an apparatus that measures current strength using electromagnetic action.

galvanopalpation, the testing of nerve sensibility of the skin by galvanic current.

galvanopuncture, the use of needles to complete an electric current.

galvanoscope, a device which detects the direction of a galvanic current.

gamete, a male or female reproductive germ cell that unites to form an offspring; the spermatozoon or ovum.

gametocyte, an oocyte or spermatocyte.

gametogenesis, the formation of gametes.

gamic, sexual, especially as applied to eggs after fertilization.

gamma globulin, a blood protein containing antibodies, given by injection as a prophylactic measure against measles, poliomyelitis, and infectious hepatitis.

gamma rays, extremely short-wave length rays which penetrate radioactive material and reduce the cell nucleus; used in radiotherapy.

gamogenesis, sexual reproduction.

gamophobia, a psychoneurotic fear of being married.

ganglial, pertaining to a ganglion.

gangliectomy, ganglionectomy, surgical removal of a ganglion.

ganglioma, a tumor of a lymphatic gland; swelling which occurs in lymphoid tissue.

ganglion, a knot-like mass of nervous tissue consisting of nerve-cell bodies, located outside the brain or spinal cord; a cystic tumor which develops on a tendon, sometimes occurring on the back of the wrist due to strain.

ganglionitis, inflammation of a ganglion.

gangrene, necrosis or a gradual deterioration of an area of tissue resulting from interference of the blood supply to that part of the body.

gargle, a solution for washing the throat or mouth; to wash the mouth or throat by holding a liquid preparation in the mouth and agitating it with expired air from the lungs.

gargoylism, Hurler's syndrome, characterized by a form of dwarfism accompanied by mental deficiency, damaged vision, and grotesque facial features.

garrot, a form of tourniquet.

gaseous, having the nature of gas.

gastralgia, periodic pain in the stomach without gastric lesion.

gastrectomy, surgical removal of part or the whole of the stomach.

gastric, pertaining to the stomach.

gastric ulcer, a peptic ulcer of the stomach.

gastrin, a hormone secreted by the glands in the pyloric end of the stomach which stimulates the secretion of gastric acid and pepsin in the cardiac end of the stomach; it is a weak stimulant of pancreatic enzymes and gallbladder contraction.

gastritis, inflammation of the stomach mucous membranes.

gastrocele, hernia of the stomach.

gastrocnemius, the large muscle in the calf of the leg.

gastrocolic, pertaining to the colon and the stomach.

gastrocolic reflex, the peristaltic waves produced in the colon by the ingestion of food into an empty stomach.

gastrocolitis, inflammation of the stomach and colon.

gastrocolostomy, surgical joining of the stomach to the colon.

gastroduodenal, pertaining to the stomach and the duodenum.

gastroduodenitis, inflammation of the stomach and the duodenum.

gastroenteric, pertaining to the stomach and the intestine.

gastroenteritis, inflammation of the stomach and the intestine.

gastroenteroptosis, displacement downward of the stomach and the intestines.

gastroenterostomy, a surgical joining of the stomach wall to the small intestine.

gastroesophageal, pertaining to the stomach and the esophagus.

gastrogavage, feeding through a tube passed into the stomach.

gastrointestinal, pertaining to the stomach and the intestines.

gastrojejunostomy, surgical joining between the stomach and jejunum.

gastrology, the study of structures, functions, and diseases of the stomach.

gastromalacia, a softening of the walls of the stomach.

gastronephritis, inflammation of both the stomach and the kidneys at the same time.

gastroparalysis, paralysis of the stomach.

gastropathy, any disorder of the stomach.

gastrophrenic, referring to the stomach and the diaphragm.

gastroplegia, see gastroparalysis.

gastroptosia, abnormal falling of the stomach, usually involving the displacement of other organs.

gastrorrhagia, excessive bleeding from the stomach.

gastroscope, an instrument for examining the interior of the stomach.

gastroscopy, examination of the stomach and abdominal cavity with a gastroscope.

gastrosia, excessive secretion of hydrochloric acid in the stomach.

gastrostaxis, an oozing of blood from the mucosa of the stomach.

gastrostomy, incision of the abdominal or stomach wall.

gatophobia, fear of cats.

gauze, a thin fabric used as a bandage applied to wounds.

gavage, a tube passed through the nares, pharynx, and esophagus into the stomach for feeding purposes, or forced pumping of the stomach contents.

gene, a unit of heredity located at a specific position on a chromosome which determines characteristics in the offspring from a parent.

generic, pertaining to a genus of a drug name, not a trademark.

genetic, pertaining to the science of genetics; referring to genes.

genetics, the science concerned with individual differences of related organisms and the study of heredity.

genial, pertaining to the chin.

genicular, pertaining to the knee.

geniculate, bent as a knee; pertaining to the ganglion of the facial nerve.

genitals, genitalia, organs of the reproductive system, especially the external organs.

genitourinary, pertaining to the genital and urinary organs.

genotype, the basic hereditary constitution of the individual in a combination of genes.

gentian violet, a dye derived from coal tar used as a stain in bacteriology, cystology, and histology; therapeutic uses include an anti-infective and an anthelmintic agent.

genupectoral position, knee-chest position.

genu varum, bowleg.

genyplasty, plastic surgery on the chin.

geotragia, practice of eating earth, clay, or chalk.

gereology, the science concerned with old age.

geriatrics, the branch of medicine concerned with the problems and diseases of aging.

germ, a microorganism that causes disease; an early embryonic stage.

German measles, rubella, a viral infection with a rash and fever of short duration.

germicide, an agent destructive to germs.

germinal, pertaining to a germ or reproductive cells, egg or sperm; germination.

germinal disk, blastoderm, or disk of cells from which the embryo develops.

germination, the stage of development of an impregnated ovum into an embryo.

germ layer, one of three embryonic layers of cells: ectoderm, endoderm, mesoderm.

gerontology, the scientific study of the aging process.

gestation, period of fetal development in the womb.

gestosis, any disorder of pregnancy such as toxemia.

giantism, gigantism, abnormal growth or development of the body or its parts.

giddiness, dizziness, vertigo, or a sensation of reeling.

gingivitis, inflammation of the gums.

girdle, an area around the waist; cingulum; a structure which resembles a belt or band.

glabella, the flat surface of the frontal bone or the area of the face between the eyebrows.

glabrous, smooth and bald.

gland, specialized secretory cells in a structure or organ; a gland may be ductless or endocrine whose secretions directly enter the blood or lymph system, or a gland maybe exocrine, having ducts which transport the secretions to an epithelial surface.

glanders, a contagious disease found in horses which is communicable to man.

glandular, consisting of, or pertaining to glands.

glans, bulbous end of the penis; head of the clitoris; goiter; a gland.

Glauber's salt, a crystalline salt used as a purgative.

glaucoma, an eye disease characterized by increased intraocular pressure resulting in degeneration of the optic nerve and gradual loss of vision.

gleet, a purulent discharge from the urethra resulting from chronic gonorrhea.

glenoid, resembling a socket.

gliadin, a protein found in the gluten of wheat or rye.

glial, pertaining to glia or neuroglia.

glioma, a tumor consisting predominantly of neuroglia.

globin, a protein formed from hemoglobin.

globulin, a simple protein insoluble in water.

globus hystericus, a sensation of a lump in the throat occurring in hysteria or other neuroses.

glomerulitis, inflammation of the glomeruli.

glomerulonephritis, nephritis with inflammation of the capillary loops in the renal glomeruli which may frequently follow other infections.

glomerulus, a small rounded mass of capillary loops eclosed within the Bowman's capsule of a renal tubule and which serves as a filter in the formation of urine.

glossa, tongue.

glossal, pertaining to the tongue.

glossitis, inflammation of the tongue.

glottis, an opening at the upper part of the trachea and between the vocal cords responsible for the modulation of the voice; the vocal apparatus of the larynx.

glucagon, a hormone secreted by the alpha cells of the islets of Langerhans in the pancreas which functions in response to hypoglycemia and to stimulate the growth hormone.

glucogenic, producing glucose.

glucohemia, sugar in the blood.

glucose, a monosaccharide or dextrose found in certain foods such as nuts; an end product in the metabolism of carbohydrates and the chief source of energy for the body.

glucosuria, excessive amount of sugar in the urine.

glutamic acid, an amino acid formed in the hydrolysis of proteins; in the form of monosodium glutamate it is used as a salt substitute.

gluteal, pertaining to the buttocks, or gluteal muscles.

gluten, protein found in cereals and bread.

glycemia, sugar or glucose present in the urine.

glycerin, a clear, syrupy liquid, soluble in alcohol and water, used in medication preparation.

glycerol, transparent, syrupy liquid formed by hydrolysis of fats.

glycine, a crystalline amino acid derived from gelatin and from other proteins.

glycogen, a storage form of carbohydrate found in the liver and muscles.

glycogenesis, the formation of glycogen from glucose in the body.

glycolysis, the breakdown of carbohydrates in living organisms by enzymatic action.

glycolytic, pertaining to the hydrolysis of sugar.

glyconeogenesis, formation of carbohydrates from fat or protein.

glycosemia, excessive sugar in the blood.

glycoside, a substance derived from plants which hydrolyze into sugars.

glycosuria, sugar in the urine.

gnathalgia, pain in the jaw.

gnathitis, inflammation of the jaw.

goiter, an enlargement of the thyroid gland causing a swelling to the front part of the neck.

gomphosis, a conical process which is inserted into a socket in an immovable joint.

gonad, female or male reproductive gland that produces gametes; the sex glands in the embryo before differentiation.

gonadal, pertaining to a gonad.

gonadotrophin, gonad-stimulating hormone.

gonarthritis, inflammation of knee joint.

gonococcus, organism causing gonorrhea, Neisseria gonorrhoeae.

gonorrhea, a contagious, catarrhal disease of the genital mucous membranes of both males and females.

gonorrheal, pertaining to gonorrhea.

goose flesh, erection of skin papilae resulting from exposure to cold, shock, or fear.

gout, a metabolic disease characterized by acute arthritis and inflammation of the great toe, diagnosed by excessive accumulation of uric acid in the bloodstream.

graft, a section of skin, muscle, bone, or nerve tissue inserted into a similar substance by surgical means.

gram, basic unit of mass, equivalent to 15.432 grains.

gramicidin, an antibiotic obtained from soil bacillus, effective against gram-positive bacteria.

gram-positive, pertaining to organisms that will retain the gentian violet color when stained; gram-negative organisms will not retain the violet color when stained.

Gram's method, a method for staining organisms for identification under a microscope.

grand mal, severe epileptic attack characterized by convulsions, stupor, and temporary loss of consciousness.

granulation, new tissue formed in the process of healing; granular projections formed on the surface of an open wound.

granule, a very small grain-like body or structure.

granulocyte, a white blood cell or granular leukocyte.

granuloma, a granular growth consisting of epithelial and lymph cells which occur in diseases such as leprosy, yaws, and syphilis.

granulomatosis, multiple granulomas.

granulose, soluble part of starch.

graphobia, unusual fear of writing.

graphorrhea, the writing of meaningless words or phrases.

gravel, small calculi of crystalline dust which form in the kidneys or bladder.

gravid, being pregnant.

gravida, a pregnant woman.

gray matter, a grayish color nervous tissue; the term is applied to the gray portions of the central nervous system which include the cerebral cortex, basal ganglia, brain nuclei, and the gray spinal cord columns.

green sickness, anemia found in adolescent girls resulting from a poor diet.

gripe, grippe, sudden onset of an infectious disease characterized by fever, fatigue, headache, back pain, and phlegm from the respiratory tract.

gripes, severe intermittent pain in the bowels.

gristle, cartilage.

groin, the hollow on either side of the body between thigh and trunk; inguinal region.

growth, to develop or increase in size; abnormal cell or tissue growth, as in a tumor.

gullet, the esophagus; passage to the stomach.

gum, fleshy tissue covering the jaws' alveolar parts and the necks of the teeth.

gumboil, a gum abscess.

gumma, a soft tumor characteristic of the tertiary stage of syphilis.

gustation, taste sensation stimulated by gustatory nerve endings in the tongue.

gustatory, pertaining to sense of taste.

gut, bowel; intestine.

gutta, a drop.

guttate, a drop-like spot, as in certain skin lesions.

guttur, throat.

guttural, pertaining to the throat.

gymnophobia, unusual aversion to looking at a naked body.

gynecologist, a specialist in gynecology, or who specializes in diseases of women.

gynecology, the science of the diseases of women, especially of the genital, urinary, or rectal organs.

gynecomania, abnormal sexual desire in the male.

gynecomastia, unusually large breasts in the male.

gynephobia, aversion to female companionship.

gyrus, one of the ridges or convolutions of the cerebral hemisphere of the brain.

H

habit, a pattern or action which becomes automatic following constant repetition; a predisposition or characteristic of a person's mental makeup; clothing characteristic of a function, as a priest; bodily temperature; an addiction to drug, alcohol, or tobacco usage.

habit chorea or spasm, voluntary spasmodic movement of muscles that has become involuntary, as blinking of the eyes, coughing, or scratching.

habitual, acting in a repeated manner from force of habit.

habitus, attitude or physical appearance that indicates a tendency to certain diseases or abnormal conditions.

hachement, massaging with chopping strokes with the edge of the hands.

hacking, strokes with the edge of the hand.

hair, threadlike outgrowth from the skin.

hairball, a mass of hair in the stomach.

halation, blurring of vision due to a strong light shining in one's eyes from the direction of the object being viewed.

halazone, a disinfectant for drinking water.

Haldol, trademark for haloperidol, a psychotropic drug used in treatment of psychosis.

half-life, the time in which the radioactive atoms associated with an isotope are reduced by half through decay.

halisteresis, the lack of calcium in bones.

halitosis, foul or offensive breath.

halitus, exhalation of vapor; the breath.

hallucination, false sensory perception in the absence of an actual external cause.

hallucinogen, a chemical substance or narcotic used to produce fantastic visions and hallucinations.

hallucinogenic, pertaining to a hallucinogen.

hallucinosis, an abnormal condition marked by persistent hallucinations.

hallux, the great toe.

hallux flexus, see hammer toe.

hallux valgus, great toe displacement toward other toes.

hallux varus, great toe displacement away from other toes.

halogen, any of the group of elements astatine, bromine, chlorine, flourine, and iodine which form salt when combined with metal.

haloid, resembling salt in composition.

halothane, used as a general anesthetic.

ham, the region behind the knee; commonly used for buttock, hip, or thigh in which the hamstring muscles are located.

hamartoma, a benign tumor composed of a new growth of mature cells on existing blood vessels; a tumor resulting from faulty development of the embryo.

hammer, common name for malleus, a bone in the middle ear.

hammer toe, deformity of the toe due to abnormal dorsal flexion.

hamstring, one of three muscles on the posterior part of the thigh which flex the leg and adduct and extend the thigh.

hamulus, a hooked-shaped structure.

hand, terminal part of the arm attached to the wrist.

hangnail, a partly detached piece of skin at the base or side of the fingernail.

haphalgesia, sensation of pain when touching objects.

haphephobia, an aversion to being touched by others.

haploid, having half the normal number of chromosomes following the division of germ cells in gametogenesis.

hairlip, a congenital defect resulting from faulty fusion of the vertical fissure in the upper lip, often involving the palate; cleft lip.

haunch, hips and buttocks.

haut-mal, grand mal seizure at its height.

hay fever, an allergy to airborne pollens marked by inflammation of mucous membranes of the nose and upper air passages, catarrh, watery eyes, headache, asthmatic symptoms, and other symptoms similar to a head cold.

head, caput; the part of the body above the neck containing the brain.

headache, diffused pain in the head.

heal, to cure or restore to health; to make whole.

healing, the process of restoring to a normal or improved condition.

health, a state of having a sound or active body and mind; a sense of well-being and the absence of disease.

healthy, enjoying or being in a state of good health.

hearing, the ability to perceive sound.

hearing aid, a small device to amplify sound waves for those with impaired hearing.

heart, a hollow muscular organ that maintains the circulation of blood throughout the body, consisting of four chambers: the lower chambers are the left and right ventricles and the upper chambers are the left and right auricles.

heart attack, a sudden decrease in the flow of blood to the heart muscle resulting in impaired heart functioning often caused by an embolism or by chronic high blood pressure.

heart block, an impairment of the conductile tissue of the heart, specifically the S-A node, A-V node, bundle of His, and Purkinje fibers which fail to conduct normal impulses resulting in altered heart rhythm.

heartburn, a sensation of burning in the esophagus behind the lower part of the sternum, sometimes accompanied by an acid-tasting liquid in the mouth.

heart disease, any pathological or abnormal condition of the heart.

heart failure, an inability of the heart to maintain sufficient circulation resulting in cessation of the heart beat.

heart-lung machine, an apparatus through which the circulation of the blood is maintained and oxygenated while the heart is opened during surgery.

heart murmur, an abnormal heart sound which is detected by a stethoscope, usually indicating either a functional or structural defect.

heat, a warm sensation; high temperature; a form of energy; sexual excitement in lower animals; to make hot.

heat exhaustion, a condition caused by prolonged exposure to high temperatures combined with fatigue; characterized by dizziness, faintness, nausea, sweating, and general weakness.

heatstroke, a condition due to excessive exposure to high temperatures or the sun, occurs especially with those who are debilitated or who have been drinking alcoholic beverages, resulting in symptoms of dizziness, nausea, weakness, spots before the eyes, ringing in the ears, reddened and dry skin, rapid pulse, and collapse.

hebephrenia, a schizophrenic disorder characterized by disorganized thinking, regressive behavior, giggling, hypochondrial complaints, and bizarre delusions and hallucinations.

hebephrenic, pertaining to hebephrenia.

hebetic, pertaining to puberty.

hebetude, mental slowness; dullness.

hebosteotomy, an enlargement of the pelvic diameter by surgery to facilitate delivery.

hectic fever, a fever that occurs with an organic disease such as pulmonary tuberculosis or kidney or liver abcess.

hedonism, preoccupation with pleasure.

helcoid, resembling an ulcer.

helicoid, resembling a helix or spiral.

heliencephalitis, inflammation of the brain due to sunstroke.

heliotherapy, therapeutic application of sunlight in treatment of disease.

helix, the whole circuit of the external ear structure.

helminth, worm-like animal including flatworms, spiney-headed worms, threadworms or roundworms, and segmented or tapeworms.

helminthiasis, the presence of parasitic worms.

helminthic, pertaining to worms; that which expels worms.

helminthicide, a worm-expelling agent.

helminthology, the study of intestinal parasitic worms.

helminthophobia, a pathological dread of worms, or delusion of being infested by worms.

heloma, callosity, or corn.

helosis, having corns.

helotomy, removal of corns by surgery.

hemacytometer, hemocytometer, an apparatus for counting blood corpuscles.

hemadostenosis, contraction of blood vessels.

hemal, pertaining to the blood or blood vessels.

hemangioma, a tumor consisting of blood vessels.

hemarthrosis, the effusion of blood into a joint.

hematemesis, the vomiting of blood.

hematherapy, the infusion of fresh blood in the treatment of disease.

hematic, referring to blood; a treatment for anemia.

hematidrosis, excreting bloody sweat.

hematimeter, an apparatus used in counting blood corpuscles in a cu. mm. of blood.

hematin, the reddish iron-containing pigment of hemoglobin.

hematinic, pertaining to blood; a medicine which increases the hemoglobin level in the blood.

hematinuria, hematin in the urine.

hematocolpos, blood accumulation in the vagina.

hematocrit, a centrifugal apparatus used to determine the percentage of red blood cells in whole blood; the volume percentage of erythrocytes or red blood cells in blood.

hematodyscrasis, pathological blood condition.

hematogenesis, the formation of blood corpuscles.

hematogenous, produced by the blood; disseminated by means of the blood stream.

hematology, the branch of medicine concerned with blood diseases.

hematoma, a swelling of blood which occurs in an organ or tissue resulting from ruptured blood vessels.

hematometra, hemorrhage in the uterus.

hematomyelia, hemorrhage of blood into the spinal cord.

hematoperitoneum, effusion of blood into the peritoneal cavity.

hematophobia, abnormal fear of the sight of blood.

hematopoiesis, formation of red blood cells.

hematorrhea, profuse bleeding.

hematosalpinx, retained menstrual flow in the fallopian tube.

hematoscopy, blood examination.

hematosis, the development of red blood cells in the formation of blood; blood oxygenation in the lungs.

hematospermia, bloody semen.

hematostatic, arresting the flow of blood in a hemorrhage; retaining blood in a part.

hematothorax, presence of blood in the chest cavity.

hematozoon, a parasitic organism in the blood.

hematuria, blood in the urine.

heme, hematin.

hemeralopia, day blindness; difficulty in seeing during the day.

hemialgia, pain in one-half of the body.

hemic, pertaining to blood.

hemicrania, affecting one side of the head, usually a migraine headache.

hemiplegia, paralysis affecting one side of the body.

hemisphere, either of two sides of the cerebellum or cerebrum.

hemispheric, pertaining to a hemisphere.

hemocytoblastoma, a tumor consisting of embryonic blood cells.

hemocytology, the scientific study of blood cells.

hemocytometer, an instrument used to determine the number of blood cells in the blood.

hemoglobin, the red oxygen-carrying pigment of red blood cells.

hemolysin, an agent or substance in a serum which dissolves red blood corpuscles.

hemolysis, destruction of red blood corpuscles with the liberation of hemoglobin.

hemophilia, an inherited blood disease of males characterized by defective coagulation and an abnormal tendency to bleed.

hemophiliac, a person afflicted with hemophilia.

hemophobia, morbid fear of the sight of blood.

hemophthalmia, hemophthalmus, escape of blood inside the eye.

hemoptysis, the spitting of blood; blood-stained sputum.

hemorrhage, excessive or profuse bleeding; an abnormally heavy flow of blood from a ruptured blood vessel.

hemorrhagenic, producing hemorrhage.

hemorrhagic, pertaining to hemorrhage.

hemorrhoid, a swelling or dilated blood vessel in the anal area.

hemorrhoidectomy, surgical excision of hemorrhoids.

hemostasis, interruption of blood flow; a stopping of bleeding; stagnation of blood.

hemostat, a device or drug which stops the flow of blood.

hemostatic, checking bleeding or hemorrhage.

hemostypic, an astringent to stop bleeding.

hemothorax, a blood fluid present in the pleural cavity due to inflammation of the lungs, as in pneumonia.

hepar, the liver.

heparin, a complex blood anticoagulant present in many body tissues, especially in the liver and lungs; an agent used in prevention and treatment of embolism and trombosis, obtained from domestic animals.

heparinize, therapeutic treatment with heparin to prolong blood clotting time.

hepatic, pertaining to the liver.

hepatitis, inflammation of the liver.

hepatogenic, being produced in the liver.

hepatography, liver roentgenography.

hepatologist, one who specializes in diseases of the liver.

hepatology, the study of the liver and its diseases.

hepatoma, a tumor of the liver.

hepatomegaly, an enlargement of liver.

hepatopathy, liver disease.

herbivorous, a vegetarian living on plants; an animal that eats plants.

hereditary, genetically transmitted from one's ancestry.

heredity, the genetic transmission of individual traits and characteristics from parent to offspring.

hermaphrodite, having genital and sexual characteristics of both male and female.

hermaphroditism, a condition characterized by the presence of both male and female sexual characteristics and genitalia.

hernia, a protrusion of an organ or part of an organ through the cavity wall that encloses it; rupture.

hernial, pertaining to a hernia.

herniated disk, the protrusion or rupture of a disk between the vertebrae, especially involving the lumbar vertebrae of the spinal column.

herniation, development of a hernia.

heroin, a morphine derivative altered to increase its potency and used to relieve pain and induce sleep; an addictive narcotic.

herpes, an inflammation of the skin and mucous membranes marked by vesicles or blisters appearing in clusters, which often spreads.

herpes simplex, a viral disease which produces clusters of blisters around the mouth or genital regions that cause itching and localized congestion. The lesions dry up within a 10-14 day period and form yellowish crusts that shed.

herpes zoster, an infectious, inflammatory skin disease; shingles.

herpetic, pertaining to herpes.

herpetiform, resembling herpes.

herterogenous, differing species or sources; dissimilar elements in contrast to homogeneous.

heterologous, consisting of abnormal cell tissue.

heterology, an abnormality; differing from the normal structure of growth.

heteropathy, an abnormal reaction to an irritation.

heterophasia, the expression of nonsensical words instead of those intended.

heterophthalmia, a difference in the color of the iris of each eye.

heteroplasty, the procedure of grafting with skin tissue from another person or animal to repair skin lesions.

heterosexual, having sexual desire for the opposite sex.

heterosexuality, sexual attraction for the opposite sex.

heterotopy, displacement of an organ or a portion of the body.

heterotropia, a defect of the eyes; not having normal bifocal vision.

heterozygosity, the state of having one or more pairs of unlike genes.

heterozygote, a person who has one or more different alleles in regard to a given character.

hexachlorophene, a bactericidal and bacteriostatic compound used as a local antiseptic and detergent in emulsions, soaps, and other skin applications.

hexadactylism, having six fingers or six toes.

hexamine, a substance used as a disinfectant of the urinary tract.

hiatus, any natural cleft or opening, as the opening in the diaphragm for the passage of the esophagus.

hiatus hernia, a protrusion of part of the stomach upward through the esophageal hiatus of the diaphragm.

hiccough, hiccup, a spasmodic closure of the glottis following a sudden involuntary intake of breath causing an abrupt, sharp sound, or inspiratory cough.

hidrosis, excessive perspiration; profuse sweating.

high blood pressure, hypertension; abnormally high pressure in the arteries at the height of the pulse wave.

hilus, a depression or an organ at the point where ducts, nerves, or vessels enter or emerge.

hindbrain, the posterior part of the brain composing the pons, cerebellum, and the medulla oblongata.

hindgut, the embryonic entodermal tube which develops into the alimentary canal including the ileum, colon, and rectum.

hip, upper portion of the thigh; hip joint on either side of the pelvis.

hipbone, innominate bone.

hip joint, ball-and-socket joint between the femur and hipbone.

Hippocrates, ancient Greek physician referred to as "the father of medicine," born in 460 B.C.

Hippocratic oath, an oath taken by graduating physicians which embodies a practicing code of ethics.

hirsute, hairy or shaggy; roughly hairy.

hirsutism, abnormal condition marked by the excessive growth of hair, sometimes in unusual places as on the face of a woman.

histaminase, an enzyme distributed throughout the body which inactivates histamine.

histamine, a bodily substance that naturally occurs whenever there is tissue damage or allergic reactions; an amine produced by the putrefactive action of bacteria; may also be synthetically produced.

histidase, an enzyme produced in the liver that converts histidine to urocanic acid.

histogenesis, the origin and development of tissue.

histologist, one who studies the microscopic structure of tissue.

histology, the scientific study of tissue, esp. their microscopic structure.

histolysis, the disintegration and breaking down of tissues.

histone, simple proteins derived from cell nuclei which yield certain amino acids resulting from hydrolysis.

histoplasmosis, a respiratory disease caused by Histoplasma capsulatum, a fungus, which produce pulmonary calcifications, sometimes mistaken for tubercular calcifications. The usually fatal infection is marked by emaciation, irregular fever, decrease in white blood cells, and enlarged spleen.

hives, an eruption of uncertain origin marked by itchy wheals; urticaria.

hoarseness, difficulty in speaking due to a harsh, rough voice, as with cold symptoms or flu.

Hodgkin's disease, a progressive disease causing an enlargement of the lymph glands, spleen, liver, and kidneys.

holarthritis, inflammation of many of the joints; polyarthritis.

homeopathy, a method of treating a disease by administering minute doses of a drug that normally causes symptoms similar to those of the disease.

homeostasis, a state of equilibrium of the internal environment of the organism; self-regulating maintenance of the metabolic or psychologic processes which are necessary for survival.

homeostatic, pertaining to homeostasis.

homergic, having the same effect.

homicide, murder; the killing of one human being by another, involving acts of manslaughter, murder, accidental killing, and justifiable homicide.

homogeneity, state of being uniform in composition or nature.

homogeneous, having the same quality or uniformity throughout; belonging to the same kind or type.

homogenesis, the reproduction and development of offspring similar to the parents in each subsequent generation.

homogenetic, pertaining to homogenesis; having a common origin.

homograft, an organ or tissue grafted from an individual or animal to another of the same species, but of a different genotype.

homologous, any organ or part which corresponds in structure and in origin.

homology, state of being homologous, or similar in structure and origin.

homosexual, one sexually attracted to another of the same sex; a homosexual person.

homosexuality, exhibiting sexual desire toward persons of the same sex.

homozygosity, having identical alleles in referring to a given character.

homozygote, an individual possessing like pairs of genes for any hereditary characteristics.

hookworm disease, a condition produced by a nematode parasite present in the intestinal tract of man and other vertebrates causing severe anemia, listlessness, and general weakness. The most common port of entry is by walking on infected soil in bare feet, and once the microscopic worms are in the body they quickly invade the heart and lungs.

hormone, a chemical substance secreted by the endocrine glands which is conveyed throughout the body and serves to regulate the activity of certain cells or organs.

host, any organism that nourishes another organism such as a parasite.

hot flashes, a condition which occurs commonly during menopause characterized by vasodilation in the skin of head, neck, and chest with a sensation of suffocation and profuse sweating.

hot line, a 24-hour telephone service which provides assistance for people who are in a crisis situation and have a need to reach a mental health professional.

humerus, the upper bone of the arm between the shoulder and the elbow.

humor, any fluid or semifluid produced in the body.

humoral, pertaining to body substances or fluids.

humpback, a curvature of the spine; kyphosis.

hunchback, a person with kyphosis.

Huntington's chorea, an inherited disease involving the central nervous system.

hyaline, a glassy, translucent nitrogenous substance.

hyaline cartilage, the typical smooth, translucent cartilage which covers bone surfaces that articulate with other bones.

hyaline membrane, a thin membrane in lung of the newborn which interferes with mal respiration.

hyaluronic acid, mucopolysaccharide (polymer) fo in connective tissue which holds cells together and acts as a protective agent; also found in synovial fluid, skin, and vitreous humor.

hyaluronidase, an enzyme which increases connective tissue permeability by breaking down the molecular structure of hyaluronic acid; an enzyme present in the testes, other tissues, and semen.

hybrid, a heterozygous individual; the offspring of parents who differ in one or more distinct traits.

hybridization, production of hybrids.

hydatid, hydatid cyst, a cystlike structure formed in the tissues by tapeworm larva, especially in the liver of man and certain animals.

hydatid mole, hydatidiform mole, a degenerative process occurring in the chorionic villi, characterized by many cysts resembling a bunch of grapes, and rapid growth of the uterus with hemorrhage.

hydradenitis, inflammation of a sweat gland.

hydradenoma, a tumor of a sweat gland.

[partial text at top left, fragmentary]

...g a wa-
...in the
...acts
...g a wa-
...of the

...osis, serous accu-
...ion in a joint cavity,
...th swelling.

...ydrated, chemical combination of a substance with water.

hydration, act of hydrating.

hydremia, excess of watery fluid in the circulating blood.

hydriatics, the application of water in treatment of disease.

hydroa, a chronic skin disease with bullous eruptions.

hydrocarbon, a compound made up of hydrogen and carbon.

hydrocele, an accumulation of serous fluid in a saccular cavity, especially the scrotum.

hydrocephalus, an abnormal enlargement of the head due to an increased accumulation of cerebrospinal fluid resulting from developmental anomalies, infection, injury, or brain tumors.

hydrochloric acid, an aqueous solution of hydrogen chloride, a strong highly corrosive acid which is used in industry and medicine; found in gastric juices in the stomach in a diluted and neutralized form which converts pepsinogen into pepsin.

hydrocortisone, an adrenal cortical steroid which has life-maintaining properties; used in synthetic preparations for inflammations, allergies, pruritus, shock, bursitis, rheumatoid arthritis, and many other diseases.

hydrogen peroxide, a colorless liquid with an irritating odor used as a mild antiseptic, germicide, and cleansing solution.

hydrolysis, any reaction produced by combining water with a salt to produce an acid and a base, or a chemical decomposition in which a substance is broken down into simpler compounds by taking up elements of water, as the conversion of starch into maltose.

hydrometer, an apparatus which measures the specific gravity of fluids.

hydromyelocele, a protrusion of a membranous sac containing cerebrospinal fluid through a spina bifida.

hydronephrosis, an accumulation of urine in the kidney causing swelling due to an obstruction of the ureter, with atrophy of the kidney.

hydropericarditis, serous effusion around the heart with inflammation.

hydroperitoneum, an accumulation of fluid in the abdominal cavity.

hydrophobia, rabies, a disease resulting from a rabid animal bite; abnormal fear of water.

hydrops, edema or dropsy.

hydrotherapy, the application of water in treatment of disease.

hydrothorax, increased swelling of the chest due to the effusion of serous fluid into the pleural cavity.

hydroureter, an accumulation of urine or fluid causing distention of the ureter due to obstruction.

hydruria, increased water content of urine with decreased solids; polyuria.

hygiene, the study and practice of certain rules or principles for the purpose of maintaining health and cleanliness.

hygenic, pertaining to hygiene.

hygienist, a specialist in hygiene, as in the dental profession.

hygroscopy, determination of the quantity of moisture in the atmosphere by a hygroscope.

Hygroton, trademark for chlorthalidone, a diuretic.

hymen, a membranous fold of tissue covering the vaginal orifice.

hyoid, the U-shaped bone between the root of the tongue and larynx.

hyosine, scopolamine in some sedative medication.

hyoscyamine, an anticholinergic alkaloid obtained from solanaceous plants used as a sedative, mydriatic, antispasmodic, and analgesic.

hyperacidity, excessive gastric acidity.

hyperactive, pertaining to hyperactivity or hyperkinetic.

hyperactivity, abnormal and excessive activity; hyperkinesia.

hyperacusis, having an exceptionally acute sense of hearing.

hyperalgesia, extreme sensitivity to pain.

hyperkinesia, excessive motor activity.

hyperaphia, extreme sensitivity to touch.

hyperbilirubinemia, an excessive amount of bilirubin in the blood.

hypercalcemia, an excessive amount of calcium in the blood.

hyperchromic, excessive pigmentation.

hyperchromia, an abnormal increase in the hemoglobin in each red blood cell, with a decrease in the number of red blood cells.

hyperemesis, an abnormal amount of vomiting.

hyperemesis gravidarum, toxemia of early pregnancy marked by excessive vomiting.

hyperemia, an unusual amount of blood or congestion in a part which gives rise to reddened areas on the skin.

hyperesthesia, an increased sensibility to external stimuli, an oversensitivity to pain, touch, cold, or heat.

hyperglocosuria, excessive sugar in the urine.

hyperglycemia, excessive increase of blood sugar, as in diabetes.

hyperinsulinism, an excessive amount of insulin in the blood, producing hypoglycemic symptoms.

hyperinvolution, a reduction in size below normal of the uterus after parturition; a reduction in size below normal of an organ following hypertrophy.

hyperkeratosis, an overgrowth of the cornea; excessive development of the horny layer of the skin; keratosis.

hypermenorrhea, abnormal flow or frequency of menstrual periods.

hypermetropia, farsightedness; hyperopia.

hypermyatrophy, abnormal muscle wasting.

hypermyotonia, excessive muscle tonus.

hypernephroma, malignant tumor of the kidney.

hypernoia, excessive imagination or mental activity.

hyperopia, defect in eyesight in which the focal point falls behind the retina resulting in farsightedness.

hyperosmia, hypersensitivity to odors.

hyperparathyroidism, overactivity of the parathyroid glands.

hyperpiesia, having extremely high blood pressure.

hyperpituitarism, excessive pituitary gland activity resulting in increased growth hormone which produces gigantism and acromegaly.

hyperplasia, increased size of a tissue or organ due to excessive proliferation of cells.

hyperpnea, increased respiratory rate with deeper breathing or panting, such as a normal state after exercise.

hyperpyretic, pertaining to elevated body temperature; hyperpyrexia.

hyperpyrexia, a high fever.

hypersecretion, an excessive increase in secretion.

hypersensitivity, an abnormal sensitivity to a stimulus, as in drug reactions; allergic.

hypertension, persistently high arterial blood pressure.

hyperthermia, an unusually high body temperature.

hyperthymia, having excessive emotion, or morbid sensitivity.

hyperthyroidism, excessive thyroid gland activity characterized by goiter, increased metabolic rate, rapid pulse, psychic disturbances, excitement, and other symptoms.

hypertonia, an abnormal tension of the muscles or arteries.

hypertonicity, excess tonus of the muscle; intraocular pressure.

hypertrichiasis, an abnormal growth of hair.

hypertrophy, an enlargement of an organ or structure as a result of functional activity and not due to an increase in the number of cells.

hypervitaminosis, a condition caused by an excessive ingestion of vitamins, especially Vitamin A and D.

hyperventilation, an increased or forced respiration which results in carbon dioxide depletion with accompanied symptoms of lowered blood pressure, vasoconstriction, and faintness.

hypesthesia, a lessened sensation to touch.

hyphidrosis, a decrease in the amount of perspiration.

hypnagogic, inducing sleep; pertaining to dreams just before loss of consciousness.

hypnogenesis, producing sleep.

hypnogenic zones, certain areas on the body which produce sleep when stimulated, as in the elbow.

hypnoidal, pertaining to a mental state between sleep and waking, similar to sleep.

hypnolepsy, irresistible sleep; narcolepsy.

hypnophobia, pathological aversion to falling asleep.

hypnosis, a subconscious state of mind accompanied by an abnormal sensitivity to respond to impressions or verbal suggestions which allows the subject to be induced into a trance or dream state.

hypnotic, any agent that induces sleep, or dulls the senses.

hypnotism, the science concerned with hypnosis.

hypnotist, one trained in hypnosis.

hypoblast, inner cell layer or entoderm.

hypochondria, an abnormal concern about health issues and false belief of being afflicted with some disease.

hypochondriasis, preoccupation with the body and abnormal fear of diseases.

hypochondrium, the abdominal portion beneath the lower ribs on each side of the epigastrium.

hypocythemia, a deficiency in the number of red blood cells.

hypodermic, administered beneath the skin such as an injection into the subcutaneous tissue.

hypodermic syringe, a hollow tube, usually with a hollow needle used to inject a solution or medication under the skin; it may be administered subcutaneously, intramuscularly, intraspinally, or intravenously.

hypodermis, subcutaneous tissue.

hypogastric, pertaining to the hypogastrium.

hypogastrium, the area below the naval and between the right and left inguinal areas.

hypogenitalism, underdeveloped genital organs.

hypoglossal, underneath the tongue.

hypoglossal nerve, a mixed nerve which carries afferent and efferent impulses that give rise to tongue movements.

hypoglycemia, a deficiency of blood sugar marked by fatigue, restlessness, malaise, irritability, and weakness.

hypohidrosis, diminished perspiration or sweating.

hypokalemia, abnormal depletion of potassium in the circulating blood producing muscle weakness, tetany, and postural hypotension.

hypokinesia, diminished motor activity.

hypomania, a mild degree of mania without behavioral change.

hypomenorrhea, a deficient menstrual flow.

hypometropia, myopia; shortsightedness.

hypophyseal, referring to the pituitary gland.

hypophysectomy, excision of the hypophysis or pituitary gland.

hypophysis, the pituitary body.

hypophysitis, inflammation of the pituitary gland.

hypopituitarism, a condition resulting from diminished pituitary secretion of hormones.

hypoplasia, incomplete development of an organ or tissue.

hypopnea, abnormally slow depth and rate of respiration.

hypopyon, a condition seen in corneal ulcer in which purulence occurs in the anterior chamber of the eye in front of the iris.

hyposecretion, diminished amount of secretion.

hyposensitive, exhibiting reduced ability to respond to external stimuli.

hypostasis, a sedimentation; poor circulation in a body part or organ.

hypostatic, pertaining to hypostasis.

hypotension, abnormally low blood pressure.

hypothalamus, part of the diencephalon; the gray matter in the floor and walls of the third ventricle of the brain.

hypothermia, subnormal body temperature, below 37°C, or between 78 and 90°F.

hypothymia, a decreased emotional response.

hypothyroidism, a condition caused by a thyroid secretion deficiency marked by lowered basal metabolism, and cretinism.

hypotonia, reduced muscle tone or activity.

hypotonic, pertaining to decreased muscle tone or tension.

hypovolemia, a diminished blood supply.

hysterectomy, surgical excision of the uterus, either through the abdominal wall or through the vagina.

ysteria, a psychological state characterized by lack of control over emotion, abnormal self-consciousness, anxiety, simulated bodily symptoms, and impairment of both motor and sensory functions.

ysterogenic, producing hysteria.

ystero-oophorectomy, surgical excision of the uterus and one or both ovaries.

ysterotomy, incision of the uterus; a caesarean operation.

I

tric, pertaining to medicine or the physician.

atrogenic, caused by the treatment of a physician, resulting in an adverse condition in a patient.

trology, medical science.

hor, a watery, fetid discharge from an ulcer or a wound.

horrhemia, septic blood poisoning caused by ichorous matter.

hthyol, trademark, used as an astringent, antiseptic, and to relieve pruritis.

hthyosis, any of many skin disorders characterized by dryness, and scaliness, giving rise to eczema; a congenital skin disorder characterized by a thick, scaly skin resembling fish-skin.

TH, interstitial cell stimu-

lating hormone, a male hormone which stimulates testosterone production in the interstitial cells of the testes.

icteric, pertaining to jaundice.

icteroid, resembling jaundice.

icterus, bile pigments causing jaundice in the tissues, membranes, and secretions of the body.

id, in Freudian theory, the unconscious part of the personality that deals with instinctive desires or libinal energy of the individual; a biological germ structure carrying hereditary qualities.

idea, a concept, or mental imge.

ideation, the thinking process, or the formation of mental images.

identical twins, twins exactly alike which originate from a single fertilized ovum.

identification, a defense mechanism, usually unconscious, by which a person identifies himself with another, such as a hero.

idiocy, mental deficiency; severe mental retardation.

idiopathic, pertaining to idiopathy.

idiopathy, usually in reference to disease without a known cause; a spontaneous disease.

idiosyncrasy, individual peculiarities; a quality which makes a person react differently and distinguishes him from others; an unusual susceptibility to a drug.

idiosyncratic, pertaining to idiosyncrasy.

idiot, severe mental retardation; an uncouth or foolish person.

idiot savant, one who is severely mentally retarded, yet has an outstanding mental ability developed to an unusually high degree, as in mathematics or music.

ileac, pertaining to the ileum.

ilectomy, excision of the ileum.

ileitis, inflammation of the ileum.

ileocecal, pertaining to the ileum and cecum.

ileocecum, referring to both the ileum and cecum.

ileocolic, relating to the ileum and colon.

ileocolostomy, surgical forming of a passage between the ileum and the colon.

ileostomy, the creation of a passage through the abdominal wall into the ileum by a surgical procedure.

ileum, the lower third portion of the small intestine between the jejunum and the cecum.

ileus, an obstruction of the small intestine.

iliac, pertaining to the ileum.

ilium, the haunch bone, or the wide upper part of the innominate bone; hip bone.

illness, having an ailment, or a deviation from a normal healthy state.

illusion, an inaccurate perception, or the misinterpretation of a real experience or sensation.

illusory, based on deceptive perception.

image, a mental picture with a likeness to a real object.

imagery, imagination; mental images that are products of the imagination.

imago, the unconscious idealized mental image of an important person from one's early childhood.

imbalance, lack of balance, as in glands or muscles.

imbecile, mental deficiency, having an intelligence quotient between 25 and 50 of about age seven.

immature, not fully developed; having not reached full growth potential.

immiscibility, state of being immiscible.

immiscible, that which can not be mixed together such as liquids, especially oil and water.

immobilization, a part or limb that is immovable; fixed; to immobilize.

immobilize, to restrain movement, as by a cast on the arm or leg.

immune, able to resist disease; protected from certain diseases by vaccination.

immunity, having resistance or being immune to injury, poisons, foreign proteins or certain invading organisms.

immunization, the process of obtaining immunity to a specific disease; active immunity with a specific agent to stimulate an immune response, or passive immunity by administering serum from immune persons.

immunize, to render immune.

immunochemistry, the study of immunology as it relates to physical chemical aspects.

immunogenetics, the study of genetic factors which control individual immune responses, and how it affects succeeding generations.

immunogenic, inducing immunity to a particular disease.

immunology, the scientific study of immunity to specific diseases.

immunosuppressive, being capable of inhibiting immune responses, as the rejection of a transplant by the body.

immunotherapy, passive immunization of an organism by the administration of antibodies in serum or gamma globulin.

immunotoxin, an antitoxin.

immunotropic, enhancing immune response mechanisms.

impacted, a firmly wedged tooth in the jawbone which prevents it from emerging from the gum; in obstetrics referring to twins being wedged firmly together preventing complete enlargement of either before delivery; accumulation of feces in the rectum.

impaction, condition of being impacted.

impalpable, not detectable by the touch.

imparidigitate, having an uneven number of fingers or toes.

impedance, self-induced resistance.

imperception, inability to perceive; faulty perception.

imperforate, having no opening.

impermeable, not allowing the passage of fluids; impenetrable.

impetigo, an inflammatory skin disease which may be highly contagious, marked by pustules that become crusted and rupture.

implant, a tissue graft, a pellet of medicine, or a radioactive substance.

implantation, the attachment of a blastocyst to the lining of the uterus which occurs within six to seven days after fertilization of the ovum; the grafting of an organ or tissue into the body.

impotence, the inability of male copulation.

impotent, unable to copulate; sterile.

impregnate, to fertilize or make pregnant; to saturate.

impregnation, the fertilization of an ovum.

impression, a depression in the surface; the effect produced upon the mind; a dental imprint of the jaw and teeth.

impulse, an instinctual urge; neural transmission through nerve fibers by electro-chemical process.

impulsive, impelling emotional or involuntary behavior.

inactivate, to render inactive.

inactivation, destruction of biological activity.

inactive, being out of use or sluggish; not active; inert.

inanition, a condition of exhaustion due to lack of nourishing food which is essential to the body.

inappetence, lack of appetite or craving for nourishment.

inarticulate, unable to express oneself verbally; not jointed.

in articulo mortis, at the time of death.

inassimilable, unable to be used as nourishment by the body.

inborn, innate characteristics which are inherited or acquired before birth; congenital or being acquired during fetal development.

inbred, producing offspring closely related.

incest, sexual intercourse between close blood relations.

incidence, the number of new cases of a disease or other condition in a given population and within a specific time period.

incipient, beginning, or about to appear.

incise, to cut into with a surgical instrument.

incision, surgical process of cutting with a knife.

incisor, one of the eight cutting teeth located in the upper and lower jaw.

inclusion, being enclosed.

inclusion bodies, stainable bodies present in the nucleus or cytoplasm of a viral-infected cell; negri bodies.

incoherent, not understandable or disorganized and rambling, as in thoughts or language.

incompatible, not capable of being mixed in solution; antagonistic or mutually unsuited.

incompetence, inability to function realistically or properly; a legal status determined by the court.

incontinence, unable to control the elimination of feces or urine.

incoordination, inability to produce rhythmic and co-ordinated muscular movements due to disturbances in tone or harmony between muscle groups.

incrustation, the formation of crusts or scabs.

incubation, the period between infection of a disease and the appearance of symptoms.

incubator, an apparatus for regulating and maintaining a suitable temperature, oxygen, etc. for the survival of premature infants; apparatus for cultivating bacteria or for artificially hatching eggs.

incubus, a nightmare; a heavy burden.

incurable, not able to be cured; an individual with terminal cancer.

incus, the middle of three ossicles in the ear that is shaped like an anvil.

index, the forefinger; a ratio between a given measurement compared with a fixed standard.

indication, a sign that points to the cause or treatment of a disease.

indigestion, failure of complete digestion usually marked by abdominal discomfort after meals.

indisposition, a disorder or temporary illness.

indole, a crystalline compound found in feces that is largely responsible for odor.

indolent, sluggish; inactive.

induced, to cause or produce, as in induced labor.

induction, the process of inducing, as an abortion; electric current generated by electricity when near a charged body; the interaction between an embryonic cell and inductive cells adjacent to it.

indurate, to become hardened; callous.

induration, the act of hardening; a specific area of hardened tissue.

inebriant, something that intoxicates.

inebriate, intoxicate; to make drunk.

inebriation, state of being intoxicated; drunkenness.

inert, inactive; sluggish.

inertia, inactivity; tendency to remain in repose.

in extremis, near death; reaching the point of death.

infant, a child under two years of age.

infanticide, the killing of an infant.

infantile, pertaining to infancy.

infantile paralysis, poliomyelitis.

infantilism, failure of development pertaining to the mind and body; failure to attain maturation.

infarct, a necrotic area of tissue following cessation of the blood supply.

infarction, the development of an infarct, as in myocardial infarction.

infect, to contaminate with pathogenic organisms.

infection, the condition in which the body is penetrated by a pathogenic agent such as a virus.

infectious, pertaining to a disease which is capable of being transmitted due to a microorganism, either by direct or indirect contact.

infectious hepatitis, inflammation of the liver caused by a virus which produces jaundice, nausea, and abdominal pain.

infectious mononucleosis, a contagious viral disease characterized by constant fatigue, and other symptoms which include fever, headache, sore throat, swollen glands, jaundice, and stomach irritability.

infecundity, sterility in women.

inferior, beneath; lower placement.

inferiority complex, manifested feelings of inferiority either real or imagined evolved from physical or social inadequacies that produce anxiety.

infertile, not productive; unable to produce offspring.

infertility, being sterile or barren.

infestation, harboring parasites which do not multiply within the body in contrast to infection which does multiply and spread.

infirm, feeble, or weak.

infirmary, a hospital or a place for the care of the sick or infirmed.

infirmity, having an illness or debility; state of being infirmed; feebleness or weakness.

inflammation, a tissue or organ reaction to injury or irritation characterized by pain, heat, swelling, redness, and possible loss of function.

inflammatory, a sudden onset marked by inflammation and heat.

influenza, a contagious viral infection marked by head and back pain, catarrh of the respiratory or gastrointestinal tract; grippe.

infra-auxillary, below the axilla, or armpit.

infraclavicular, below the collarbone.

infracostal, below a rib.

infraction, incomplete fracture of a bone in which the two parts do not become displaced.

inframammary, below the mammary gland.

infraorbital, beneath the orbit of the eye.

infrapubic, below the pubis.

infrared rays, invisible heat rays beyond the red end of the visible spectrum.

infrascapular, below the shoulder blade.

infrasternal, below the sternum.

infundibulum, a funnel-shaped passage; a tube which connects the frontal sinus cavity with the middle nasal cavity.

infusion, introduction of a solution into a vein.

ingesta, substances taken into the body through the mouth such as food.

ingestion, the process of taking food into the gastrointestinal tract.

ingrowing, growing inward.

inguinal, pertaining to the groin region.

inhalant, a medicinal preparation which may be inhaled.

inhalation, the process of breathing medicated vapors or oxygen into the nose and lungs; act of drawing in of breath.

inhalator, an apparatus used for administering vaporized medication by inhalation, or for breathing in oxygen.

inherent, belonging to something naturally; intrinsic.

inheritance, hereditary factors transmitted and blended in the offspring.

inherited, characteristics received from one's ancestors.

inhibition, the act of repressing or the state of being restrained; commonly applied to the unconscious defense against the sex instinct; suppression.

inhibitor, something which inhibits.

inject, to introduce a solution into the body tissue or cavity with a syringe.

injection, forcing a fluid or liquid into a body tissue or cavity using a sterile needle and syringe; injections into the skin may be subcutaneous, intramuscular, or intravenous.

inlet, a passage which leads to a cavity.

innate, inborn, or hereditary.

innervate, the supply of nerves to an organ or part of the body; to stimulate through the nerves.

innervation, stimulating a body part through the action of nerve fibers, or nervous energy; the functioning of the nervous system.

innocent, benign, not malignant.

innocuous, harmless; inoffensive.

innominate artery, the right artery arising from the aortic arch.

innominate bone, the hip bone consisting of the ilium, ischium, and pubis which form the pelvis.

innominate veins, the right and left vein from the jugular and subclavian veins which form the superior vena cava.

inoculability, being susceptible of infection transmitted by inoculation.

inoculate, to inject a virus or bacteria into the body to cause a mild disease as a prevention against certain diseases and to build immunity.

inoculation, the act of injecting serum to induce antibody formation.

inoculum, a substance introduced into the body by inoculation.

inoliomyoma, a tumor consisting of smooth muscle tissue.

inoma, a fibrous tumor.

inoperable, unsuitable for excision without danger of death.

inquest, postmortem examination to determine legally the medical cause of death; act of inquiry.

insane, unsound mind; mentally deranged.

insanitary, unhealthy; pertaining to filth.

insanity, a legal term for mental derangement or mental illness; mental incompetence; unable to distinguish "right from wrong".

insatiable, incapable of being satisfied.

insemination, discharge of seminal fluid into the vagina; fertilization of an ovum.

insensibility, the state of being insensible.

insensible, unconscious; incapable of sensory perception.

insensitive, lacking feeling or physical sensation.

insertion, the place of muscle attachment to a bone allowing movement; the act of implanting.

insidious, a gradual and deliberate development; a slow developing disease that does not exhibit early symptoms.

insight, self-understanding.

insipid, without taste; lacking animation or spirit.

in situ, in its normal position.

insolation, exposure to the rays of the sun for brief periods, as a treatment of certain skin disorders; heat therapy; heat- or sunstroke.

insoluble, incapable of being dissolved.

insomnia, disturbances in sleep patterns; chronic inability to sleep.

inspection, to visually examine the external surface of the body.

inspersion, sprinkling with powder or a solution.

inspiration, inhalation; pertaining to breathing air into the lungs; a state of being inspired.

inspiratory, pertaining to breathing in, or inspiration.

inspissate, to thicken by absorption of liquid content or by evaporation.

inspissated, being thickened by absorption, evaporation, or dehydration.

inspissation, the process of diminishing fluidity and increasing thickness.

instep, the upper surface of the foot or the arch, in front of the ankle.

instillation, dispensing a liquid drop by drop.

instinct, an inborn drive or innate urge characteristic of a species necessary for self-preservation, and which satisfies basic biological needs.

instinctive, unlearned responses determined by instinct.

instrumentation, the use of instruments, or work resulting from their use.

insudation, an accumulated substance derived from the blood, as in a kidney.

insufficiency, being inadequate for its function or purpose.

insuffiate, to blow a medicated substance into a cavity such as lungs; to blow air into the lungs.

insuffiation, the process of insuffiating.

insuffiator, a device used for insuffiation.

insula, any round cutaneous body.

insulin, a pancreatic hormone secreted by the beta cells of the islets of Langerhans essential for oxidation and utilization of blood sugar. A sterile preparation of insulin is used in the treatment of diabetes mellitus.

insulinemia, the presence of too much insulin in the blood.

insulin shock, a condition resulting from an overdose of insulin which causes the blood sugar level to drop below normal, producing symptoms of hypoglycemia such as increased hunger, thirst, excitability, rapid pulse, flushing, pallor, sweating, fainting, convulsions, and coma.

insuloma, a tumor of the islets of Langerhans.

insusceptibility, having immunity.

integration, constituting a whole; assimilation.

integument, a covering such as skin; the skin.

integumentary, pertaining to a covering consisting of dermis or epidermis.

intellect, having the mental capacity to comprehend ideas and to exercise judgment; the capacity for knowledge.

intellectual, pertaining to the mind, or possessing intellect.

intellectualization, a defense mechanism that uses reasoning as a defense against conscious confrontation with unconscious conflict and its distressing mental tension.

intelligence, having the capacity to learn, to comprehend relationships, and to reason with facts and propositions.

intelligence quotient, (I.Q.), a numerical rating of intelligence, determined by dividing one's mental age, derived through intelligence test scores, by one's chronological age, then by multiplying by 100.

intemperance, excessive usages of anything.

intensive, relative to the degree or extent of activity.

interaction, the process of two or more things acting on each other.

interarticular, situated between two joints.

interatrial, situated between the atria of the heart.

interbrain, diencephalon.

intercellular, between the cells.

interchondral, between the cartilage.

interclavicular, between the clavicles.

intercostal, between the ribs.

intercourse, coitus; the sexual act; social contacts.

intercurrent, intervening; a disease that occurs during another illness.

interdental, between the teeth.

interdigital, between the fingers or toes.

interdigitation, fingerlike processes that interlock.

interfemoral, between the thighs.

interlobar, between lobes.

intermenstrual, between menstrual periods.

intermission, a temporary cessation of symptoms of a disease.

intermittent fever, an absence of symptoms between attacks of fever, as in malaria.

intermittent pulse, a pulse in which a beat is dropped at intervals, as in cardiac exhaustion.

intermuscular, between muscles.

intern, interne, a medical graduate assisting in a hospital as a resident physician or surgeon.

internal medicine, the branch of medicine concerned with diseases not usually treated by surgery.

internist, one concerned with internal diseases, and not a surgeon.

internuncial, serving as a connecting medium.

interosseous, between bones.

interosseus, a muscle lying between bones.

interpalpebral, between the eyelids.

interparietal, between walls; between the parietal bones; between the parietal lobes on the cerebrum.

intersex, a person having both male and female characteristics.

interspace, an area between two similar parts, as between ribs.

interstice, a gap or space in a tissue or an organ.

interstitial, placed between; pertaining to interstices or gaps between the cellular structures.

interventricular, between two ventricles.

intervertebral, between two adjacent vertebrae.

intestinal, pertaining to the intestine.

intestinal juice, a chemical liquid produced by the intestinal mucosa.

intestine, the alimentary canal which is divided into the small intestine and the large intestine extending from the pylorus to the anus.

intima, the innermost lining of a structure, as a blood vessel.

intolerance, the inability to endure pain; the side effects of drugs or foods.

intoxicant, an agent which intoxicates.

intoxication, the state of being intoxicated or drunk; being poisoned by a toxic substance.

intra-abdominal, within the abdomen.

intra-arterial, within the arteries.

intra-articular, within a joint.

intra-atrial, within the atrium of the heart.

intracellular, within cells.

intracranial, within the skull.

intracutaneous, within the substance of the skin or layers.

intracutaneous test, a test to determine allergic sensitivity.

intradermal, between the layers of the skin.

intradural, within the dura matter.

intraglandular, within a gland.

intra-intestinal, within the intestine.

intramammary, within the breast.

intramastoiditis, inflammation of the antrum and mastoid process.

intramural, within the substance of a wall or hollow cavity.

intramuscular, within a muscular substance.

intranasal, within the nasal cavity.

intraocular, within the eyeball.

intraoral, within the mouth.

intraorbital, within the orbit of the eye, or eye socket.

intraosseous, within the substance of a bone.

intraperitoneal, within the peritoneal cavity.

intrapleural, within the pleural cavity.

intrapsychic, originating within the mind such as conflicts; mental origin or basis.

intrapulmonary, within the lung.

intrathoracic, within the thorax.

intratracheal, introduction into the trachea.

intrauterine, within the uterus.

intravascular, within a blood vessel.

intravenous, within a vein.

intraventricular, within a ventricle.

intravital, occurring during life.

intrinsic, belonging within or pertaining essentially to a part.

intrinsic factor, a substance produced from gastrointestinal mucosa of animals which increases the absorption of Vitamin B complex in humans.

introitus, an opening into a cavity such as the vagina.

introjection, a defense mechanism in which external objects are taken within oneself symbolically.

introspection, looking into one's own mind.

introversion, a preoccupation with oneself with little interest in the outside world; turning inside out of a part or organ.

introvert, one whose interests are turned inward and away from reality.

intubation, the introduction of a tube into a body cavity, as into the larynx.

intumesce, to swell or enlarge.

intumescence, the process of enlarging.

intussusception, the prolapse of one part of the intestine into another part adjacent to it; a growth of new cells by receiving nutrients and its transformation into protoplasm.

intussuscipiens, that part of the intestine which contains the intussusceptum.

inulin, a starch of certain plants which yield fructose upon hydrolysis, used in renal function testing.

in utero, within the uterus.

invagination, folding of one part within another structural part, as in intestines; intussusception.

invalid, a weak and sickly person.

inversion, the turning inside out of an organ, especially the uterus; homosexuality; a chromosomal aberration resulting in a change in the sequence of genes.

invertase, an enzyme found in intestinal juice.

invertebrate, having no backbone.

in vitro, observable in a test tube or within an artificial environment.

in vivo, within a living organism.

involuntary, working independently of conscious control.

involution, a turning inward; the process of decreasing the size of the uterus after delivery; a degeneration of the internal organs with the aging process.

iodide, a compound of iodine.

iodine, a chemical element composed of a black, crystalline substance, essential to the body for synthesis of thyroxine, a thyroid hormone.

iodism, a poisonous condition occurring with prolonged use of iodine or its compounds.

iodoform, a yellowish crystalline substance with an offensive odor used as an antiseptic.

iodopsin, photosensitive violet pigment present in the retinal cones which are important for color vision.

ipecac, dried roots of the plant impecacuanha used in treatment against amebic dysentery; other uses are as an expectorant, emetic, and diaphoretic.

iridemia, hemorrhaging from the iris.

iridocyclectomy, surgical removal of part of the iris and of the ciliary body.

iridocystectomy, surgical procedure to form an artificial iris.

iridotomy, surgical incision of the iris without removal of a piece.

iris, the pigmented contractile membrane forming the portion of the eye containing the pupil.

iritis, inflammation of the iris.

iron, a chemical element essential for the formation of hemoglobin in the body, and the prevention of certain forms of anemia.

irradiate, to treat with radiation.

irradiation, the therapeutic use of roentgen rays, radium rays, ultraviolet and other radiation for healing purposes.

irrational, lacking reason or understanding.

irrigate, to wash out with water or solution.

irrigation, to cleanse a canal or cavity with the injection of fluids.

irritability, the state of being excitable; a condition in which an organism, organ, or body part responds excessively to stimuli.

irritant, that which causes irritation; an agent which produces local inflammation and gives rise to irritation.

irritation, a condition which produces unusual sensitivity in part of the body.

ischemia, temporary and localized anemia due to restricting circulation to a part.

ischial, pertaining to the ischium.

ischium, the lower portion of the hip bone.

ischuria, suppression or retention of urine.

islets of Langerhans, clusters of beta cells which produce insulin in the pancreas.

isoagglutinin, an antibody serum which agglutinates blood cells.

isogamete, a gamete or sex cell which conjugates with a similar cell and reproduces; a gamete of the same size as another with which it unites to form a zygote.

isoleucine, an amino acid containing fibrin and other proteins essential in the diets of man.

isomer, a compound which has the same molecular formula in each chemical substance but differing in chemical and physical properties resulting from different arrangements of the atoms in the molecule.

isomeric, pertaining to isomer arrangements.

isometric, pertaining to, or having equal dimensions.

isometric exercises, physical exertion of muscles that does not involve motion, achieved by setting one muscle against another.

isometropia, having the same refraction in the two eyes.

isosthenuria, a decreased variation of specific gravity of urine in renal dysfunction.

isothermal, having an equal degree of heat.

isotonic, of equal tone or tension, as in muscles; pertaining to a solution in the body having the same osmotic pressure.

isotope, a chemical element having the same atomic number as another, but differing in atomic mass.

isotropic, possessing the same properties in every direction such as conduction.

isthmitis, inflammation of the throat or fauces.

isthmus, a narrow connection between two cavities.

itch, an irritation of the skin that induces a desire to scratch; pruritus; scabies.

iter, a tubular passageway.

ivy poisoning, a dermatitis caused by poison ivy contact with the skin.

ixodic, caused by ticks.

J

jacket, a covering for the trunk or thorax made of plaster of Paris or leather bandage, used to immobilize the spine or to correct certain deformities.

jactition, extreme restlessness marked by tossing to and fro during an acute illness; convulsive movements.

jargon, chattering, unintelligible language or speech pattern; paraphasia.

jaundice, a yellow tinge to the skin and sclera of the eyes caused by an increase in bile pigment resulting from excess bilirubin in the blood due to obstruction of the bile ducts, excessive red blood cell destruction, or disturbances in liver cell function.

jaw, one of two bones that form the framework of the mouth.

jecur, the liver.

jejunectomy, surgical removal of part or all of the jejunum.

jejunitis, inflammation of the jejunum.

jejunocolostomy, surgical creation of a communication between the jejunum and the ileum.

jejunoileitis, inflammation of the jejunum and ileum.

jejunojejunostomy, surgical joining between two portions of the jejunum after the removal of the diseased part.

jejunotomy, surgical incision of the jejunum.

jejunum, the middle section of the small intestine extending from the duodenum to the ileum.

jerk, an abrupt muscular movement; reflex action to a stimulus.

joint, a junction or union between two bones such as at the elbow; an articulation between two bones or cartilage.

Jolles test, a test to determine the presence of biliary pigments in urine.

jugal, pertaining to the malar or zygomatic or bony arch of the cheek.

jugular, pertaining to the throat.

jugular veins, the large veins at the front of the throat which receive the blood from the head, brain, and face and returns it to the heart.

jugulate, to quickly stop or arrest a process or disease by therapeutic intervention such as a tracheotomy.

juice, body secretions.

junction, coming together of two parts as a nerve with a muscle.

junctura, an articulation or suture of bones.

juvenile, pertaining to youth; immature; young.

juxtaposition, a side by side position.

K

Kahn's test, a blood test for detecting syphilis.

kakotrophy, malnutrition.

kalium, potassium.

kaliuresis, presence of potassium in the urine.

kaolin, a mineral clay used as an adsorbent in the coating of pills and in kaolin mixture with pectin.

karyogenesis, the formation and development of a cell nucleus.

karyokinesis, division of the nucleus of a cell at an early stage of mitosis.

karyoplasm, the substance of the nucleus in a cell.

karyosome, chromatin mass within the nuclear network.

karyotype, complete characteristics of a cell's nucleus including its size, form, and chromosome number.

katabolism, catabolism, the opposite of anabolism.

katotropia, the tendency for the eyeball to drop downward; a turning downward.

keloid, scar formation consisting of dense tissue.

keloidosis, a formation of keloids.

kelotomy, operation for a strangulated hernia through the tissues of the constricting part or neck.

kenophobia, extreme fear of empty spaces.

keratalgia, a neuralgia of the cornea.

keratectasia, the conical protrusion of the cornea of the eye.

keratectomy, surgical excision of part of the cornea.

keratiasis, the formation of multiple horny warts on the skin.

keratin, a scleroprotein present in skin, hair, nails, and horny formations.

keratitis, inflammation of the cornea.

keratoconjunctivitis, inflammation of the cornea and the conjunctiva of the eye.

keratoderma, the horny layer of the skin; the cornea.

keratodermatitis, inflammation of the horny layer of the skin.

keratodermia, hypertrophy or thickening of the horny layer of the skin, especially on the palms of the hands and soles of the feet.

keratogenous, producing horny tissue development.

keratoid, resembling horn or corneal tissue layer of the skin.

keratoma, a callosity, or horny growth of tissue.

keratome, a surgical knife for incising the cornea.

keratometer, a device for measuring the curves of the cornea.

keratonosis, any disease of the horny layer of skin which is nonflammatory.

keratoplasty, plastic surgery on the cornea.

keratosis, any growth of horny tissue development on the skin.

keratotomy, surgical incision of the cornea.

kernicterus, a form of jaundice, icterus neonatorum, occurring in infants due to high levels of bilirubin in the blood resulting in severe neural symptoms and degeneration of parts of the brain.

ketamine, a general anesthetic which is rapid-acting.

ketoacidosis, acidosis caused by an accumulation of ketone bodies in the blood.

ketogenesis, the production of ketones or acetone within the body, especially in diabetes.

ketol, an organic compound formed in the intestine and pancreas during digestion and decomposition of protein.

ketone, a substance or an organic compound containing the carbonyl group (CO), as acetone.

ketone bodies, any acetone, B-hydroxybutyric acid, or acetoacetic acid produced during the oxidation of fatty acids and found in the blood and urine, especially in diabetics.

ketosis, an accumulation of ketone bodies in the body.

kidney, one of two glandular, bean-shaped organs situated at the back of the abdominal cavity which excrete urine (consisting of 95% water and 5% of solids).

kinanesthesia, the loss of perceptive power in sensations of movements.

kinesalgia, painful muscular movement.

kinesia, motion sickness.

kinesis, motion.

kinesthesia, sense of muscle movement.

kinetotherapy, treatment that employs active and passive movements, as in physiotherapy.

kinesiology, the science concerned with anatomy and muscular movement.

kinesioneurosis, a functional disorder manifested by tics and spasms which affect external muscles.

kleptomania, impulsive stealing

kleptomaniac, one afflicted with kleptomania.

klieg eye, inflammed conjunctiva, increased lacrimation and photophobia due to long periods of exposure to intense lights.

Kline test, a microscopic test for the presence of syphilis.

knee, pertaining to the knee joint between the thigh and the lower leg.

kneecap, the patella.

knee jerk reflex, a contraction of the quadriceps muscle which causes an involuntary kick when a sharp striking blow to the ligament patellae is applied by an instrument.

knock-knee, inward curvature of the legs which cause the knees to knock together when walking.

knuckle, the rounded end of the phalangeal joint of a finger.

Korsakoff's syndrome, a disease characterized by psychosis, polyneuritis, delirium, insomnia, illusions and hallucinations, as a sequel to chronic alcoholism.

kraurosis, a dryness and hardening of the skin and mucous membranes.

kymograph, a device for recording variations in motion and blood pressure changes.

kyphosis, a humpback; an abnormal backward curving of the spine.

kyphotic, humpback or hunchbacked.

kysthitis, inflammation of the vagina.

kysthoptosis, a prolapse of the vagina.

L

labia, lips; the lips of the vulva.

labial, pertaining to lips.

labia majora, two folds of adipose tissue covered with pigmented skin and hair on the outer surface and free from hair on the inner surface which lie on either side of the vaginal opening.

labia minora, two thin folds of mucous membrane located within the labia majora on either side of the vaginal opening.

labile, unsteady; fluctuating.

labium, a lip-like structure; lip.

labor, delivery; parturition; childbirth.

labyrinth, the inner ear consisting of the vestibule, the cochlea, the semicircular canals or bony labyrinth, and the membranous labyrinth.

labyrinthectomy, surgical removal of the labyrinth.

labyrinthine, pertaining to the labyrinth; intricate.

labryrinthitis, inflammation of the labyrinth.

lac, any milklike medical substance.

lacerate, to tear, or to make a ragged gash of the flesh.

laceration, the process of tearing, as a tearing injury to the vaginal opening by childbirth.

lacrima, pertaining to tears or tearing.

lacrimal, characterized by tears, or pertaining to organs that produce tears.

lacrimal gland, a gland which secretes tears, located in the orbit of the eye.

lacrimation, a discharge of tears.

lacrimonasal, pertaining to the lacrimal sac and nose.

lacrimotomy, surgical incision of the lacrimal duct or gland.

lactagogue, galactagogue, a substance that stimulates alveoli of the mammary glands to secrete milk.

lactalbumin, a protein in human milk.

lactation, secretion of milk; breast feeding.

lacteal, pertaining to milk; relating to intestinal lymphatics which transport chyle.

lactescense, becoming milky, or resembling milk.

lactic, pertaining to milk.

lactic acid, a syrup-like, colorless substance formed by fermentation of sugars by microorganisms which occur naturally in sour milk; it is also formed during muscular activity by breaking down glycogen; medical uses of lactic acid are found in antiseptics and dietary products.

lactiferous, the process of secreting and conveying milk.

lactiferous ducts, referring to the ducts of the mammary gland.

lactifuge, an agent used to cause cessation of milk secretion in the mammary glands.

lactin, pertaining to lactose, a sugar of milk.

lactobacillus, a rod-shaped, gram-positive bacteria that produce lactic acid from carbohydrates and which cause milk to sour.

lactogenic, inducing lactation, the secretion of milk.

lactose, a sugar derived from milk which yields glucose and galactose upon hydrolysis, used as a sweetening substance in foods.

lactosuria, milk sugar in the urine.

lacuna, a minute hollow found in bones where osteoblasts lie; a gap found in cartilage or bone consisting of bone cells.

lacus lacrimalis, the inner portion of the eye where tears accumulate.

lagophthalmos, lagophthalamus, incomplete closure of the eyelids.

la grippe, an acute infectious respiratory or gastrointestinal disease; influenza.

laliatry, speech disorder therapy.

lallation, infantile speech or babbling; stammering; the constant use of ''i'' instead of ''r.''

lalopathy, any speech disorder.

lalophobia, extreme reluctance to communicate verbally due to stammering.

laloplegia, a paralysis caused by a stroke which affects speech muscles but not tongue action or movements.

lalorrhea, an abnormal flow of speech.

lamella, a gelatinous disk inserted under the lower eyelid used as a medicinal application to the eye.

lamina, a thin layer of membrane; pertaining to either flattened side of the vertebral arch.

laminectomy, surgical removal of the posterior vertebral arch.

laminitis, inflammation of the lamina.

lance, a surgical instrument; to incise with a lancet.

lancet, a pointed surgical instrument with two sharp edges.

lanolin, a greasy, purified substance obtained from sheep's wool used as a base in ointments or lotions that are beneficial to the skin.

lanuginous, a lanugo or wooly covering, as in the human fetus immediately after birth.

lanugo, a downy hair covering the body of a fetus.

lapactic, cathartic; laxative.

laparocystotomy, surgical incision through the abdomen for removal of a cyst or an extrauterine fetus.

laparoenterostomy, a surgical creation of an opening through the abdominal wall into the intestine.

laparotomy, an abdominal operation; surgical opening of the abdomen.

laryngalia, neuralgia of the larynx.

laryngeal, pertaining to the larynx.

laryngectomy, surgical removal of the larynx.

laryngismus, laryngeal spasm.

laryngitic, pertaining to or resulting from laryngitis.

laryngitis, inflammation of the larynx.

laryngography, a description of larynx movements as recorded by a laryngographic device.

laryngologist, a specialist in laryngology.

laryngology, the branch of medicine concerned with the treatment of diseases of the larynx.

laryngoparalysis, paralysis of the muscles of the larynx.

laryngopharyngeal, pertaining to both the larynx and the pharynx.

laryngopharyngitis, inflammation of both the larynx and the pharynx.

laryngopharynx, the lower part of the pharynx which extends into the larynx and esophagus.

laryngoplasty, surgical repair of a defect of the larynx.

laryngoscope, an instrument with a tiny light used to examine the larynx.

laryngoscopy, an examination of the interior of the larynx by an instrument.

laryngospasm, spasm of the muscles of the larynx.

laryngostomy, operation to make a permanent opening through the throat into the larynx.

laryngotomy, surgical operation of the larynx.

laryngotracheotomy, a surgical procedure in which upper tracheal rings and the larynx are incised to form an artificial airway.

larynx, the enlarged upper portion of the trachea or organ of voice, composed of nine cartilages and the vocal cords.

laser, a device that transfers light frequencies into an extremely intense beam of radiation which is capable of emitting immense heat when focused, used in surgery, in diagnosis, and in research.

Lasix, trademark for furosemide used as a diuretic and to prevent the accumulation of fluid in the body.

lassitude, weakness; listlessness; exhaustion.

latent, hidden; present in a concealed form but capable of becoming manifest; potential.

latent content, the unconscious meaning associated with thoughts or actions, especially applied to dreams or fantasies.

latent period, the period in disease from the time of infection to the appearance of symptoms∞ psychoanalytic theory, a period of psychosexual development.

lateral, situated to the side, or directed to the side.

lateroflexion, flexion or bending to one side.

lateropulsion, the tendency to fall to one side involuntarily due to cerebellar and labyrinthine disease.

lateroversion, a tendency to turn to one side.

laudanum, tincture of opium.

laughing gas, nitrous oxide gas.

lavage, the washing out of a cavity or organ, as in the stomach in poisoning.

lax, without tension.

laxative, a gentle purgative or cathartic.

lead colic, severe abdominal pain due to lead poisoning.

lead poisoning, an acute condition of poisoning from large doses of absorbed lead, as in children who eat paint chips, the absorbed lead affects the brain, nervous and digestive systems, and the blood; a condition among workers exposed to lead products in industry.

lecithin, derived from glycerin, a fatty substance found in the blood, bile, brain, egg yolk, nerves, and animal tissue and which yield stearic acid, glycerol, phosphoric acid, and choline upon hydrolysis.

leech, a blood-sucking water worm once used as a means of blood- letting, now abandoned; a device used for drawing blood.

leg, the lower extremity; that part of the body extending from the knee to the ankle.

leiomyoma, a smooth muscle tissue tumor.

leiomyosarcoma, a malignant smooth muscle tumor.

lema, the dried secretion of the meibomian glands which collects in the inner corners of the eye.

lens, the crystalline lens behind the pupil of the eye that focuses light rays on the retina; a piece of glass or other transparent material so shaped as to converge or scatter light rays.

lenticular, lens shaped; pertaining to a lens.

lentiginous, a freckle; covered with tiny dots.

lentitis, inflammation of the crystalline lens of the eye.

leper, one afflicted with leprosy.

leprosy, an infectious disease caused by a microorganism, once believed to be incurable, marked by a gradual onset of symptoms such as general malaise, headache, chilliness, mental depression, numbness in various body parts, ulcerations, tubercular nodules, and loss of fingers and toes.

leprous, afflicted with leprosy.

leptocephalus, one possessing an abnormally small head.

leptomeninges, the two delicate structures that cover the brain and spinal cord.

leptopellic, having an abnormally narrow pelvis causing labor to be difficult or impossible indicating need for cesarean section.

Leptospira, disease infecting spirochetes which are thin, hooked- end, aerobic bacteria that sometimes infect man.

leptospirosis, a condition resulting from Leptospira infection, marked by lymphocytic meningitis, hepatitis, and nephritis occurring in combination or separately.

lesbian, a female homosexual.

lesion, an abnormal localized tissue formation; a wound resulting from disease or injury.

lethal, causing death; fatal; deadly.

lethargic, relating to lethargy; sluggish; stupor; inclined to sleep.

lethargy, a condition characterized by drowsiness, indifference or inattention.

leucine, an amino acid derived from protein digestion which is present in all body tissue and is essential for normal growth and metabolism.

leucinuria, the presence of leucine in the urine.

leucitis, inflammation of the sclera.

leucovorin, folinic acid used in treatment of megaloblastic anemias caused by a deficiency in folic acid.

leukanemia, leukemia existing with anemia.

leukemia, a progressive and fatal disease characterized by rapid and abnormal growth of leukocytes in the blood-forming organs of the body such as bone marrow, spleen, and lymph nodes, and the presence of immature white blood corpuscles in the circulating blood; cancer of the blood.

leukemic, pertaining to leukemia.

leukemoid, resembling leukemia symptoms but caused by another condition.

leukoblast, a cell that gives rise to a leukocyte.

leukoblastosis, an excessive growth of immature white blood corpuscles.

leukocyte, white blood cells or corpuscles of which there are two types: granulocytes, containing granules in cytoplasm, and agranulocytes, lacking granules in cytoplasm. The leukocytes are scavengers and are essential to fight invading bacteria within the body.

leukocythemia, a condition marked by excessive white blood corpuscles in the body, and an enlarged spleen, lymphatic glands, and bone marrow; leukemia.

leukocytic, pertaining to leukocytes.

leukocytogenesis, the formation of white blood corpuscles or leukocytes.

leukocytolysis, the dissolution or destruction of white blood cells.

leukocytopenia, an abnormally low white blood cell number in the circulating blood.

leukocytosis, an increased number of white blood cells in the blood usually indicating an infection, or it may occur due to hemorrhage, surgery, coronary occlusion, malignant tumors, some intoxications, pregnancy, and toxemias.

leukoderma, usually an acquired condition marked by a localized deficiency of pigmentation in the skin rendering a patchy effect.

leukoma, a white, corneal opacity.

leukopenia, an abnormal decrease in white blood cells, below 5,000 per cu. mm.

leukoplakia, white patches which form on the mucous membranes of the cheek or tongue that may become malignant.

leukorrhea, an abnormal condition marked by a white or creamy- yellowish discharge from the vagina resulting from acute inflammation and infection by Trichomonas vaginalis.

leukosis, excessive growth of leukocyte-producing tissue.

levator, a muscle that raises a body part; an instrument used to lift depressed portions such as part of the skull.

levitation, a sensation that one is being lifted gently or moving through the air without physical support, as in a dream state.

levulose, fruit sugar; fructose which is present in honey and many fruits, used in medicinal preparations.

libidinous, marked by intense sexual desire or lust; salacious.

libido, sexual drive; innate drives and instincts that motivate human behavior; the energy force associated with pleasure seeking and sexual instinct.

lichen, any of various forms of eruptive skin diseases which have small, firm, and closely set papules.

lid, eyelid.

Lieberkuhn crypts, tubular glands present in the intestinal wall.

lien, the spleen.

lienitis, inflammation of the spleen.

lientery, diarrhea with undigested food in the fecal matter.

ligament, a strong fibrous band of connecting tissue which binds the articular ends of bones to limit motion or to hold body organs in place.

ligamentous, pertaining to a ligament.

ligate, to apply or bind, as with a ligature.

ligation, the application of a ligature.

ligature, any material that binds, such as a band, thread, or wire, used for tying blood vessels; the process of tying.

limb, an extremity, an arm or leg; a limblike appendage of a structure.

limbus, the rim or edge of a part.

limen, the edge, or threshold.

liminal, barely noticeable; pertaining to the threshold, as in consciousness.

lingua, the tongue, or resembling a tongue.

lingual, pertaining to the tongue.

liniment, a liquid medicine containing oil, alcohol, or water for external use, applied by friction to the skin as treatment for sprains.

linin, a threadlike substance that connects the chromatin granules in the cell nucleus.

linitis, an inflammation of the gastric cellular tissue.

linkage, in genetics, two or more genes which tend to remain together in the same chromosome in the formation of gametes.

lip, the soft structure around the mouth, or a formation bordering an opening or groove.

liparous, obese; fat.

lipase, a fat-splitting digestive enzyme occurring in the pancreas, liver, and found in the blood and which breaks down fat into fatty acids and glycerol.

lipemia, an accumulation of fat in the blood.

lipid, any group of fats which are water-insoluble.

lipidosis, a disease of faulty lipid metabolism in which an abnormal accumulation of lipids form in the body, as in Tay-Sachs disease, Gaucher's disease, and Niemann-Pick disease.

lipogenic, producing fat.

lipoid, resembling fat.

lipolysis, the dissolution or breaking down of fat into fatty acids and glycerol.

lipoma, a benign fatty tumor.

lipomatosis, excessive fat deposits in the tissues; obesity.

lipomatous, pertaining to lipoma.

lipometabolism, metabolism of fat.

lipoprotein, a simple protein combined with a lipid.

lipothymia, fainting; syncope.

lipotropic, having an affinity for fat utilization, therefore decreasing fat deposits in the liver.

lipuria, fat in the urine.

liquefacient, a liquefying drug that causes solid deposits to be converted into liquid.

liquescent, becoming liquid.

liquor amnii, referring to the amniotic fluid which is a clear, watery substance that surrounds the fetus in the amniotic sac.

lithiasis, the formation of calculi and concretions, as gallstones.

lithium, a metallic element in its salt form used in the treatment of manic and hypomanic states of excitement, as in manic-depressive illness.

lithogenesis, the formation of calculi.

litholysis, disintegration or dissolution of calculi.

lithotomy, surgical incision into the bladder for removal of a stone.

lithotripsy, the crushing of a stony formation in the bladder or urethra.

lithotrite, a device used for crushing stone in the bladder.

lithuresis, the passage of calculi or crushed stone by urination.

litmus paper, a chemically treated blue paper which turns red by acids, but remains blue in alkali solutions, used to indicate the presence of acid in urine testing.

liver, the largest organ of the body, a reddish-brown glandular structure situated on the right side beneath the diaphragm and which secretes bile and aids metabolic functioning.

livid, cyanotic or bluish color to skin; discoloration.

lividity, the condition of being discolored or livid.

lobar, pertaining to a lobe of the lungs.

lobe, the globular part of an organ with well-defined boundaries; lower portion of the ear without cartilage.

lobectomy, the removal of a lobe of any organ or gland by surgical excision.

lobotomy, incision of a lobe; the severing of nerve fibers, disconnecting the diencephalon and sectioning the white matter of the brain, used in treatment of mental disturbances.

lobular, consisting of small lobes.

lobule, a small lobe.

lochia, a discharge of blood, mucus, and tissue from the uterus during the first few weeks after childbirth.

locomotion, moving from one place to another; moving the body.

locomotor, pertaining to locomotion.

locomotor ataxia, a form of sclerosis which affects the posterior columns of the spinal cord; tabes dorsalis. Charcot's arthropathy.

loculus, a small cavity.

logagnosia, a form of aphasia; word blindness.

logagraphia, unable to express ideas in writing.

logamnesia, forgetfulness, or unable to recognize spoken or written words.

logomania, excessive and continuous flow of speech with a repetitive quality.

logorrhea, a condition marked by incoherent and excessive talking seen in the insane.

loin, portion of the back between thorax and pelvis.

lordosis, an abnormal inward curvature of the spine.

lordotic, pertaining to lordosis.

LSD, lysergic acid diethylamide.

lubricant, an agent which makes the skin soft and smooth.

lucid, clarity of mind; rational.

lues, a pestilent disease, especially syphilis.

lumbago, dull back pain across loin region caused by sudden chilling of overheated lumbar muscles.

lumbar, pertaining to the loins.

lumbar vertebrae, referring to five bones of the spinal column extending from the sacrum to the thoracic vertebrae.

lumbosacral, pertaining to both the lumbar vertebrae and the sacrum.

lumbricalis, one of the muscles of either the hand or foot resembling a wormlike structure.

lumen, the space or cavity within a tube or tubular structure or organ; a unit of light; a hollow of a tube.

lunatic, one who is insane or mad.

lungs, one of two cone-shaped structures which function as respiratory organs responsible for providing oxygen for the body and discharging waste products.

lunula, the pale crescent at the root of fingernails.

lupiform, resembling lupus.

lupus, any of the skin diseases caused by tubercle bacilli characterized by lesions with raised edges and depressed centers that become scarlike when the scales shed.

lupus erythematosus, a chronic inflammation of the skin characterized by reddish macules that scale and drop off; the lesions form a butterfly pattern over the bridge of the nose and cheeks, occurring predominantly in females between puberty and menopause.

luteal, pertaining to the corpus luteum, the cells, or the hormone.

lutein, a yellowish pigment from the corpus luteum, lipochromes, fat cells, and egg yolk.

luteinization, the process involving the development of the corpus luteum within the ruptured graafian follicle.

luteinizing hormone, a substance secreted by the pituitary gland that stimulates the reproductive organs and the development of the corpus luteum.

luteoma, a tumor of the ovary containing lutein cells.

luxation, a dislocation.

lying-in, puerperal period; puerperium; confinement.

lymph, a transparent, opalescent liquid composed of plasma and white cells found within the lymphatic vessels. The fluid is collected from the body tissues and returned to the blood through the lymphatic system.

lymphadenitis, inflammation of the lymph nodes or glands.

lymphatic, pertaining to lymph, or the lymphatic vessels.

lymph cell, a lymphocyte.

lymph node, lymph gland, a rounded body of glandular tissue found at intervals throughout the lymphatic system, varying in size from a pinhead to an olive, which produce lymphocytes and monocytes.

lymphoblast, immature cells that become lymphocytes.

lymphocyte, a white blood corpuscle or leukocyte which participates in the body's immunity.

lymphocytic, referring to lymphocytes.

lymphocytoma, a malignant lymphoma or tumor.

lymphocytosis, a condition in the blood that involves an excess of lymphocytes above normal range.

lymphogranuloma, Hodgkin's disease; inflamed lymph nodes, as in venereal disease.

lymphogranulomatosis, infection of the lymphatic system; Hodgkin's disease.

lymphoid, resembling lymph or tissue of the lymphatic system.

lymphoma, any malignant disorder of the lymphoid tissue.

lymphopoiesis, the formation of lymphocytes or lymphatic tissue.

lymphosarcoma, a malignant tumor of lymphoid tissue, but not including Hodgkin's disease.

lyse, to cause disintegration of cells; the process involving lysis.

lysergic acid, a crystalline ergot derivative composing the base of LSD.

lysine, an amino acid derived from protein digestion, essential for growth and repair.

lysis, gradual decline of a fever or disease, opposite of crisis; destruction to a cell or substance by an influencing agent.

Lysol, trademark, used as a disinfectant and antiseptic.

lysozyme, an antibacterial enzyme present in tears, saliva, and various body fluids.

M

macerate, to soften by soaking or steeping.

maceration, the softening of a solid or tissue by soaking.

macrocardius, abnormal heart enlargement.

macrocephaly, an excessively large head.

macrochelia, excessively large lips.

macrocolon, megacolon, enlargement of the colon.

macrocyte, an abnormally large red blood corpuscle.

macrocytic, pertaining to a macrocyte.

macrocytosis, an excess of macrocytes, being greater in number than normal.

Macrodantin, trademark for nitrofurantoin used in treatment of urinary tract infection caused by Escherichia coli.

macrodontia, abnormally large size of one or more teeth.

macrogamete, the larger female gamete which is fertilized by the smaller male gamete; pertaining to the female reproductive cell.

macroglossia, excessively large tongue.

macromastia, excessively large breasts.

macrophage, a large phagocytic cell derived from monocytes present in loose connective tissues and various body organs which become active when stimulated by inflammation.

macroscopy, examination of an object with the naked eye.

macula, macule, a small colored spot on the skin.

maculation, the development of macules on the skin.

maculopapular, having both macules and papules.

mad, mentally deranged; irrational; suffering from rabies.

madarosis, the loss of eyelashes or eyebrows.

magnesium, a mineral element found in soft body tissue, muscle, bone and teeth essential to the proper functioning of the body. An excellent source of magnesium is found in nuts, whole-grain products, dry beans and peas, and dark green vegetables.

maidenhead, hymen.

mal, sickness or a disorder.

mala, cheek; cheekbone.

malacia, abnormal softening of body tissue or organs.

maladjusted, an inability to adjust one's desires or needs to the environment often causing anxiety.

malady, illness.

malaise, generalized uneasiness or discomfort, as a preliminary condition of disease; morbid discontent.

malar, pertaining to the cheekbone, or cheek.

malaria, a febrile, infectious disease caused by a protozoan parasite found in red blood cells, injected by a mosquito bite and characterized by periodic attacks of chills, fever, sweating, which may cause progressive anemia and enlargement of the spleen.

malformation, deformity or abnormal structure, especially congenital.

malign, malignant.

malignancy, condition of being malignant.

malignant, virulent and becoming worse, or resisting treatment, as in cancerous growths which threaten to produce death.

malinger, to pretend to be ill, usually to gain sympathy or to escape work.

malleal, pertaining to the malleus.

malleolus, the projections on either side of the ankle joint.

malleus, one of the three bones in the middle ear shaped like a hammer.

malnutrition, insufficient or faulty nutrition due to lack of necessary food ingestion, improper absorption, or any other disorder of nutrition.

malocclusion, imperfect closure or meeting of opposing teeth caused by abnormal growth of the upper or lower jaw.

malodor, an offensive stench or odor.

malodorous, ill-smelling, fetid, or putrid.

malpighian layer, the innermost layer of the epidermis which replaces the outer cells of the skin.

malposition, an abnormal placement of a body part.

malpractice, wrong and injurious treatment implying neglectful or illegal performance of duty by one in a practicing position, as a physician, surgeon, lawyer, or public servant.

malpresentation, an abnormal position of the fetus over the pelvic inlet, as in breech, or scapula.

Malta fever, brucellosis, an infectious disease transmitted from animals to man, marked by swelling of joints and spleen, excessive perspiration, weakness, and anemia.

maltase, a salivary and pancreatic enzyme which converts maltose to glucose by hydrolysis.

maltose, a disaccharide found in malt, malt products, and seed sprouts, formed by the hydrolysis of starch; primarily used as a sweetener.

mamma, mammary glands, or breasts.

mammary, pertaining to the breasts or glands which secrete milk formed in the lactiferous ducts during lactation.

mammilla, the nipple of the breast; a nipple-like process or proturberance.

mammillary, resembling a nipple, or concerning a nipple.

mammogram, radiography of the mammary gland.

mammography, a study of the mammary structures by X-ray photography to detect cancer.

mammotomy, surgery of a breast.

mandible, the lower portion of the jaw.

mandibular, pertaining to the lower jaw bone.

manducation, chewing of food, mastication.

maneuver, a skillful procedure, as in manipulation of the fetus and placenta to aid in delivery.

mania, intense excitement; madness; violent passion or desire.

manic-depressive, one afflicted with alternating attacks of mania and depression; cyclic affective psychosis.

manifestation, the appearance of symptoms of a disease that determine diagnosis.

manifest content, the remembered content of a dream including events and images.

manubrium, the upper portion of the sternum which articulates with the clavicle and the first pair of costal cartilages.

manus, hand.

manustupration, masturbation.

marasmus, emaciation or wasting of flesh, especially in infants.

marijuana, marihuana, an intoxicating drug usually in cigarette form, illegally used in the U.S.

marrow, soft tissue consisting of red or yellow marrow occupying the inner cavities of long bones responsible for blood cell and hemoglobin production.

masculine, having male characteristics.

masochism, sexual perversion in which pleasure is derived from physical or psychological pain inflicted upon another, or being abused; any pleasure obtained from the abuse of another which gives sexual gratification to the recipient.

masochist, one addicted to masochism.

massage, methodical manipulation of the body applied by kneading or rubbing the bare skin to stimulate circulation or increase flexibility.

masseter, the principle muscle of the mouth which is used in mastication and closing of the mouth.

masseur, a man trained in massage techniques.

masseuse, a woman trained to practice massage.

mastadenitis, inflammation of the mammary gland.

mastadenoma, a benign breast tumor.

mastalgia, breast pain.

mastectomy, surgical excision of the breast.

mastication, chewing of food.

masticatory, pertaining to mastication; a substance chewed to promote salivary secretion.

mastitis, inflammation of the breast occurring mostly in women during lactation.

mastodynia, pain in the breast.

mastoid, pertaining to the mastoid process located in the temporal bone behind the ear.

mastoidal, pertaining to the mastoid.

mastoidalgia, pain in the mastoid.

mastoidectomy, surgical removal of mastoid cells.

mastoiditis, inflammation of any of the mastoid process.

mastopexy, surgical correction of large, drooping breasts.

mastoptosis, pendulous or sagging breasts.

masturbation, manustupration, self production of an orgasm by manipulation of the genitals.

materia medica, scientific study concerned with all drugs used in the treatment of diseases, their origin, ingredients, preparation, dosage, and uses.

maternal, pertaining to a mother.

maternity, the state or condition of motherhood.

matter, pus; any substance that occupies space such as gas, liquid, or solid.

maturation, maturing or ripening, as a graafian follicle.

mature, fully developed.

maturity, the state of being mature.

maxilla, the upper jawbone.

maxillary, referring to the jawbone.

M.D., Doctor of Medicine.

measles, a highly infectious viral disease, usually occurring in childhood, characterized by reddish skin eruptions appearing on the face which rapidly increase in size and spread to the trunk and extremities, elevation of temperature, loss of appetite, and bronchitis; rubeola.

meatus, a passage or opening; a duct in the body; opening of the nose or ear.

meconium, the first fecal discharge of a newborn infant, usually tarry colored, consisting of salts, mucilaginous amnii, mucous, bile, and epithelial cells; also: opium.

media, medium, pertaining to the middle, as in the wall of an artery.

mediad, in the median line of the body, or central plane.

medial, median, pertaining to the middle.

mediastrinum, a median partition of the chest cavity from the sternum backward; a septum between two main portions of an organ; the pleural folds and space between the right and left lung.

mediate, between two parts or sides.

medicable, expectation of cure; treatable.

Medicaid, medical aid for the disabled or needy of any age not eligible for social security benefits, sponsored by federal, local, and state governments.

medical, pertaining to medicine.

medicament, a remedy or substance for healing wounds; medication.

Medicare, a Federal insurance program financed by social security which provides medical care for the aged.

medication, the administration of remedies, medicine, or drugs for the treatment of diseases or the healing of wounds.

medicine, any drug or remedy; the science of diagnosis and treatment of diseases and care of the injured; nonsurgical means of treatment of diseases; the science of preserving health.

medulla, the marrow; medulla oblongata; the inner surface of an organ or part of an organ.

medulla oblongata, the lower portion of the brain stem, or enlarged part of the spinal cord in the cranium.

medullary, pertaining to the marrow or inner portion.

megacardia, an enlargement of the heart.

megacephalic, enlargement of the head.

megacephaly, the condition of having an enlarged head or megacephalic.

megacolon, extreme enlargement of the colon.

megalomania, a mental disorder characterized by extreme preoccupation with delusions of power, greatness, or goodness.

meiosis, the process of nuclear cell division of mature reproductive cells in which the number of chromosomes are reduced to half their original number before the cell divides in two, or from diploid to the haploid.

melancholia, a major affective disorder characterized by worry, anxiety, agitation, great depression, severe insomnia, and inhibition of activity; many of the observable symptoms are similar to the depressed phase of manic-depressive psychoses.

melancholy, an abnormal state of despondency or dejection; an overelaboration of sadness and grief.

melanemia, an unnatural dark pigment in the blood.

melanidrosis, black colored sweat.

melanin, the black or brown compounds which are the chief pigments produced by melanoblasts located in the deepest layers of the skin. Many factors influence skin melanin pigments such as exposure to the sun, radiation therapy, hormone deficiency, and some types of Vitamin B deficiency.

melanism, excessive amounts of black or dark pigment in the skin, hair, and eyes.

melanoleukoderma, having mottled skin.

melanoma, any tumor which is composed of melanin-pigmented cells; a malignant melanoma.

melanomatosis, the formation of widespread melanomas on or beneath the skin.

melanopathy, a diseased condition of the skin marked by dark pigmented areas.

melanosis, an abnormal deposit of black pigments in the skin found on different parts of the body.

melanosis lenticularis, a very rare skin disorder which appears in early youth marked by various pigmented areas, ulcers, and atrophy.

melanotic, blackish discoloration; pertaining to melanosis.

malenuria, dark pigments present in urine.

melissophobia, abnormal aversion or fear of bee or wasp stings.

melitemia, the presence of sugar in the blood; glycemia.

melitis, inflammation of the cheek.

membrane, a thin layer of tissue which lines a cavity or canal, covers organs, or separates one structure from another.

membranoid, resembling a membrane.

membranous, pertaining to a membrane, or relating to the nature of a membrane.

membranous labyrinth, the inner ear which is also called labyrinth because of its complicated shape. The membranous labyrinth within the bony labyrinth consists of the utricle and saccule inside the vestibule, the cochlear duct inside the cochlea, and the membranous semicircular canals inside the bony structures.

menarche, the onset of menses, normally between ages 10--17.

Mendel's laws, the fundamental rules which govern the transmission of genetic traits based on experiments with the common garden pea (Pisum sativum).

Meniere's disease, a usually progressive disease of the labyrinth characterized by a hearing loss, ringing in the ears, dizziness, and a sensation of fullness or pressure.

meningeal, pertaining to the meninges.

meninges, relating to the three membranes enveloping the spinal cord and brain including the dura mater, pia mater, and the arachnoid.

meningioma, a tumor in the meninges.

meningitis, inflammation of the membranes of the brain or spinal cord, especially of the arachnoid or pia mater.

meningocele, congenital hernia in which the meninges protrude through an opening of the skull or spinal column.

meningococcus, the microorganism, Neisseria meningitidis, that causes cerebral meningitis.

meningoencephalitis, inflammation of both the brain and its membranes.

meningoencephalomyelitis, inflammation of the brain, the spinal cord, and their membranes.

meningomyelitis, inflammation of the spinal cord and its membranes.

meniscectomy, surgical removal of meniscus cartilage of the knee.

meniscus, a crescent-shaped interarticular fibrocartilage found in joints, as in the knee joint; concavo-convex lens.

menopausal, pertaining to menopause.

menopause, the cessation of the menses; climacteric, or change of life for women between ages 45--50.

menorrhagia, excessive or profuse bleeding during the menstrual period.

menorrhea, normal menstruation; free flowing menstruation.

menses, monthly menstruation; monthly flow of blood from the female genital tract.

menstruate, the process of discharging blood from the uterus.

menstruation, the periodic discharge of blood and mucus from the uterus occurring at regular intervals of approximately 28 days during a woman's life from puberty to menopause.

menstruum, a solvent or a medium.

mensuration, the act of measuring.

mental, relating to the mind.

mental age, the age of a person's mental ability which may be determined by mental tests.

mental deficiency, mental retardation; subnormal intellectual functioning, present at birth or which may develop during early childhood, affecting areas of learning, social adjustment, and maturation.

mentality, one's mental capacity or mental power; intellectuality.

mentum, the chin.

meperidine, a synthetic narcotic used as an analgesic and sedative.

meprobamate, a tranquilizing drug used to relieve anxiety and mental tension.

merbromin, trademark Mercurochrome, used as an antiseptic and a germicide.

mercuric chloride, a compound of mercury, highly poisonous, useful as a disinfectant, fungicide, antiseptic, and preservative.

mercuric oxide, a yellowish powder used in ointments.

mercury, a metallic element soluble in hydrochloric acid, useful in two salt forms, mercurous and mercuric, in germicides.

mercury poisoning, acute poisoning due to ingestion marked by severe abdominal pain, vomiting, watery and bloody diarrhea, diminished urinary output, and digestive tract ulceration; chronic form of mercury poisoning due to absorption through the skin and mucous membranes by inhalation, and ingestion which causes inflammed tongue, bleeding gums, loosening of teeth, tremors, incoordination and other various symptoms.

Merthiolate, trademark for thimersol used as an antiseptic and germicide.

mesarteritis, inflammation of the middle coat of an artery.

mescaline, a crystalline alkaloid drug obtained from mescal cactus which causes hallucinations.

mesencephalon, the middle portion of the brain, or midbrain.

mesenchyme, a network of embryonic mesodermic cells that develop into connective tissues, blood and lymphatic systems, heart, and cartilage and bone.

mesenteric, pertaining to the msentery.

mesenteritis, inflammation of a mesentery.

mesentery, a fold of membranous tissue which attach and support various organs to the body wall such as the peritoneal fold connecting the small intestine to the posterior abdominal wall.

mesial, pertaining to the middle.

mesial plain, a median plane or division of the body longitudinally into symmetrical parts.

mesmerism, an early term for hypnosis, named after Anton Mesmer (1733--1815) which now means therapeutic hypnotism.

mesmerize, to hypnotize; to facinate.

mesoblast, the mesoderm, or an early stage in the development of the middle layer of the mesoderm.

mesocardia, a location of the heart in the middle plane of the thorax.

mesocolic, pertaining to the mesocolon.

mesocolon, the mesentery or peritoneal fold that connects the colon to the posterior wall of the abdomen.

mesoderm, the middle layer of the primary embryonic layers lying between the ectoderm and the entoderm.

mesometritis, inflammation of the uterine muscular structures.

mesomorph, a body type which is well-proportioned, muscular, and of medium height.

mesomorphic, having characteristics of mesomorphs.

mesonephroma, a malignant tumor found in the female genital tract, or in the ovary.

mesonephros, an excretory organ of the embryo.

mesosternum, the middle portion of the sternum.

mesothelium, a layer of cells derived from the mesoderm which forms the lining of the embryonic cavity.

metabolic, pertaining to metabolism.

metabolism, all physical and chemical changes within the organism involving energy and material transformations, and including two fundamental processes, anabolism (building-up process), and catabolism (breaking down process).

metabolite, any product of metabolic functions.

metabolize, to be transformed by metabolism.

metacarpal, pertaining to the metacarpus; a bone of the hand between the fingers and wrist.

metacarpus, the bony structure of the hand between the fingers and the wrist.

metaphase, the second stage of mitosis or cell division in which chromosomes align across the equatorial plane of spindle fibers prior to separation.

metaplasia, a change of one kind of tissue into a form that is abnormal for that tissue.

metamorphosis, a change in form or structure; in pathology, a change that is degenerative.

metapsychology, speculative psychology concerned with mental processes that reach beyond empirical verification.

metastasis, the movement of bacteria or diseased body cells from an organ or body part to another part of the body, usually applied to malignant cells spread by the lymphatics or blood stream.

metastatic, pertaining to metastasis.

metatarsal, a bone of the metatarsus or foot.

metatarsus, the portion of the foot between the tarsus or ankle and the phalanges or toes; including the five bones of the foot.

metencephalon, anterior portion of the hindbrain which consists of the cerebellum and pons; that part of the brain vesicles formed by a specialization of the hindbrain in the development of the embryo.

meteorism, formation of gas or flautus resulting in distention of the abdomen or intestines.

methadone, a synthetic compound with actions similar to morphine which is habit-forming; the hydrochloride is used as a potent analgesic and weak sedative, also used as an antitussive in tuberculosis, bronchiectasis, whooping cough, bronchogenic carcinoma, and congestive heart failure; used in treatment of addiction as a withdrawal substitute for morphine.

methemoglobin, present normally in the blood in small amounts, but becomes toxic when a larger portion of hemoglobin is converted into methemoglobin by the oxidation of iron, giving the blood a dark-brown color and decreasing its function to carry oxygen.

methenamine, a urinary antiseptic.

methionine, an essential amino acid important to nutrition.

metopic, pertaining to the forehead.

metopian, that part of the forehead between the frontal eminences.

metra, the uterus.

metralgia, pain in the uterus.

Metrazol, trademark for pentamethylenetetrazol used in treating certain heart conditions and as a respiratory stimulant.

metrectomy, surgical excision of the uterus; hysterectomy.

metritis, inflammation of the uterus.

metrocarcinoma, cancerous uterine tumor.

metrocystosis, the formation of many uterine cysts.

metropathy, any uterine disease.

metroptosis, a dropped uterus.

metrorrhagia, excessive or profuse bleeding from the uterus not associated with menses.

microbe, a microorganism, bacteria, or germ which produces disease.

microbic, referring to microbes.

microbiologist, a specialist in microbiology.

microbiology, the scientific study of microorganisms.

microcephalic, pertaining to a small head below 1350 cc.

microcephaly, microcephalism, an abnormal small head, a congenital anomaly, as seen in idiocy.

micrococcus, belonging to gram-positive bacteria of the Micrococcaceae family which are globular or oval and produce certain diseases in man.

microcyte, a small red blood cell less than 5 microns in diameter occurring in certain anemias.

micron, measurement of a unit of length equal to one millionth of a meter.

microorganism, a bacteria, or minute living structure which cannot be seen with the naked eye.

microscope, an optical apparatus which magnifies minute structures and microorganisms.

microscopic, pertaining to a microscope; visible only by means of a microscope.

microscopy, a microscopic examination, as in viewing specimens under a glass slide.

microsome, a minute particle or granule present in cell protoplasm.

microtome, a device for cutting thin sections of tissue for microscopic examination.

micturate, to discharge urine; urinate.

micturition, urination, or voiding of urine.

midbrain, mesencephalon, which lies below the inferior surface of the cerebrum and above the pons, consisting mainly of white matter.

middle ear, consisting of the tympanic membrane and a cavity containing the incus, malleus, and stapes.

midriff, the diaphragm.

midwife, a woman who practices midwifery; one who assists at childbirth.

midwifery, the art of assisting at childbirth or delivery.

migraine, sudden attacks of headache which usually affect the vision and may cause nausea, vomiting, constipation or diarrhea, resulting from constriction of the cranial arteries affecting one side of the head.

miliaria, an acute inflammation of the sweat glands causing vesicles to appear on the skin due to obstruction and the retention of sweat.

miliaria rubra, prickly heat, or heat rash.

miliary, resembling millet seeds; small nodules on the skin due to excessive exposure to heat.

milieu, pertaining to environment.

milium, a tiny pink and white vesicle or nodule appearing beneath the skin due to the retention of a fatty secretion of the sebaceous gland.

milk, an opaque white secretion of the mammary glands for feeding the young.

milk fever, a fever appearing with the beginning of lactation following childbirth, resulting from an infection.

milk leg, an inflammation of the iliac or femoral vein which causes pain and swelling, often a complication of childbirth.

milk tooth, a temporary or deciduous tooth occurring in childhood.

milligram, one-thousandth of a gram; abbreviated mg.

millimeter, one-thousandth meter; abbreviated mm.

millicron, one-thousandth of a micron; one-millionth of a millimeter.

mind, the psyche; having integrated brain functioning resulting in one's ability to perceive, comprehend, reason, and process information in an intelligent manner.

miosis, an abnormal contraction of the pupils.

miotic, an agent that produces contraction of the pupil.

misanthropy, hatred of mankind.

miscarriage, spontaneous abortion; referring to the interruption of pregnancy usually between the fourth month and viability.

miscegenation, marriage or sexual union between mixed races; inbreeding between different races.

miscible, having mixing capability; able to be mixed with separation.

misogamy, a hatred or fear of marriage.

misogyny, an aversion to women.

misologia, hatred for mental work.

misoneism, an aversion to new ideas; conservatism.

misopedia, an abnormal dislike for children.

mithridate, an antidote against poisoning.

mithridatism, acquiring immunity to a poison by taking small amounts and gradually increase dosages.

mitochondria, threadlike structures in cell cytoplasm.

mitosis, indirect cell division involving complex changes in the nucleus in a continuous process divided into four phases: prophase, metaphase, anaphase, and telephase.

mitotic, pertaining to mitosis.

mitral, pertaining to the bicuspid valve in the heart that prevents the blood in the left ventricle flowing back to the left auricle.

mittelschmerz, pain between menstrual periods at the time of ovulation.

modality, a method of application of any therapeutic agent.

molar, broad surfaced tooth for grinding, one of three on both sides of the upper and lower jaw.

mole, nevus; a congenital discolored spot on the skin which is slightly elevated.

molluscum, any slightly infectious skin disease marked by the formation of cutaneous tumors.

mongolism, Down's syndrome, a congenital mental deficiency.

mongoloid, a person with characteristics of mongolism.

moniliasis, candidiasis; an infection of the mucous membranes or skin caused by yeastlike fungi.

moniliform, resembling a string of beads.

monoamine, a molecule from one amino group, as serotonin, dopamine, and norepinephrine.

monocular, affecting one eye; pertaining to a single lens.

monocyte, a phagocytic leukocyte with a nucleus shaped like a kidney which is formed in bone marrow and which constitutes part of the important defense mechanism of the body.

monocytosis, having an excess of monocytes in the blood.

monodactyly, having only one digit on a foot or hand.

monomania, a mental illness marked by a morbid preoccupation with one idea or activity.

monomaniac, a person afflicted with monomania.

monomelic, affecting only one limb.

mononuclear, having a single nucleus.

mononucleosis, having an excess of monocytes in the blood stream; an infectious mononucleosis is an acute disease caused by the Epstein-Barr virus marked by fever, sore throat, general lymph node enlargement, and an abnormal increase of mononuclear leukocytes.

monoparesis, paralysis of one part of the body.

monophobia, pathological fear of being alone.

monoplegia, paralysis of one limb or one group of muscles.

mons pubis, the pubic eminence.

morbid, pertaining to, or being affected by disease; referring to an unhealthy mental state.

morbidity, the state of being diseased.

morbiliform, resembling measles with skin eruptions.

morgue, a public mortuary where dead bodies are held until identified or buried.

moribund, dying, or a state of dying.

morning sickness, nausea and vomiting that affects some women during the early stages of pregnancy.

moron, an adult who is feebleminded or mentally deficient, whose mental intellect corresponds to that of a normal child between ages 7–12 years.

morose, a gloomy or sullen disposition.

morphia, morphine.

morphine, an alkaloid found in opium used as an analgesic and sedative.

morphinism, habitual or excessive use of morphine which results in a morbid disposition.

morphinomania, madness resulting from the habitual use of morphine; a morbid and uncontrolled desire for morphine.

morphogenesis, various changes occurring during the development of an organism or part of the body.

morphology, the study of structure and form of organisms without regard to function.

mortal, causing death; destined to die; human.

mortality, state of being mortal; statistical death rate.

morula, a solid mass of cells formed by cleavage of a fertilized ovum.

mosaic, in genetics, a person exhibiting mosaicism.

mosaicism, two or more cell lines which are distinct karyotypically or genotypically and are derived from a single zygote.

motility, having spontaneity of movement; capable to perform voluntary movements.

motion sickness, a condition marked by nausea, vomiting, and dizziness caused by rhythmic, irregular, or jerky movements, as in sea sickness.

motor, a muscle, nerve, or center that conveys an impulse which produces movement.

Motrin, trademark for ibuprofen used as an anti-inflammatory agent, and possesses analgesic and antipyretic properties.

mouth, the cavity or first portion of the digestive system, consisting of the hard palate, teeth, tongue, and cheeks; essential part for speaking, and is an alternate breathing passage.

mouth-to-mouth resuscitation, a life-saving procedure to induce artificial respiration of an apneic victim by pressing the nostrils together to close the airway and at the same time blowing directly into the mouth and lungs using short, repeated, and regular breaths.

movement, motion or the act of moving; evacuation of the bowels.

mucilage, a gummy, aqueous preparation or glue used as an adhesive.

mucin, a glycoprotein which is the chief component of mucous secretions.

mucocutaneous, pertaining to an area where the skin and mucous membranes come together.

mucoid, a glycoprotein which is similar to mucin but differing in solubility.

mucoprotein, protein, containing polysaccharides, which is present in all connective and supporting tissues in the body.

mucopurulent, containing mucous and pus.

mucosa, referring to mucous membrane.

mucoserous, composed of both mucous and serum.

mucosin, mucin present in viscous, and sticky mucus.

mucous, resembling or pertaining to mucus; secreting mucus.

mucous membranes, membranes that secrete mucus.

mucoviscidosis, the disease cystic fibrosis of the pancreas.

mucus, a viscid secretion of the glands and mucous membranes, consisting of mucin, leukocytes, various salts, and desquamated cells.

multigravida, a woman pregnant for the third time or more.

multipara, a woman who has had two or more viable fetuses.

multiparous, having borne more than one child.

multiple sclerosis, MS, a progressive and degenerative disease of the central nervous system which is not contagious, marked by tremors, muscular weakness, speech disturbances, and visual complaints.

mumps, an acute contagious disease occurring mainly in childhood marked by swelling of the large salivary glands in front of the ears, but may involve the meninges and testes in postpubertal males.

mural, pertaining to the wall in any cavity of the body.

murmur, an abnormal heart sound which has a blowing or rasping quality.

muscle, an organ which produces body movement within an animal by contraction, composed of bundles of fibers of different lengths, breaths, and thicknesses.

muscular, pertaining to muscles; composed of muscle; having well-developed muscles.

muscular dystrophy, a progressive disease in which deterioration and atrophy of the muscles cause wasting and symmetrical weakening, believed to be inherited.

musculature, involving the muscular arrangement of the body or of a part.

musculoskeletal, comprising the skeleton and the muscles.

mutant, a living organism that is a product of genetic mutation.

mutate, to alter or change.

mutation, a permanent change in genetic material; an individual exhibiting such a change.

mute, one who is unable to speak.

myalgia, having muscle pain; muscular pain.

myasthenia, muscular debility or weakness.

myasthenia gravis, a neuro-muscular disorder without atrophy, characterized by progressive fatigue and exhaustion of the muscular system.

myatrophy, muscle wasting.

mycete, a fungus.

Mycobacterium, a gram-positive bacteria found in swimming pools which causes granuloma.

mycology, the scientific study of fungi.

mycosis, a disease caused by fungi.

mycotic, pertaining to mycosis.

Mycostatin, trademark for nystatin used for fungus infections.

mydriasis, dilatation of the pupils.

mydriatic, an agent that dilates the pupil of the eye.

myelencephalitis, inflammation of the brain and the spinal cord.

myelencephalon, the posterior part of the embryonic hindbrain from which the medulla oblongata and the lower portion of the fourth ventricle develop.

myelin, the whitish fatlike substance that surrounds the axon of myelinated nerve fibers.

myelinic, pertaining to myelin.

myelinization, the formation of the myelin sheath around the axon.

myelin sheath, a segmented wrapping of a double layer of Schwann cells surrounding some nerve fibers.

myelitis, inflammation of the spinal cord or bone marrow.

myelocyte, a cell intermediate between a promyelocyte and a metamyelocyte in development of leukocytes found in red bone marrow.

myeloencephalitis, inflammation of the spinal cord and brain.

myelography, radiography of the spinal cord after an injection of a radiopaque substance into the subarachnoid space.

myeloid, pertaining to or resembling bone marrow; referring to the spinal cord; resembling myelocytes but not developing from bone marrow.

myeloma, a tumor originating in hematopoietic cells of bone marrow.

myocardiograph, an instrument for tracing heart movements.

myocarditis, inflammation of the myocardium.

myocardium, the thickest and middle layer of the wall of the heart, or muscle of the heart.

myogenic, originating in muscle.

myoglobin, a protein of hemoglobin in muslces, composed of one polypeptide chain and one hemp group, and carrying more oxygen and less carbon monoxide.

myograph, an apparatus used to measure muscular contraction.

myology, the study of muscles and their accessory structures such as bursae and synovial membrane.

myoma, a tumor consisting of muscular tissue.

myomatous, pertaining to a myoma.

myoneural, concerned with both muscles and nerves.

myopia, nearsightedness; defective vision in which objects can only be seen clearly when very close to the eyes.

myopic, pertaining to myopia.

myositis, inflammation of voluntary muscle tissue.

myospasm, spasm of a muscle or group of muscles.

myotomy, dissection of muscular tissue.

myringa, tympanic membrane.

myringitis, eardrum inflammation.

myringoscope, a device used to examine the eardrum.

myxedema, a condition causing nonpitting edema with abnormal deposits of mucin in the tissues, accompanied by a blunting of the senses and intellect due to hypothyroidism.

myxoma, a tumor consisting of connective tissue cells and mucous.

myxorrhea, an excessive flow of mucus.

myxovirus, a group of related viruses which produce influenza, mumps, and measles.

N

nacreous, a pear-like, iridescent luster in certain bacterial clusters.

nail, the horny cutaneous cell structure on the dorsal end of fingers and toes forming flat plates.

nalorphine, used as an antagonist of morphine and in treatment of narcotic overdose.

nanism, dwarfism; an abnormal small stature.

nape, the back of the neck.

naprapathy, a treatment of disease based on the assumption that an illness is due to faulty ligament functioning which may be corrected or adjusted by massage and manipulation of joints and muscles.

narcissism, self-love, or being interested in one's self, as opposed to the love of another person. An excess of narcissism interferes with relationships, but some degree of self-love if considered normal.

narcolepsy, an uncontrollable desire to sleep for brief periods.

narcosis, a state of unconsciousness, stupor, or insensibility produced by a chemical or narcotic drug.

narcotic, a drug which produces sleep; used in moderate doses, a central nervous system depressant which relieves pain and induces sleep; used in excessive doses, produces unconsciousness, stupor, coma, and even death.

narcotized, to become unconscious under the influence of a narcotic.

naris, nares; nostril or nostrils.

nasal, pertaining to the nose.

nascent, having just come into existence; being born.

nasofrontal, pertaining to the nasal and frontal bones.

nasolabial, pertaining to the nose and lip.

nasolacrimal, pertaining to the nose and tear ducts and glands.

nasology, the study of the nose and its diseases.

nasopalatine, pertaining to both the nose and palate.

nasopharyngeal, pertaining to the nose and pharynx.

nasopharyngitis, inflammation of the nasopharynx.

nasopharynx, that portion of the pharynx situated above the soft palate.

natal, pertaining to birth.

natality, birth rate.

nates, the buttocks.

natural selection, Darwin's theory of evolution which accounts for the origin of species. Because of limited food supply and a struggle for existence those genetic species which have particular characteristics tend to survive.

naturopathy, the therapeutic use of natural forces such as air, heat, light, massage, and water.

nausea, having an upset stomach and the inclination to vomit.

nauseant, causing one to feel nauseated; affecting nausea.

nauseate, to cause nausea.

nauseous, affecting or producing nausea, disgust, or loathing.

navel, the depression in the center of the abdomen; the umbilicus.

navicular, boat-shaped; a wrist or ankle bone.

nearsightedness, myopia; seeing clearly only objects that are near.

nearthrosis, an artificial joint due to a broken bone.

nebula, a corneal opacity; an oily liquid prepared for atomizer usage.

nebulizer, an apparatus which produces a fine spray such as an atomizer.

neck, that part of the body which connects the head to the trunk; a constricted part of an organ.

necrobiosis, a gradual degeneration and death of certain tissues or cells.

necrophilia, a pathological attraction to dead bodies or death.

necrophobia, morbid fear of death or dead bodies.

necropsy, autopsy; examination of a corpse.

necrose, to become necrotic.

necrosis, death of cells or bone caused by enzymatic degradation surrounding tissues which are healthy.

necrotic, pertaining to death of a portion of tissue.

negative, lacking confirmation of a disease by testing results, as a negative diagnosis; showing resistance.

negativism, opposition to advice; an opposite behavior to one appropriate in a specific situation.

Neisseria, a gram-positive bacteria, causing gonorrhea.

nematode, a roundworm belonging to Nematoda, a parasitic phylum whose hosts may be man, animals, or domestic plants.

nematology, the study of nematodes.

Nembutal, trademark for pentobarbital sodium used as a hypnotic and sedative prior to anesthesia and to control convulsions.

neoantigen, an intranuclear antigen present in cells which are infected by oncogenic viruses.

neogenesis, regeneration of tissues.

neomycin, a broad-spectrum antibiotic effective against various gram-negative organisms, used in skin infections, wounds, burns, and ulcers which form in the urinary tract, ear, eye, skin, and for preoperative preparation of the skin.

neonatal, pertaining to the newborn infant.

neonate, a newborn infant.

neophobia, an aversion to all unknown things or new scenes or circumstances.

neoplasia, the formation of new tissues or a neoplasm.

neoplasm, any new abnormal growth of tissue in the body; a tumor.

neoplastic, pertaining to neoplasm.

neoplasty, surgical restoration of tissue or parts.

Neo-synephrine hydrochloride, trademark for phenylephrine useful in raising blood pressure, as a decongestant, and as a mydriatic.

nephralgia, pain in a kidney.

nephralgic, pertaining to renal pain.

nephrectomy, excision of a kidney.

nephric, pertaining to the kidney or kidneys.

nephrism, various symptoms caused by chronic kidney disease.

nephritic, pertaining to nephritis; referring to a kidney.

nephritis, inflammation of the kidney.

nephrolith, a stone or calculus in the kidney.

nephrolithiasis, the presence of renal calculi.

nephrolithotomy, surgical removal of a kidney stone.

nephroma, a tumor of the kidney or its tissue.

nephron, the structural and functional unit of the kidney, approximately a million and a quarter nephrons in each kidney.

nephropathy, kidney disease.

nephrosis, a kidney disease marked by degenerative lesions of the renal tubules without inflammation.

nerve, a white cord-like structure comprising nerve fibers which conduct and convey impulses from the brain and spinal cord throughout the body.

nerve cell, a neuron.

nerve fiber, an enlongated thread-like process, or axon, which conducts impulses.

nerve impulse, an excitatory process occurring in nerve fibers by the introduction of a stimuli.

nervous, easily excited or agitated; pertaining to a nerve.

nervous breakdown, signifying any mental disorder that affects an individual's normal activities such as depression, psychosis, or neurosis.

nervousness, excitability or mental unrest.

nervous system, consisting of a network of nerve cells responsible for controlling body functions including ganglia, spinal cord, nerves, and brain; CNS, or central nervous system which acts to regulate and coordinate bodily activities and initiate responses that help the body to adjust to environmental changes.

neural, pertaining to a nerve or nerves; the nervous system.

neuralgia, sharp pain along the course of a nerve or several nerves.

neural tube, a tubular formation of nerve tissue in the embryo from which the brain and spinal cord develop.

neurasthenia, a condition following depressed states from prolonged emotional tension marked by weakness, exhaustion, headache, sweating. polyuria, ringing ears, vertigo, double vision, fear, irritability, poor concentration, insomnia, and many other symptoms.

neuraxitis, encephalitis.

neurectomy, excision of a nerve or part of a nerve.

neurectopia, an abnormal position of a nerve.

neurilemma, a thin membranous sheath surrounding a nerve fiber.

neurinoma, a peripheral nerve tumor.

neuritis, inflammation of a nerve or nerves accompanied by impaired reflexes.

neuroblastoma, a hemorrhagic malignant tumor involving nerve ganglia.

neurocirculatory, pertaining to circulation and the nervous system in the body.

neurocrine, relating to hormonal influence on nervous activity.

neurodermatitis, severe irritation and itching of the skin due to a nervous disorder.

neurodynia, pain in a nerve.

neurofibril, any of the delicate fibrils found in nerve cells which extend into the axon and dendrites.

neurofibroma, a tumor of peripheral nerves found in connecting nerve tissue.

neurofibromatosis, a conditioned marked by various sizes of tumors on peripheral nerves, muscles, bones, and skin.

neurogenic, beginning in a nerve or nerve tissue.

neurogenous, developing in the nervous system.

neuroglia, delicate connective tissue which supports the structure of nervous tissue in the central nervous system.

neuroglial, pertaining to neuroglia.

neuroglioma, a tumor consisting of neuroglial tissue.

neuroleptic, an antipsychotic drug.

neurologist, a specialist in neurology.

neurology, the branch of medicine concerned with the nervous system.

neurolysin, an agent which destroys neurons.

neurolysis, the cutting of a nerve sheath to relieve tension; stretching a nerve to reduce tension; dissolution of nerve tissue.

neuroma, a new growth composed of nerve cells and nerve fibers.

neuromalacia, an abnormal softening of the nerves.

neuromuscular, pertaining to both nerves and muscles.

neuromyopathic, affecting the nervous system and muscles including the heart.

neuron, a nerve cell, or any of the conductive cells of the nervous system.

neuronal, relating to neurons.

neuropathology, the study of the diseases of the nervous system.

neuropathy, any disease of the peripheral nervous system.

neuropharmacology, the science concerned with the effects of drugs on the nervous system.

neurophysiology, the physiology of the nervous system.

neuroplasty, surgical repair of nerves.

neuropsychiatry, the branch of medicine concerned with both neurology and psychiatry.

neurosis, an emotional disorder characterized by anxiety arising from unresolved and unconscious conflicts, considered to be less severe than psychoses because personality disorganization and distortion of reality are not manifested.

neurosurgery, surgery performed on the nervous system.

neurosyphilis, syphilis involving the central nervous system.

neurotherapy, treatment of nervous disorders.

neurotic, pertaining to one affected with neurosis; relating to nerves; an unusually nervous person.

neurotomy, surgical cutting of nerves.

neurotoxin, a poisonous substance which is destructive to nerve cells and tissue.

neurotripsy, crushing of a nerve by surgery.

neurovascular, pertaining to the nervous and vascular systems.

neutral, neither acid or alkaline.

neutrophil, a leukocyte that stains readily with neutral dyes.

nevocarcinoma, a malignant melanoma developing from a mole.

nevoid, resembling a nevus.

nevose, marked with nevi or moles.

nevus, a congenital circumscribed malformation of the skin which is not caused externally; a birthmark.

newborn, recently born infant.

Niacin, trademark for nicotinic acid essential to the body.

nicotine, a poisonous alkaloid found in tobacco used as an insecticide, and in veterinary preparations as an external parasitic.

nicotinic acid, from the complex Vitamin B group consisting of a crystalline compound occurring in various animal and plant tissues, used for its curative property in pellagra, poor peripheral circulation, and high cholesterol levels in the blood.

nictitation, the act of winking; blinking of the eyelids.

night blindness, defective vision in the dark due to lack of visual purple in the rods of the retina, or to regenerative slowness after being exposed to light.

nightmare, a terrifying and anxiety provoking dream.

nightwalking, somnambulism; a state of walking habitually in one's sleep.

nipple, mammilla papilla, a protuberance from the mammary gland from which the lactiferous ducts discharge milk in the female; any similarly shaped structure.

nit, the egg of a louse.

niter, potassium nitrate or sodium nitrate.

nitrate, a salt of nitric acid.

nitric acid, a corrosive, poisonous liquid in concentrated form widely used in industry and in the manufacture of medicinal preparations.

nitrogen mustard, used in therapeutic mustard compounds important in treating some diseases.

nitroglycerin, a vasodilator used in treatment of angina pectoris; also used in making dynamite or rocket propellants by treating glycerol with nitric and sulfuric acids.

nitrous oxide, a gas used as a general anesthetic and analgesic, especially during dental procedures and surgery; laughing gas.

noctalbuminuria, an excessive amount of albumin voided in urine at night.

nocturia, excessive urination at night; enuresis or bedwetting.

node, a knot or swelling; a constricted area; a tiny rounded structure; a lymph gland.

nodose, knotlike projections at intervals; having nodes.

nodular, resembling nodules.

nodule, a tiny node; an aggregation of small cells.

nodulose, having nodules or small knots.

nodus, a node.

noma, a progressive gangrenous condition of the mouth and cheek spreading from the mucous membranes to cutaneous surfaces, occurring in malnourished children.

nomenclature, classified system of anatomical structures, organisms, and names signifying the genus and species of animals and plants.

nonipara, a woman who has delivered nine viable fetuses.

nonunion, the failure of a fracture to heal, especially the ends of a bone that do not unit.

nonviable, not capable of living; inadequate development.

norepinephrine, a hormone secreted by the adrenal glands, a powerful vasopressor, and used to restore blood pressure in hypotensive conditions.

normal, a standard; natural and proper functioning.

nose, the projection on the face that contains the nares, the nasal cavity, olfactory nerve endings, and functions in speech, respiration, and sense of smell.

nosebleed, epistaxia.

nosology, scientific classification of diseases.

nosomania, an assumption that one has some special illness or disease; hypochondriasis.

nosomycosis, a fungal disease; mycosis.

nosophobia, morbid fear of sickness.

nostril, one of either of the nares.

notalgia, back pain.

notochord, a rod-shaped primitive groove of the embryo which develops into the vertebral column.

Novocain, trademark for procaine hydrochloride used as a local anesthetic.

noxious, injurious to health; hurtful.

nubility, being able to marry or marriageable, said of a girl at puberty; the final stage of sex development.

nucleate, having a nucleus.

nucleic acid, an organic compound found in cells, especially the nucleus, which is important to heredity and the control of cell metabolism. It is composed of phosphoric acids, bases from purines or pyrimidines, carbohydrates, and sugars.

nucleolus, a small rounded body within the cell nucleus in which the synthesis of RNA takes place.

nullipara, a female who has never given birth to an infant.

nulliparous, having never borne an infant.

numb, having no feeling or sensation in a body part.

numbness, a state of lacking sensation in a part of the body; lacking the power to move; state of being numb.

nurse-midwife, a person trained in the two disciplines of nursing and midwifery, and having received certification from the American College of Nurse-Midwives.

nutation, involuntary nodding of the head.

nutrient, a substance that provides nourishment, as in a component of food.

nutriment, nourishment that serves to sustain the body by promoting growth and replacement of worn-out cells.

nutrition, the process of ingesting food and utilizing it in the growth, repair, and maintenance of body activities.

nutritionist, one who specializes in scientific study of nutrition.

nutritious, providing nourishment.

nutritive, pertaining to nutrition and the process of assimilating food substances.

nyctalgia, pain occurring during the night.

nyctalopia, poor vision in a faint light or at night; night blindness.

nyctophilia, an unusual preference for night.

nyctophobia, morbid fear of darkness.

nympha, small fold of mucous membrane which form the inner lips of the vulva.

nymphomania, an abnormal and excessive need for sexual intercourse in females.

nystagmus, involuntary rapid eye movements.

nyxis, paracentesis, or puncturing the abdominal cavity for the removal of fluid to relieve the pressure of ascites; piercing.

O

oarialgia, pain in an ovary.

obduction, scientific examination of a dead body to learn cause of death; autopsy.

obese, extremely corpulent; fat; overweight.

obesity, a condition of the body in which an abnormal amount of fat accumulates beyond body requirements.

oblique, a slanting or diagonal direction; involvement of two muscles of the eye, the abdomen, the head, and the ears which run at an angle, not laterally.

obsession, an uncontrollable need to dwell on a thought or an emotion, or to behave in a specific way.

obsessive, pertaining to obsession.

obstetric, pertaining to obstetrics or midwifery.

obstetrician, a physician who attends women during pregnancy, labor, and puerperium.

obstetrics, the branch of medicine concerned with prenatal care and puerperium.

obstipation, extreme constipation which is resistive to treatment and cure, usually caused by an obstruction.

obturate, to obstruct or to close.

obturator, any obstruction that closes an opening, as a plate or disk that closes an abdominal opening.

obtusion, a deadening of normal sensations.

occipital, pertaining to the occiput or the back part of the head.

occipital bone, concerning the bone in the lower posterior portion of the skull between the parietal and temporal bones in the head.

occipitocervical, pertaining to the occiput and the neck.

occipitofacial, relating to both the occiput and face.

occipitomental, pertaining to the occiput and chin.

occipitoparietal, pertaining to the occiput and parietal bones.

occipitotemporal, pertaining to the occiput and temporal bones.

occiput, the back part of the skull.

occlusion, the state of being occluded or closed; referring to closely fitting opposing teeth in the upper and lower jaw.

occlusive, pertaining to occlusion or closing up.

occult, hidden or concealed from view, as a hemorrhage.

occult blood, a minute amount of blood that can only be detected by a microscope or chemical means.

occupational disease, a functional disease caused by one's occupation, such as writer's cramp.

occupational therapy, a method of rehabilitative treatment using activities to encourage a physically or mentally disabled person to aid his own recovery by performing light work, physical exercise, creative arts, cooking, crafts, or vocational training.

ochlophobia, abnormal fear of crowds.

ocular, pertaining to the eye; concerned with the eye or vision; the eyepiece of a microscope.

oculist, one who specializes in diseases of the eye; ophthalmologist.

oculomotor, referring to movements of the eye.

oculomotor nerve, the third cranial nerve which originates in the ventral part of the midbrain and extends to the external eye muscles.

oculomycosis, any of the fungal eye diseases.

oculus, the eye.

adontalgia, a toothache.

odontectomy, excision or the removal of a tooth.

odontitis, inflammation of a tooth.

odontoblast, connective tissue cells that line the tooth pulp outer surface and form deposits of dentin on teeth.

odontoid, resembling a tooth.

odontologist, a dentist or dental surgeon.

odontology, dentistry; the study of teeth, as they relate to health, growth, diseases and structure.

odontoma, a tumor arising from dental tissues.

odontonecrosis, extensive tooth decay.

odontopathy, diseases of teeth.

odontophobia, unusual aversion to the sight of teeth; morbid fear of dental surgery.

odontorrhagia, hemorrhaging from a socket after tooth extraction.

odontosis, development or eruption of teeth.

odontotherapy, special treatment of diseased teeth.

oedipal, pertaining to the Oedipus complex.

Oedipus complex, Freudian concept; abnormal intense love of a child for a parent of the opposite sex manifested by envy and aggressive feelings toward the parent of the same sex, most commonly love of a son for his mother.

oikomania, a nervous disorder caused by unhappy home surroundings.

oikophobia, an abnormal dislike of the home.

ointment, a soft fatlike substance used in external preparations and having an antiseptic quality.

olecranal, pertaining to the olecranon.

olecranoid, resembling the olecranon or elbow joint.

olecranon, the large bony projection of the ulna forming the elbow joint.

olfaction, the process of smelling; the sense of smell.

olfactology, the study of the sense of smell.

olfactory, referring to the sense of smell.

olfactory nerves, the first pair of cranial nerves consisting of sensory fibers which conduct impulses from the mucosa of the upper part of the nasal cavity to the brain.

olfactory organ, the nose consisting of hair cells with receptors in the mucosa of the upper part of the nasal cavity which are extremely sensitive to delicate odors.

oligemia, deficiency of blood volume in the body.

oligocholia, a lack of bile.

oligocythemia, decreased number of red blood cells than normal.

oligogalactia, a deficient milk secretion.

oligohemia, an insufficiency of circulating blood in the body.

oligohydramnios, an abnormal small amount of amniotic fluid.

oligohydruria, urine that is highly concentrated.

oligopnea, having infrequent respirations.

oligospermia, a deficient number of spermatozoa in seminal fluid.

oliguria, insufficiency in the amount of urine produced.

omental, pertaining to the omentum.

omentectomy, surgical removal of a portion of the omentum.

omentitis, inflammation of the omentum.

omentum, a double fold of peritoneum which extends from the stomach to the abdominal viscera.

omphalic, pertaining to the umbilicus.

omphalitis, inflammation of the umbilicus.

omphalocele, a protrusion of a portion of the intestine through an abdominal defect in the wall at the umbilicus occurring at birth.

omphalos, umbilicus or navel.

omphalotomy, cutting the umbilical cord at birth.

onanism, coitus interruptus, or withdrawal during intercourse before ejaculation; masturbation.

oncogenesis, producing tumors.

oncology, the branch of medicine concerned with the study of tumors.

onychauxis, nail hypertrophy.

onychectomy, surgical removal of a finger or toe nail.

onychia, inflammation of a nail bed frequently causing nail loss.

onyx, a fingernail or toenail.

onyxis, ingrown nails.

oocyte, an early stage of the ovum before maturation.

oogenesis, the formation and development of the ovum after a series of cell divisions beginning with the primordial germ cells in the ovary.

oogenetic, pertaining to oogenesis.

oophorectomy, excision or surgical removal of an ovary; ovariectomy.

oophoritis, inflammation of an ovary.

operable, subject to surgical treatment with a reasonalbe chance of safety.

ophidism, poisoning caused by snakebite.

ophthalmalgia, pain the eye.

ophthalmia, inflammation of the eye or its membranes.

ophthalmic, belonging to the eye.

ophthalmologic, pertaining to ophthalmology.

ophthalmologist, a medical physician who practices ophthalmology.

ophthalmology, science of the eye; study of eye anatomy, physiology, and diseases.

ophthalmopathy, any of the eye diseases.

ophthalmoplasty, plastic surgery of the eye or the surrounding appendages.

ophthalmoplegia, paralysis of the eye musculature.

ophthalmoscope, an instrument used to examine the interior of the eye or the retina.

opiate, any medicine derived from opium; sleep inducing.

opiomania, an abnormally intense craving for opium.

opisthotonos, a tetanic spasm in which the feet and head are bent backwards and the body arched forward, sometimes seen in meningitis and tetanus.

opium, dried juice obtained from unripe poppy capsules, used in medicine for its narcotic and analgesic effect.

opsonin, an antibody that causes bacteria to become more susceptible to phagocytic destruction.

optic, pertaining to the eyes.

optical, pertaining to vision.

optic disk, optic disc, the area in the retina known as the blind spot where the optic nerve enters.

optician, a specialist who makes optical lenses or eyeglasses for correcting visual defects.

optic nerve, the second cranial nerve which functions as the sense of sight, one of a pair.

optics, the scientific study of light and vision.

optometer, an instrument which measures the eye's refractive power.

optometrist, one trained to measure the eye's refractive powers and to fit eyeglasses to correct defects in vision.

optometry, an examination and measurement of refractive powers of the eye and the correction of visual defects with eyeglasses.

oral, pertaining to the mouth.

oralogy, the study of oral hygiene and diseases of the mouth.

orbit, the bony cavity which holds the eyeball.

orbital, concerning the orbit of the eye.

orchialgia, pain in the testis.

orchidectomy, surgical removal of a testicle.

orchioplasty, plastic surgery of a testis or testes.

orchitis, inflammation of a testis.

orderly, a male hospital employee who attends especially to male needs.

organ, a body part that performs a specific function.

organelle, a specialized part of cell strucutre, such as a mitochondrion or ''power plant'' within a cell.

organic, pertaining to an organ; having an organized structure; pertaining to substances produced by living organisms; denoting chemical materials containing carbon.

organism, any living plant, animal, or unicellular bacteria, yeasts, or protozoa.

organoplexy, the reattachment of an organ by surgical fixation.

organotherapy, treatment of diseases by endocrine gland preparations and extractions from animals.

orgasm, a state of culminated sexual excitement; the apex of sexual intercourse.

orientation, the ability to comprehend one's self with regard to time, place, and person.

orifice, the entrance or outlet of a body cavity; foramen, meatus, or opening.

Orinase, trademark for tolbutamide used to treat uncomplicated, mild, or stable diabetes mellitus that has some functioning islet cells.

ornithosis, a disease found in birds and domestic fowl which may be transmitted to man.

oropharynx, the space between the soft palate and the upper epiglottis.

orthocephalic, having a head with a height and length index between 70--75.

orthodontia, the science of dentistry concerned with correcting teeth irregularities, malocclusion, and facial abnormalities.

orthodontist, a dentist who specializes in orthodontia.

orthogenics, eugenics, or the science that is concerned with the improvement of hereditary qualities in the human race.

orthognathics, the study of the causes and treatment of malposition of jaw bones.

orthopedics, the branch of surgery dealing with the skeletal system in preservation and restoration of its articulations, and structures.

orthopedist, an orthopedic surgeon.

orthopnea, difficulty in breathing except in an erect sitting position or standing, associated with cardiac diseases, pulmonary edema, severe emphysema, pneumonia, angina pectoris and several other conditions that affect respiration.

orthopsychiatrist, one specialized in orthopsychiatry.

orthopsychiatry, the branch of psychiatry concerned with the study and treatment of human behavior in the clinical setting and which emphasizes preventive techniques that provide healthy emotional growth of children.

orthoptic, promoting normal binocular vision.

orthoptics, treatment with ocular exercises to correct strabismus.

orthoscope, an apparatus for examining the eyes which uses a layer of water that neutralizes corneal refraction.

orthoscopic, pertaining to the correction of vision.

orthoscopy, an examination using an orthoscope.

orthotonos, orthotonus, muscular spasm which fixes the head, body, and limbs in a straight and rigid line.

os, a body opening; the mouth; a bone.

oscheitis, inflammation of the scrotum.

oscillograph, an instrument which records electric vibrations of the heart activity or blood pressure.

oscillography, a process which records alternating current waves.

oscilloscope, an electronic instrument that presents visual changes of electrical variations on the fluorescent screen of a cathode-ray tube.

osmics, the science concerned with the sense of smell.

osmidrosis, a condition in which body perspiration has a strong offensive odor.

osmose, subject to osmosis.

osmosis, the movement or diffusion of a solution through a selectively permeable, or a semipermeable membrane from an area of higher density to an area of lesser density. In the human body the cell membranes are selectively permeable which permits oxygen, blood, and nutrients to pass through cells by the process of osmosis. Waste products are removed from the blood in the kidneys through the same process of osmosis.

ossa, bones.

osseous, bonelike, or bony.

ossicle, a small bone, as in the middle ear.

ossicula auditus, the three small bones in the middle ear: incus, malleus, and stapes.

ossiculectomy, surgical excision of one of the ossicles of the middle ear.

ossiferous, forming or producing bone; bonelike tissue.

ossify, to form bone, or to turn into bone.

osteal, pertaining to bone.

ostectomy, surgical removal of a bone or part of a bone.

osteectopia, displacement of a bone.

osteitis, inflammation of bone.

osteoarthritis, a degenerative disease of the joints, especially those which bear the bodies weight.

osteoarthropathy, any disease of the joints or bones.

osteoarthrosis, a chronic bone disease which is noninflammatory.

osteoblast, arising from a fibroblast cell which matures and produces bone.

osteoblastic, pertaining to the bone-forming osteoblast.

osteclasis, the fracture or refracture of a bone by surgical means to correct deformity in the bone.

osteoclast, a large multinuclear cell present in growing bone and which functions to absorb and remove osseous tissue in the formation of canals; an instrument used for refracturing bone.

osteodermia, formation of bony tissue in the skin.

osteodystrophia, bone development that is defective.

osteodystrophy, defective bone formation.

osteogen, a substance from which bone is formed within the inner periosteal layer.

osteoid, resembling bone.

osteology, the branch of anatomy concerned with bones and the structure of bones.

osteoma, a bony tumor, or a bone-like structure which develops on a bone.

osteomalacia, softening of the bones.

osteometry, study of bone measurements.

osteomyelitis, inflammation of the bone marrow, or of both the bone and marrow.

osteopath, one trained in osteopathy.

osteopathic, pertaining to osteopathy.

osteopathy, any bone disease; the branch of medicine based on the theory that the body is able to make its own remedies against disease with favorable environmental conditions and good nutrition; its therapeutic procedure involves manipulation of the bony framework and muscles for correction or cure.

osteophyte, a bony outgrowth from the surface of a part.

osteophytic, pertaining to an osteophyte.

osteoplastic, pertaining to bone repair.

osteoplasty, plastic surgery of the bones to correct a defect.

osteoporosis, loss of bone calcareous matter and increased bone porosity.

osteosclerosis, abnormal density or hardening of the bone.

osteoseptum, the bony portion of the septum of the nose.

osteotome, a bevelled chisel for surgical cutting through bones.

osteotomy, surgical procedure for cutting through a bone, or excising part of it.

ostium, ostial, a mouth, orifice, or a small opening.

otalgia, pain in the ear.

otantritis, inflammation of the mastoid antrum.

otectomy, surgical removal of the middle ear contents.

otic, pertaining to or concerning the ear.

otitis, inflammation of the ear.

otocleisis, an occlusion of the auditory tube.

otolaryngologist, a specialist in otology, rhinology, and laryngology.

otolaryngology, the division of medicine concerned with the ear, nose, and throat.

otolith, a minute calcareous body in the inner ear composed of calcium carbonate.

otologist, one trained in diseases of the ear.

otology, the science of the ear, its diseases, and functions.

otopharyngeal, pertaining to both the ear and the pharynx.

otopharyngeal tube, eustachian tube, the passage between the tympanic cavity and the pharynx.

otosalpinx, referring to the eustachian tube or otopharyngeal tube.

otoscope, an instrument used for an ear examination.

otoscopy, the auscultation of the ear with an otoscope.

ovarian, pertaining to the ovary.

ovariectomy, excision of an ovary or part of it; oophorectomy.

ovariohysterectomy, surgical removal of the ovaries and uterus.

ovariotomy, incision into an ovary, as in an ovarian tumor procedure to excise it.

ovaritis, inflammation of an ovary.

ovary, one of two reproductive glands in females which produce ova and sex hormones.

overexertion, excessive physical activity to the point of exhaustion.

overextension, hyperextension; extension beyond a reasonable point.

overriding, having one end of a fracture slipping past the other part.

overweight, exceeding one's normal weight by 10--15%; obese.

oviduct, fallopian tube, one of two tubes which extend laterally from the ovary to the uterus and which transport the ovum from the ovary to the uterus.

ovular, pertaining to an ovum.

ovulate, to release an ovum from one of the ovaries.

ovulation, the periodic process of ovulating.

ovule, an immature ovum within a graafian follicle.

ovum, an egg, or female reproductive cell, capable of developing into a new organism of the same species after fertilization.

oxygen, an odorless, colorless gas essential to respiration of most plants and animals, which constitutes approximately 20% of the atmosphere's total volume, and is necessary to support combustion.

oxygenate, to saturate or combine with oxygen.

oxygen tent, an air-tight enclosure that allows the oxygen content of air to be raised above normal to aid the respiration of a patient.

oxygen therapy, the administration of oxygen for treating conditions resulting from a lack of oxygen such as arterial anoxia from pneumonia, pulmonary edema, breathing obstruction, or congestive heart failure.

oxyhemoglobin, the combined arterial blood of hemoglobin and oxygen.

oxytocic, an agent used to accelerate childbirth; a drug which stimulates uterine contractions.

oxytocin, a pituitary hormone that stimulates uterine contractions.

ozena, a disease of the nose marked by a thick muco-purulent discharge with an offensive odor.

ozone, a form of oxygen with three atoms to a molecule which is irritating and toxic to the respiratory system.

ozostomia, a foul breath; halitosis.

P

pabulum, food or nourishment.

pacemaker, the sinuauricular node which sets the pace of cardiac rhythm situated in the right atrium which controls the heartbeat; an artificial cardiac pacemaker, as a small electronic device.

pachycephaly, abnormal thickness of the skull bones.

pachydermatous, having an unusual thickness of the skin.

pachydermia, excessive thickening of the skin; elephantiasis.

pachymeningitis, inflammation of the dura mater in the brain.

pachyvaginitis, a chronic condition of the vaginal walls in which they become abnormally thickened.

packing, the filling of a wound or cavity with gauze or similar material.

pagetoid, resembling Paget's disease.

Paget's Disease, Osteitis Deformans; a progressive, chronic disorder of bone metabolism which causes a thickening of bones, predominantly in the skull and shin.

pain, a sensation of agony, or suffering due to the stimulation of certain nerve endings; emotional suffering such as grief.

painful, a feeling of pain; distressing.

painter's colic, a condition marked by colic accompanying lead poisoning resulting in vomiting, abdominal pain, prostration, paralysis, and collapse.

palatable, savory, or agreeable to taste.

palatal, pertaining to the palate.

palate, the partition which separates the nasal and oral cavities in the roof of the mouth.

palatitis, inflammation of the palate.

palatoglossal, pertaining to the palate and tongue.

palatognathous, a congenital cleft palate.

palatoplasty, plastic repair of the palate to correct a cleft.

palatoplegia, paralysis the musculature structure of the palate.

palatum, palate.

palilalia, an abnormal condition in which words and phrases are repeated with increasing rapidity.

palindromia, a relapse, or recurrence of an illness or disease.

palingraphia, an abnormal condition in which written letters or words are repeated.

palinphrasia, an abnormal repetition of words and phrases in speaking.

pallial, pertaining to the cerebral cortex or brain.

palliate, to sooth; to relieve symptoms.

palliative, a drug that affords relief; something that soothes pain.

pallid, having no color; pale; wan.

pallidum, the globus pallidus of the cerebral hemisphere.

pallium, the cerebral cortex.

pallor, a paleness to the skin.

palm, the hollow surface of the hand.

palmar, referring to the palm of the hand.

palmar reflex, a grasping reflex found in newborn infants which is more developed in some than in others. It persists for 4 or 5 months then gradually disappears.

palpable, able to be touched, or easily perceived.

palpation, the act of examining with the hand; the application of fingers to the surface of the body to assist in diagnosing its condition.

palpebra, the eyelid.

palpebral, pertaining to the eyelid, or situated near it.

palpitate, to cause to throb or pulsate intensely, especially associated with the heart; abnormally rapid throbbing or fluttering involving the heart.

palpitation, an abnormal rapid or irregular heart beat, usually subjective.

palsy, a temporary or permanent paralysis or loss of ability to control movement; a person so disabled.

paludism, malaria; swamp fever.

panaris, infection and inflammation around a fingernail, or toenail.

panacea, a solution or remedy to cure all diseases; a cure-all.

panarthritis, inflammation in all joints.

pancreas, an elongated gland situated behind the stomach which secretes digestive enzymes and produces insulin.

pancreatalgia, pain in the pancreas.

pancreatectomy, surgical excision of the pancreas or a portion of it.

pancreatic, pertaining to the pancreas.

pancreatic juice, contains digestive enzymes produced in the tubuloacinar units of the pancreas, important in carbohydrate metabolism.

pancreatin, a substance derived from the pancreas of hogs and cattle containing the enzymes amylase, protease, and lipase which is used as an aid to digestion.

pancreatitis, inflammation of the pancreas.

pandemic, pertaining to an epidemic of a disease which affects a major portion of a country or the world.

panagenesis, a theory by Darwin, now abandoned, which states that each cell of a parent is represented in the reproductive cell, and is capable of reproducing itself in the offspring.

panhidrosis, panidrosis, perspiration over the entire body surface.

panhysterectomy, surgical removal of the entire uterus including the cervix uteri.

panic, an overwhelming fear that produces extreme anxiety; a sudden unreasonable, contagious fear that produces mass flight.

pannus, superficial vascular tissue growth arising from the conjunctiva into the cornea of the eye.

panophobia, panphobia, a fear of everything; a vague apprehension.

pansinusitis, inflammation involving all the nasal sinuses.

pant, to gasp or breathe quickly, especially after physical exertion; pant or panting during the second stage of labor under direct supervision of a trained person which allows the woman to have some control over expulsion of the fetus.

pantalgia, pain felt over the whole body.

papilla, a tiny nipple-shaped protuberance found on the elevations of the tongue and on the fingertips; the mesodermal papilla surrounding the hair bulb; the optic disc.

papillary, resembling or referring to a papilla; pertaining to the nipple of the breast.

papillectomy, surgical excision of a papilla.

papillitis, inflammation and swelling of the optic disc.

papilloma, a benign skin tumor consisting of hypertrophied papilla.

papillomatosis, the condition of having multiple papillomas.

Pap Smear, a microscopic examination of cells collected from the vagina for early detection of cervical or uterine cancer.

papule, a small elevated lesion of the skin.

papulopustular, having both papules and pustules.

papulosis, marked by multiple papules.

para, a woman who has given birth to one or more viable offspring.

para-anesthesia, the loss of feeling in the lower part of the body, or two corresponding sides of the body.

parabiosis, the union or fusion of two individuals, as conjoined twins.

paracentesis, a puncture of a cavity for the aspiration of fluid, as in dropsy.

paracephalus, a congenital defective head and imperfect sense organs in a fetus.

parachlorophenol, used in dentistry as a local anti-infective.

parachromatopsia, color blindedness.

paracusis, defective sense of hearing.

paracystitis, inflammation of the tissues surrounding the urinary bladder.

paradenitis, inflammation in tissues surrounding a gland.

parageusia, dysfunction in the sense of taste.

parahepatitis, inflammation of parts adjacent to the liver.

paralalia, an abnormal speech defect marked by producing a vocal sound different from one desired, or speaking with sound distortion.

paralambdacism, unable to sound the letter "l" and substituting another letter for it.

paraldehyde, a colorless liquid polymer characterized by an unpleasant odor used as a sedative and hypnotic in medicinal preparations.

paralexia, a condition in which one is unable to comprehend printed or written words and transposes words or syllables into meaningless combinations; dyslexia.

paralogia, a disorder of reasoning ability; psychosis.

paralysis, an impairment of motor function in one or more parts of the body due to a lesion; an impairment of sensory function which causes a loss of voluntary motion.

paralysis agitans, a progressively slow form of Parkinson's disease marked by masklike facies, fine hand tremors, slowing of voluntary muscle movement, shuffling gait, peculiar posturing, weakness, and other symptoms.

paralytic, pertaining to paralysis; a person with paralysis.

paralyze, to affect with paralysis, or to cause a temporary or permanent loss of muscular movement or sensation.

paramastitis, inflammation surrounding the breast.

paramedic, one who performs adjunctive professional medical duties.

paramenia, an abnormal or difficult menstrual period.

paramnesia, the sensation of remembering something which has never actually existed or occurred.

paranephritis, inflammation of the adrenal gland; inflammation of connective tissues which surround the kidney.

paranephros, one of two adrenal glands.

paranesthesia, see para-anesthesia.

paranoia, a rare mental disorder marked by elaborate and systematized delusions of grandeur and persecution, a condition which does not appear to interfere with the rest of a person's thinking and personality.

paranoiac, one affected with paranoia.

paranoid, a term applied to persons who are overly suspicious and who harbor grandiose or persecutory delusions, or ideas of reference; resembling paranoia.

paranoid schizophrenia, a mental disorder characterized primarily by persecutory or grandiose delusions, but frequently associated with hallucinations.

paraphasia, a type of aphasia in which wrong words are employed in senseless combinations.

paraphobia, mild form of phobia.

paraphonia, an unusual weakness in the sound of one's voice; a partial loss of the voice.

paraphrasia, a disordered arrangement of spoken words.

paraplegia, paralysis of the lower trunk and the lower limbs.

paraplegic, pertaining to paraplegia; one affected with paraplegia.

parapsoriasis, slow developing, persistent skin disorder marked by scaly red lesions.

parapsychology, the study of metapsychic phenomena which deal with psychical actions and experiences that fall outside the scope of physics or physical law, as telepathy, clairvoyance, etc.

parasalpingitis, inflammation of the tissues around a fallopian tube.

parasite, any animal or plant that lives inside or upon the body of another living organism, often at a disadvantage to the host; symbiosis.

parasitic, concerning a parasite.

parasitism, the condition of being infected with parasites.

parasitize, to infect or be infected with a parasite.

parasitology, the scientific study of parasites.

parasitosis, a disease resulting from parasitism.

parastruma, an enlargement of the parathyroid gland resulting from a goiterlike tumor.

parasympathetic nervous system, a subdivision of the autonomic nervous system. Fibers which originate from nuclei in the midbrain, medulla, and sacral region of the spinal cord, pass through the cranial and sacral nerves. Some of the effects of the parasympathetic system are: constriction of pupils, slowing of heart rate, contraction of smooth muscles, increased glandular secretions, and the constriction of bronchioles.

parasynovitis, inflammation of tissues surrounding the synovial sac.

parathyroid, one of four tiny endocrine glands, pea-size, located on the lower back portion of the thyroid gland that secretes the hormone parathormone responsible for calcium-phosphorous metabolism.

paprathyroidal, pertaining to the parathyroid glands.

parathyroidectomy, surgical removal of one or more of the parathyroid glands.

paratyphoid, an infection resembling typhoid fever caused by bacteria Salmonella.

paregoric, a mixture containing a derivative of opium, anise oil, camphor, alcohol, benzoic acid, and glycerin, used in treatment of diarrhea.

parencephalitis, inflammation of the cerebellum.

parencephalon, the cerebellum.

parenchyma, the functioning cells of an organ.

parenteral, situated or occurring outside of the digestive tract, as by injection through an alternate route or means.

paresis, an imcomplete paralysis; a weakness of an organic origin.

paresthesia, an abnormal tactile sensation, often described as creeping, burning, tingling, or numbness.

paretic, pertaining to paresis.

paridrosis, any disordered condition involving the secretion of perspiration.

paries, parietes, the enveloping wall of any hollow organ.

parietal, pertaining to the wall of a cavity.

parietal bone, one of two bones forming the top portion and sides of the skull.

Parkinson's disease, a chronic, slowly progressive nervous disorder characterized by muscular rigidity, tremors, drooling, restlessness, peculiar involuntary movements, shuffling gait, chewing movements and protrusion of the tongue, blurred vision, and other neurological symptoms.

parkinsonism, Parkinson's disease.

parodontitis, inflammation of the tissues around a tooth.

parodynia, a difficult or abnormal delivery; labor pains.

paroniria, terrifying abnormal dreaming.

paroniria ambulans, sleepwalking.

paronychia, infection of the tissues around the base of a nail.

parorexia, a perversion of the appetite marked by a craving for strange foods.

parosmia, an abnormal sense of smell.

parotid, pertaining to the parotid gland; near the ear.

parotidectomy, surgical removal of a parotid gland.

parotid gland, one of two salivary glands on other side of the face in front of each ear.

parotiditis, inflammation of a parotid gland; mumps.

parous, having given birth to at least one offspring.

paroxysm, a sudden, intense attack, or recurrence of symptoms; a seizure or spasm.

paroxymal, pertaining to paroxysms.

parrot fever, psittacosis; a disease occurring in parrots and other domestic birds that is transmitted to man, which resembles pneumonia accompanied by fever, cough, and enlargement of the spleen; ornithosis.

parturient, pertaining to birth or giving birth, as a woman in labor.

parturition, the birth process; labor; childbirth.

parulis, an abcess of the gum, especially beneath a tooth socket.

parvule, a tiny pill, granule, or pellet.

passive,   not   active; submissive.

pasturization, a process of heating a liquid such as milk for a definite period of time and at a moderate temperature in order to destroy specific bacteria which is undesirable.

Pasteur treatment, a method of treatment for preventing rabies by a series of injections with a virus of gradually increasing strength.

pastille, a medicated lozenge for irritated mucosa of the throat and mouth; a small cone of aromatic paste used to fumigate or disinfect the air by burning it within a room.

patch test, a skin test to determine sensitivity.

patella, kneecap.

patellar, pertaining to the kneecap.

patellar reflex, an involuntary jerk of the leg following a tapping of the patellar ligament with an instrument; knee jerk reflex.

pathetic, the causing or arousing of emotions such as pity or sorrow.

pathogen, a microorganism that causes disease.

pathogenesis, the development of disease; the pathogenic reactions occurring in the development of disease.

pathogenic, causing disease.

pathogenicity, having the ability to produce morbid changes or disease.

pathognomonic, specifically characteristic of a disease; denoting one or more symptoms indicative of a disease.

pathological, pertaining to the causes of a specific disease.

pathologist, a specialist trained in pathology.

pathology, the scientific study of the nature and causes of disease, and changes in function and structure; manifestations of a disease.

pathophobia, morbid fear of disease.

patient, a person who is receiving medical treatment; one who is enduring pain without complaining.

pavor nocturnus, night terror such as nightmares during sleep occurring in children and the aged.

peccant, producing disease; morbid; pathogenic.

pectoral, pertaining to the chest or breast; an expectorant which relieves respiratory tract disorders.

pectoralgia, pain in the chest.

pectoral girdle, the arch formed by the collarbone and the shoulder.

pectoralis, pertaining to the breast or chest; one of the four muscles of the breast.

pectus, the chest; breast; thorax.

pedal, referring to the foot.

pedatropy, marasmus; a wasting disease occurring in children; Tabes mesenterica, tuberculosis of mesenteric glands in children.

pederasty, coitus between males through anal intercourse, especially with young boys; sodomy.

pediatrician, a physician who specializes in pediatrics.

pediatrics, the branch of medicine concerned with children and their development, and the care and treatment of children's diseases.

pedicle, a footlike, narrow structure; a bony process which forms the root of the vertebral arch.

pedicular, pertaining to pediculosis.

pediculosis, being infected with lice.

pedodontia, pedodontics, the branch of dentistry concerned with the teeth and mouth care of children.

pedodontist, a dentist trained in pedodontics.

peduncle, a stemlike collection of nerve fibers that attaches a new growth such as a nonsessile tumor which hangs free on a stalk; a band connecting structures of the brain.

peduncular, relating to a peduncle.

pedunculation, developing a stalk or peduncle.

pelioma, a livid cutaneous spot; ecchymosis.

peliosis, a condition marked by purple patches on the skin and mucous membranes; purpura.

pellagra, a disease caused by niacin deficiency which affects the skin, digestive system, and nervous system.

pellagrin, one afflicted with pellagra.

pellagroid, resembling pellagra.

pellicle, a thin membrane; a film which forms on the surface of liquids.

pellucid, translucent; limpid or clear.

pelvic, pertaining to the pelvis.

pelvimeter, an apparatus for measuring the pelvis.

pelvis, the lower portion of the body trunk formed by the innominate bones, the sacrum, and the coccyx.

pemphigus, a condition marked by successive crops of watery blisters eruting on the skin and mucous membranes which disappear leaving pigmented areas.

pendulous, to hang or swing freely.

penetrometer, an instrument which measures the penetrating power of x-rays and radiation.

penicillin, one of a group of antibiotics semisynthesized from various molds, especially from the genus Penicillum, effective against most gram-positive bacteria and certain gram-negative forms, also effective against some forms of mold, spirochetes, and rickettsias by inhibiting bacterial growth.

penicillium, a genus of fungi, often found in mold forms of bluish color on cheese, bread, and fruit.

penile, pertaining to the penis.

penis, the male organ for urination and copulation, a pendulous structure that is suspended from the front and the sides of the pubic arch.

penitis, inflammation of the penis.

pentobarbital, a barbiturate acid derivative, the sodium salt is effective as a hypnotic and sedative, or as an analgesic; Nembutal sodium, a trademark, reduces responsiveness to external stimuli and is often used as a sedative prior to anesthesia.

pentylenetetrazol, a bitter, white powder used in preparation of a compound that is effective as a respiratory stimulant in certain circulatory conditions, and as a convulsant analeptic.

peotomy, excision of the penis.

pepsin, the primary enzyme of gastric juice that reduces protein to proteoses and peptides; an extract obtained from the glandular layer of the stomachs of hogs, sheep, or cows, used as a digestive aid.

pepsinogen, the inactive form of pepsin, the proteolytic enzyme in gastric juice which is converted to the active form by hydrochloric acid.

peptic, concerning digestion; relating to pepsin; a medicine that aids digestion.

peptic ulcer, an ulcer found in the lower part of the esophagus, in the stomach, in the duodenum, or in the gastrojejunostomy.

peptidase, any of a group of proteolytic enzymes that hydrolyze peptides or peptones into amino acids.

peptide, the linkage of two or more amino acid units by hydrolysis.

peptone, a derived protein produced by partial hydrolysis of native protein by the action of pepsin and trypsin.

peptonize, the process of converting a native protein into peptone.

peracute, very acute.

per anum, through the opening of the anus; by way of the anus.

Percodan, trademark for a fixed preparation of oxycodone hydrochloride and oxycodone terphthalate with aspirin, caffeine, and phenacetin.

percuss, to perform percussion by tapping a body part for diagnostic purposes.

percussion, the process of striking or tapping a part of the body with quick, sharp blows in diagnosing a condition of the underlying parts by sound.

percussor, an instrument used for percussion.

percutaneous, performed through the skin, as in the application of ointment by rubbing into the skin.

perflation, the process of blowing air into a cavity in order to expand its walls or to expel its contents.

perforans, perforating or penetrating, as of nerves or muscles.

perforation, the act of puncturing a hole, as caused by ulceration; any hole made through a substance or part.

perfusion, the passage of fluids through the blood vessels of an organ; the pouring of a fluid through an organ or tissue.

periadenitis, inflammation of tissues surrounding a gland.

periarterial, surrounding an artery.

periarteritis, inflammation of the outer coats of an artery.

peribronchitis, inflammation of all tissues around the bronchi or bronchial tubes.

pericardiac, pericardial, pertaining to the pericardium.

pericardiectomy, surgical removal of part or all of the pericardium.

pericardiotomy, incision of the pericardium.

pericarditis, inflammation of the pericardium.

pericardium, the fibroserous sac that envelops the heart and the roots of the great blood vessels.

pericecal, surrounding the cecum.

pericecitis, inflammation of the tissues situated around the cecum.

perichondral, relating to the perichondrium.

perichondrium, a membrane of fibrous connective tissue covering all cartilage except at synovial joints.

pericolic, around the colon.

pericolitis, inflammation of the area surrounding the colon.

perichonchal, around the concha of the ear.

pericorneal, around the cornea of the eye.

pericranium, the periosteum or membranous covering of the skull.

pericystitis, inflammation of the tissues around the urinary bladder.

peridental, surrounding a tooth or part of it.

perihepatitis, inflammation of the peritoneal capsule of the liver and the tissues of the surrounding area.

perimeter, the outer margin of a body; a device for measuring the visual field.

perimetrium, the peritoneum covering the uterus.

perimetry, the circumference of the body; the measurement of the scope of the field of vision using a perimeter.

perineal, pertaining to the perineum.

perineorrhaphy, the repair of a laceration in the perineum following childbirth.

perineotomy, surgical incision of the perineum to facilitate childbirth.

perineum, the area between the anus and the vulva in the female, or between the scrotum and the anus in a male.

perineurium, the connective tissue sheath surrounding the bundle of fibers in peripheral nerves.

period, the menses; the time it takes for a disease to run its course.

periodic, occurring at intermittent intervals.

periodontal, pertaining to the periodontium around a tooth.

periodontics, the branch of dentistry concerned with diseases of the periodontium and their treatment.

periodontist, a dentist trained in periodontics.

periodontitis, inflammation of the periodontium.

periodontium, the surrounding supportive tissues around a tooth, including the bone and gum.

perionychia, iniflammation around a finger or toe nail.

perionychium, the epidermis bordering a finger or toe nail.

periosteal, pertaining to the periosteum.

periosteotomy, surgical incision into the periosteum.

periosteum, the fibrous membrane which forms a covering of bones containing numerous blood vessels for nouorishment, and a supporting structure for the attachment of muscles, and ligaments.

periostitis, inflammation of the periosteum.

periotic, around the ear; pertaining to certain bones that protect the internal ear, and constituting a portion of the temporal bone.

peripheral, pertaining to an outer surface.

periprostatitis, inflammed tissues surrounding the prostate gland.

perisalpingitis, inflammation of the peritoneal coat surrounding the oviduct.

peristalsis, normal contraction and relaxation of the hollow tubes of the alimentary canal which slowly moves the contents along for variable distances.

peristaltic, pertaining to peristalsis.

perisystole, the interval preceding the systole in the cardiac rhythm.

perithelioma, a tumor of the perithelial layer of the blood vessels.

perithelium, the fibrous outer layer, composed of connective tissue, of the smaller blood vessels and capillaries.

peritoneal, relating to the peritoneum.

peritoneum, the thin, serous membrane which lines the entire internal surface of the abdominal cavity and envelops the viscera.

peritonitis, inflammation of the peritoneum.

peritonsillar, around a tonsil.

permanent teeth, the teeth which develop at the second dentition that supplant the milk teeth.

permanganate, a purple salt which contains potassium, manganese, and oxygen, used in solution as a disinfectant and an oxidizer.

pernicious, fatal; destructive; very harmful.

pernicious anemia, a severe and often fatal blood disease caused by a progressive decrease in red blood cells resulting in muscular weakness, gastrointestinal disorders, and neural disturbances.

peroneal, pertaining to the fibula.

peroral, by mouth; given by mouth.

per os, by mouth.

peroxide, a compound containing more oxygen than other oxides of the element, for example, the peroxides of hydrogen, sodium, and nitrogen.

perspiration, the secretion of sweat; sweating.

perspire, to sweat; to excrete fluid of perspiration through the skin.

pertussis, an infectious disease marked by catarrh and cough; whooping cough.

perversion, deviation from normal, as in sexual perversion or desire.

pervert, one who is perverted, esp. sexually.

pervious, capable of being penetrated; permeable; passing through.

pes, resembling a foot; serving as a foot; foot.

pessary, a device placed into the vagina to support and correct the uterus or rectum; a medicated vaginal suppository; a contraceptive device.

pestiferous, infectious; producing a pestilence; noxious.

pestilence, a widespread contagious disease that is usually of epidemic proportion and deadly, specifically bubonic plague.

pestilential, producing an infectious and deadly disease; destructive.

petechia, a tiny red spot occurring on the skin caused by a small amount of escaping blood.

petrolatum, a semisolid, purified mixture obtained from petroleum used in ointment preparations which protect and soothe the skin.

petrosal, pertaining to the petrous portion of the temporal bone.

phagedena, a sloughing and eroding ulcer that spreads.

phagocyte, a leukocyte which has the ability to destroy bacteria by ingesting or absorbing the harmful cells.

phagocytic, concerning phagocytosis.

phagocytosis, the destruction and absorption of bacteria and particles by phagocytes.

phagomania, an abnormal craving for food.

phakitis, inflammation of the crystalline lens of the eye.

phalacrous, baldness.

phalangeal, pertaining to a phalanx.

phalangitis, an inflammation of one or more digits.

phalanx, any of the bones of the fingers or toes.

phallic, pertaining to the phallus, or penis.

phallitis, an inflammation of the phallus or penis.

phallus, the penis.

phantasy, daydream; imaginary possibilities.

phantom limb, an illusion that a limb still exists after amputation.

pharmaceutical, pertaining to drugs or to a pharmacy.

pharmaceutics, the science of preparing pharmaceutical preparations.

pharmacist, one licensed to prepare, sell, or dispense drugs, and to fill prescriptions of physicians.

pharmacodynamics, the scientific study of drug actions and effects upon the body.

pharmacognosy, the branch of pharmacology concerned with natural drugs and possible medicinal substitutes.

pharmacologist, one who specializes in pharmacology.

pharmacology, the science concerned with drugs, including origin, chemistry, nature, effects, and uses of drugs.

pharmacopoeia, an authoritative book on official listings of drugs and drug standards, such as the United States Pharmacopeia.

pharmacy, the branch of health science that deals with preparation, dispensing, and proper usage of drugs; a drug store.

pharyngeal, relating to the pharynx.

pharyngitis, inflammation of the pharyngitis.

pharyngology, the branch of medicine that studies the larynx and its diseases.

pharyngoparalysis, paralysis of the musculature of the pharynx.

pharynx, the membraneous tube that connects the mouth and the esophagus.

phase, a stage of development; a distinct stage in mitosis.

phenacaine, a crystalline compound used in its hydrochloridic form to anesthetize the eye for removal of foreign particles and to relieve discomfort of laceration in the cornea.

phenacetin, an analgesic.

phenobarbital, a white crystalline substance used as a hypnotic, sedative, and antispasmodic.

phenolphthalein, a crystalline compound used as a laxative.

phenoluria, excretion of phenols in the urine.

phenotype, the physical appearance of a person, or the traits exhibited.

phenylketonuria, see PKU.

phial, a vial; a small container for medicine.

phimosis, a narrowness of the preputial orifice that prevents the foreskin from being pushed back over the glans penis.

phlebitis, inflammation of a vein.

phlebotomist, one trained to open a vein for blood letting.

phlebotomy, the practice of opening a vein for the letting of blood in treatment of disease.

phlegm, a thick mucus which is secreted in respiratory passages.

phlegmatic, one sluggist in temperament; apathetic.

phlyctena, a tiny watery blister or pustule.

phlyctenular, resembling a pustule; pertaining to vesicles.

phlyctenule, a tiny blister or vesicle, as on the cornea or conjuctiva.

phobia, an abnormal or exaggerated fear, usually illogical.

phonation, the utterance of vocal sounds.

phonatory, pertaining to utterance of vocal sounds.

phonetics, the science of speech and the pronunciation of words.

phonic, concerning the voice, speech, or sound.

phosphatase, an enzyme which catalyzes the hydrolysis of phosphoric esters secreted by the liver and important to the metabolism of carbohydrates.

phosphocreatine, an important form of high-energy phosphate found in muscle tissue; the source of energy in muscle contraction.

phospholipid, any group of lipids that contain phosphorus, including lecithin and cephalin, found in living cells, especially nerve tissue.

photalgia, pain in the eye caused by intense light.

photic, pertaining to light.

photochemotherapy, treating with drugs that react to sunlight or ultraviolet radiation.

photodermatitis, an abnormal skin condition caused by overexposure to light, especially from the sun.

photophobia, an abnormal intolerance to light.

photopia, vision in day-light.

photopsia, an appearance of flashes of light, occurring in certain retinal, optic, or brain conditions.

photopsin, a protein found in the cones of the retina that combines with retinal to produce photochemical pigments responsible for color vision.

photoreceptor, a receptor, or a nerve end-organ that is sensitive to light.

photosensitive, an abnormal sensitivity to sunlight, occasionally seen in certain drug reactions.

phototherapy, exposure to the sun or artificial light rays in treatment of disease. Ultraviolet phototherapy is effective in preventing dangerous levels of bilirubin in low birth weight infants with increased jaundice conditions.

phrenalgia, pain in the diaphragm; melancholia.

phrenasthenia, mental deficiency, or feeblemindedness.

phrenic, pertaining to the mind or to the diaphragm.

phrenology, the study of the shape of the skull as supposedly indicative of mental powers and character.

phylaxis, the active bodily defense against infection.

physiatrics, the branch of medicine concerned with physical therapy, and use of light, heat, water, electricity, and massage in the diagnosis and treatment of disease; physiotherapy.

physic, the art of medicine and healing; a cathartic; general drugs; to purge.

physical, pertaining to the body; relating to material things; pertaining to physics.

physician, one trained and legally qualified to practice medicine after being licensed by an appropriate board; a doctor who practices medicine as distinguished from one specializing in surgery.

physics, the study of natural forces and phenomena, and properties of energy and matter.

physiognomy, the face or quality of countenance as indicative of moral or mental character; the facial expression and bodily appearance used in diagnosis.

physiological, pertaining to physiology; normal; concerning functions of the body.

physiologist, one who specializes in physiology.

physiology, the science concerned with the functions of the living organism, its organs, and its parts; the science of the functioning of all structures in the human body.

physiotherapy, the treatment of disease by physical therapy.

physique, the organization, development, and structures of a body; body build.

physostigmine, an alkaloid obtained from the Calabar bean, used as a topical myotic in glaucoma.

pial, pertaining to pia mater.

pia mater, the highly vascular membrane forming the innermost of the three coverings which envelop the brain and spinal cord. The inner coverings consist of membranes, called meninges, which are composed of three distinct layers of tissue: the dura matter, the arachnoid membrane, and the pia mater.

pica, an unnatural craving for substances that are not food such as clay, chalk, or ashes; a depraved appetite.

pigeon breast, an abnormal projection of the sternum and the area surrounding the sternum resulting in a malformation of the chest, often seen in rickets.

pigment, coloring substance in the tissues or cells.

pigmentary, concerning a pigment.

pigmentation, a deposit of coloring matter or pigments.

pigmented, colored by a deposit of pigment.

pilar, pilary, pertaining to the hair; covered with hair.

piles, hemorrhoids.

pill, medicine in a small globular or oval shaped mass to be swallowed; a tablet.

pilose, covered with hair; hairy.

pilosis, an excessive growth of hair.

pilosity, hairiness.

pimple, a tiny elevation of the skin with an inflamed base which may form pus; pustule.

pineal, pertaining to the pineal body.

pineal body, a small, cone-shaped body in the brain believed to be an endocrine organ which secretes a hormone that stimulates the adrenal cortex; pineal gland.

pink eye, acute conjunctivitis; contagious inflammation of the eyelids affecting man and some animals; a non-infectious, sporadic condition of the conjunctiva caused by irritation from various agents.

pinna, the auricle, or the external part of the ear.

pinnal, pertaining to the pinna.

pinworm, a nematoid worm which infects the intestines; formerly called oxyuris.

pisiform, resembling a pea, or pea-shaped bone of the wrist; the smallest carpal bone.

pitting, the formation of pits or depressions in the skin, as in smallpox.

pituitary, pertaining to the pituitary gland; a substance prepared from the posterior portion of animal pituitary glands used as an antidiuretic and as a vasoconstrictor; the hypophysis cerebri.

pituitary gland, a small, grayish colored, oval-shaped endocrine gland attached to the base of the brain which secretes a number of hormones that regulate many bodily processes including growth, reproduction, and metabolic activities; referred to as the "master gland" of the body.

pituitrin, an extract derived from posterior lobes of the pituitary glands of cattle used to stimulate contraction of blood vessels, peristalsis in intestines, and uterine contractions to facilitate labor.

pityriasis, a skin disease marked by irregular scaly patches and shedding of branlike scales, occurring in humans and some domestic animals.

PKU, phenylketonuria, a metabolic hereditary disorder resulting in faulty metabolism of phenylalanine which causes mental retardation.

placebo, an inactive preparation given merely to satisfy the patient's demand; used in experimentation and research of the effectiveness of genuine drugs in controlled studies.

placenta, the flatlike organ attached to the wall of the uterus through which the fetus receives nourishment and oxygen, and passes off metabolic waste products.

placental, pertaining to the placenta.

placentation, the formation and attachment of the placenta to the wall of the uterus; the process or events following implantation of the embryo and the development of the placenta.

placentitis, inflammation of the placenta.

plague, a widespread contagious disease with a high mortality rate; a virulent, infectious, and acutely febrile disease caused by the Pasteurella pestis bacteria, transmitted to man by fleas from rodents; bubonic plague.

planomania, pathological desire to wander and to be free of social restraints.

planta, the sole of the foot.

plantar, pertaining to the sole of the foot.

plantar wart, a painful wart occurring on the bottom of the foot.

plaque, a rounded patch on the skin or on a mucous surface; a blood platelet.

plasma, the liquid part of the blood or lymph; cell protoplasm outside the nucleus.

plasmin, a proteolytic enzyme in the blood which causes fibrin breakdown and has the ability to dissolve blood clots.

plasmolysis, the dissolution and shrinkage of cytoplasm within a living cell caused by excessive water loss by osmosis.

plaster cast, a firm dressing made of gauze and plaster of Paris which is used to immobilize an injured part of the body, as in bone fractures.

plastic, capable of building tissue; material that can be molded.

plastic surgery, surgery utilized to restore and repair external defects, malformation, injured bones, body organs, and tissue by grafts of bone or tissues.

platelet, a minute disk-shaped structure found in the blood important in clotting of the blood, and in stimulating phagocytic action of leukocytes.

platycephalic, having a wide skull with a flattened top.

platyhelminthes, a group of worms or phylum having a flattened body, including tapeworms, planarians, and flukes.

platypodia, flatfeet.

platyrrhine, having a wide nose in proportion to length.

plethora, an excess blood volume; congestion.

plethoric, pertaining to plethora.

pleura, a serous membrane lining the walls of the thorax and enclosing the lungs.

pleural, pertaining to the pleura.

pleuralgia, pain in the pleura, or in the side.

pleurectomy, surgical removal of part of the pleura.

pleurisy, inflammation of the pleura, frequently accompanied by respiratory difficulties and fever.

pleuritic, pertaining to pleurisy.

pleuropneumonia, inflammation of the pleura and of the lungs.

plexor, a small hammer with a soft rubber head used in percussion for diagnostic purposes.

plexus, a network of vessels or nerves; a complicated network of interlacing parts.

plica, a fold.

plicate, folded or braided.

plication, a process by which folds are stitched in an organ's wall to decrease its size.

plumbism, a chronic condition caused by lead poisoning.

pneumatogram, a record made by a pneumatograph.

pneumatograph, an apparatus for registering respiratory movements.

pneumatometer, an apparatus which measures the quantity of air involved in inspiration and expiration.

pneumobacillus, the bacillus Klebsiella pneumoniae which causes pneumonia.

pneumococcal, pertaining to pneumococci.

pneumococcus, bacterium Diplococcus pneumoniae which produces lobar pneumonia and various infectious diseases.

pneumoconiosis, any lung disease due to an occupation, such as by inhaling dust particles, mineral dust, or coal dust.

pneumogastric, pertaining to the lungs and the stomach; pneumogastric nerve, or vagus nerve.

pneumoencephalography, a radiographic examination of the fluid- containing structures of the brain after cerebrospinal fluid is withdrawn by a lumbar puncture and replaced by injecting air or a gas.

pneumoenteritis, inflammation of the lungs and intestine.

pneumomyelography, a radiography of the spinal canal after the withdrawal of spinal fluid and the injection of air or gas.

pneumonectomy, pneumectomy, surgical excision of part or all of a lung.

pneumonia, inflammation of the lungs caused by microbes, chemical irritants, dusts, or allergy, characterized by chills, fever, chest pain, cough, purulent sputum often spotted with blood.

pneumonic, pertaining to the lungs; having pneumonia.

pneumothorax, the presence of air or gas in the pleural space which may occur spontaneously due to trauma, or deliberately introduced in collapsing a lung.

pock, a pustule on the skin in an eruptive disease, as in smallpox.

pockmark, a depressed scar on the skin made by smallpox or other disease.

podagra, pain in the great toe caused by gout.

podalgia, pain in the feet.

podiatrist, chiropodist; one who specializes in podiatry.

podiatry, a specialized field concerned with the care or the foot, including its anatomy, medical and surgical treatment, and its diseases.

pogoniasis, an excessive growth of the beard, especially on women.

poison, an agent or substance which may cause structural damage or functional disorders when introduced into the body by ingestion, inhalation, absorption, or injection.

polio, poliomyelitis.

polioencephalitis, inflammatory lesions of the brain involving the gray matter.

poliomyelitis, a viral disease of the gray matter of the spinal cord marked by fever, sore throat, headache, vomiting, and frequently stiffness of the neck and back.

pollex, the thumb.

pollex pedis, the great toe; hallux.

pollution, the act of making foul or impure, as air, soil, or water.

polyarteritis, a condition in which the body is affected by multiple sites of inflammatory and destructive lesions in the arteries.

polyarthritis, inflammation of several joints at the same time.

polychromatic, having many colors.

polyclinic, a hospital or clinic which treats all kinds of injuries and diseases.

polycythemia, a condition in which the total cell mass of the blood is abnormally increased; excessive red blood cells; erythrocytosis.

polypolydactylism, the presence of more than normal numbers of fingers or toes.

polydipsia, abnormal thirst, or having an excessive desire to drink.

polydysplasia, abnormal development of several organs, systems, or tissues.

polyesthesia, the feeling that several points on the body were touched on application of one stimulus to a single point.

polygalactia, excessive secretion of milk.

polygenic, pertaining to the belief that humans have their origin from more than one ancestral line.

polygraph, an apparatus for recording blood pressure, pulse, respiration, and electrical resistance of the skin all at the same time; lie-detector.

polynuclear, polymorphonuclear, having many-shaped nuclei.

polyp, polypus, protruding mass of tissue growth from a mucous membrane, commonly found in the nose, uterus, and rectum; a tumor with a footlike structure.

polyphagia, excessive eating.

polyphagous, eating many different kinds of food.

polyphobia, morbid fear of many things.

polyplegia, paralysis of several muscles.

polypnea, abnormally heavy panting or breathing.

polyposis, formation of multiple polyps.

polyptome, a surgical instrument for excision of a polyp.

polyspermia, excessive secretion of seminal fluid; polyspermy.

polyspermy, the fertilization of an ovum by more than one mature male germ cell, or spermatozoon.

polythelia, the presence of more than one nipple on a mammary gland or breast.

polyunsaturated, denoting a fatty acid, or pertaining to animal or vegetable fats having more than one double bond in its hydrocarbon chain; linoleic acid.

polyvalent, multivalent, as in vaccine which has several strains of antibodies.

pons, a broad band of nerve fibers in the brain which connects the lobes of the cerebrum, medulla, and cerebellum; pons Varolio.

popliteal, pertaining to the area behind the knee; the ham.

pore, a tiny opening in skin or tissue.

porosis, the formation of cavities or pores in repair of bone fractures; callus formation in bone repair.

porosity, state of being porous.

porous, having many open spaces or pores.

porphyrin, any of a group of metal-free pyrrole derivatives, occurring in protoplasm, forming the basis of animal and plant respiratory pigments.

porphyrinemia, presence of porphyrin in the blood.

porphyrinuria, excretion of porphyrin in the urine.

portal, concerning an entrance to an organ; pertaining to the porta hepatis, or the fissure of the liver.

portal vein, the large vein which carries blood from the stomach, intestine, pancreas, and spleen to the liver.

position, a placement of the body, or a bodily posture, as in supine, prone, or standing position.

posology, the system of dosage of medicines.

postauricular, located behind the auricle of the ear.

postcibal, after eating; postprandial.

posterior, situated at the back; behind; coming after.

postmortem, subsequent to death, as an autopsy.

postnasal, occurring behind the nose, as postnasal drip.

postnatal, occurring after birth of a newborn.

postpartum, after childbirth, referring to the mother.

postprandial, after a meal; postcibal.

postulate, something taken for granted without proof; a fundamental principle.

posthumous, occurring after death, which is said of a child delivered by cesarean section after death of the mother.

postural, pertaining to or affected by posture.

posture, an attitude or carriage of the body.

potable, fit to drink.

potassium, a mineral element which is the main cation of intracellular fluid in the body. It functions with sodium and chloride to regulate osmotic pressure and acid-base balance; in combination with calcium and magnesium ions, it is essential for normal muscle excitability, especially the heart muscle; and it is necessary in the conduction of nerve impulses.

potassium permanganate, a dark crystalline compound used as a topical anti-infective, an astringent, and oxidizing agent.

potency, the quality of being strong or potent; ability to perform coitus; strength.

potion, a dose of liquid medicine.

Pott's disease, caries of the vertebrae caused by tubercular infection resulting in the destruction and compression of vertebrae marked by curvature of the spine.

pouch, a pocket-like space or sac.

poultice, a soft, moist dressing made of hot linseed, bread, mustard, or soap and oil which is applied to the skin to relieve inflammation, and to hasten the excretion of pus.

pox, an eruptive or pustular disease, usually caused by a virus, such as chicken pox.

practical nurse, a nurse who is not a graduate registered nurse but who has sufficient professional training and skills to provide care for the ill.

practitioner, one who practices medicine; physician.

preanesthetic, a drug given to ease the induction of a general anesthetic.

precancerous, preceding the development of a carcinoma.

precipitant, an agent that causes precipitation.

precipitation, the process by which a substance is made to separate from another in a solution and settle in solid particles to the bottom.

precipitin, an antibody formed in the blood that causes certain proteins to precipitate when it unites with its antigen.

precocious, exhibiting mature mental development at an unusually early age.

preconscious, in reference to thoughts that are not in immediate awareness but that may readily be recalled.

precursor, something that precedes.

predigestion, a partial digestion of food by artificial means to make it more readily digestible.

predisposition, having a tendency to develop certain diseases, acquired or hereditary.

pregnable, vulnerable.

pregnancy, state of being pregnant.

prpregnant, being with child; the condition of having a developing fetus in the womb.

prehensile, adapted for grasping or seizing.

prehension, the act of graspping.

premature, happening before the proper time, as a premature infant.

premaxilla, the incisive bone.

premaxillary, situated in front of the maxilla, or upper jaw.

premedical, pertaining to preparatory professional studies in medicine.

premedication, preliminary medication which produces narcosis prior to administering general anesthesia.

premolar, in front of a molar tooth, or teeth.

premorbid, occurring before the development of a disease.

prenatal, previous to birth.

preoperative, preceding an operation or surgery.

prepuce, foreskin.

preputium, pertaining to the prepuce.

presbyatrics, geriatrics.

presbyopia, defect of vision involving loss of accommodation in which near objects are seen less distinctly than those at a distance, occurring in advancing age.

presbyopic, pertaining to presbyopia.

prescription, a written order for dispensing medication which is signed by a physician.

presenile, resembling senility but occurring in early or middle life.

presentation, in obstetrics, the manner in which the fetus is presenting itself at the mouth of the uterus and which can be determined by the examining finger, such as breech, cephalic, or scapula.

pressor, stimulating or increasing the activity of a function, as a nerve or an elevation of blood pressure.

pressure sore, bed sore; decubitus ulcer.

presystole, the period of time before the systole of the heart beat.

preventive, pertaining to a vaccine or medicine that wards off disease; prophylactic.

prickly heat, a noncontagious eruption of the skin causing red pimples that itch and tingle, usually in hot weather.

primary lesion, an original lesion from which a second one develops.

primary sore, the initial sore or hard chancre of syphilis.

primipara, a woman who has given birth to her first child, or who is parturient for the first time.

primiparity, the condition of having given birth to only one child.

probang, a flexible slender rod with a ball, sponge, or tuft at one end used to remove matter from the esophagus or larynx or to apply medicine.

probe, a slender instrument for exploring wounds, body cavities, or passages.

procaine, a compound which uses hydrochloride salt in solution for a local anesthetic as a nerve block, and for spinal anesthesia.

process, a bony prominence or protuberance; a series of steps or events leading to a specific result.

procreant, pertaining to procreation.

procreate, to beget; to reproduce.

procreation, the act of producing offspring; reproduction.

proctalgia, pain in the anus or rectum.

proctectomy, surgical removal of the anus or rectum.

proctology, the branch of medicine dealing with rectal and anal disorders.

proctoplasty, plastic repair of the anus or rectum.

proctoscope, an instrument with illumination for inspecting the interior of the rectum.

proctoscopy, an examination of the lower intestine with a proctoscope.

proctostomy, surgical creation of an artificial opening into the rectum.

prodrome, a symptom which indicates an approaching disease.

professional nurse, one who is licensed by the state board of examiners, and who works with doctors in a hospital or various other settings. The professional nurse plays an important role as a member of a treatment or surgical team.

progeria, premature senility usually occurring in childhood, marked by wrinkled skin, baldness, and hardened arteries.

progestational, referring to changes in the uterus when the corpus luteum is preparing the endometrium for the fertilization and growth of the ovum.

progesterone, progestin, the hormone excreted by the corpus luteum which prepares the uterus for reception and development of the fertilized ovum. Some synthetic and natural agents are called progestins and are used in treatment of menstrual disorders.

prognathous, marked by jaws which project forward beyond the face.

prognosis, a prediction of the probable course and outcome of a disease.

prognostic, pertaining to prognosis.

progressive, advancing forward; gradually increasing in severity of symptoms.

prolactin, a hormone that stimulates lactation.

prolamin, any of a group of simple proteins found in the seeds of grain such as wheat or oats.

prolan, a hormone present in the urine of pregnant women which allows early diagnosis of pregnancy.

prolapse, falling down, or downward displacement of a part or an organ.

proliferation, the rapid growth and reproduction of similar forms, as cells.

proline, an amino acid made in the body necessary to protein synthesis which is a basic constituent of collagen.

promazine, a phenothiazine used in the form of hydrochloride salt as a major tranquilizer in psychomotor states of anxiety and agitation.

promontory, a projecting bodily protuberance.

pronation, the act of lying with the face downward, or in a prone position; the position of turning the hand so that the palm faces downward.

pronotor, a muscle of the forearm that pronates the palm.

prone, lying with the face downward and lying horizontally.

propagation, reproduction.

prophage, an intracellular lysogenic bacterial virus that provides protection to its host from active viruses.

prophase, the first stage in cell reduplication in mitosis.

prophylactic, an agent that wards off disease; pertaining to prophylaxis.

prophylaxis, a preventive measure or treatment; the prevention of disease.

proprietary, a medicine protected against free competition by a trademark or patent.

proprioceptor, a sensory nerve ending originating chiefly in muscles, tendons, and the labyrinth that are concerned with movements and position of the body.

protosis, a bulging of the eyes; a forward displacement of an organ.

propulsion, a tendency for the body to bend forward while walking, characteristic in paralysis agitans; festination.

prosection, a programmed dissection for the purpose of demonstration of the anatomic structures of cadavers.

prosencephalon, forebrain.

prosopoplegia, facial paralysis.

prostatalgia, pain in the prostate gland.

prostate gland, a gland that surrounds the male urethra at the neck of the bladder and which contributes to the secretion of semen.

prostatic, pertaining to the prostate gland.

prostatitis, inflammation of the prostate gland.

prostatocystotomy, incision of the bladder and prostate.

prostatomegaly, an enlargement of the prostate gland.

prostatovesiculectomy, surgical excision of the prostate gland and seminal vesicles.

prosthesis, an artificial part substituted for a missing part of the body, such as an arm or leg.

prosthodontics, the branch of medicine which constructs artificial teeth or oral structures to replace missing or injured parts; prosthodontia.

prosthodontist, one trained in prosthodontics.

prostrate, lying with the body extended; to exhaust.

prostration, extreme exhaustion, or lack of energy.

protamine, basic proteins found in the sperm of some fish used as an antidote to heparin overdosage.

protanopia, inability to distinguish reds and greens; red blindness.

protease, any proteolytic enzyme that assists in hydrolysis of peptide linkages in the digestive action on proteins; peptidase.

protein, found in all cells, and constitutes about 15% of human body weight; any of a group of complex organic compounds that contain carbon, hydrogen, oxygen, nitrogen, and sulfur.

proteinase, any enzyme that hydrolyzes proteins, as pepsin and rennin.

proteinic, pertaining to protein.

proteinuria, an excess accumulation of serum proteins in the urine.

proteolysis, the hydrolysis of protein into simpler compounds such as polypeptides.

proteolytic, pertaining to proteolysis.

proteose, a class of compounds produced by partial degradation of proteins by hydrolysis.

prothrombin, a complex globulin protein in the blood important to coagulation.

protodiastole, pertaining to the first of four phases of ventricular diastole.

protopathic, responding solely to gross stimuli such as pain.

protoplasm, the primary living matter which composes all vegetable and animal cells and tissues.

protoplasmic, pertaining to protoplasm.

protozoan, a microscopic, one-celled organism.

protozoology, the science of protozoans, a division of zoology.

proud, flesh, pertaining to flesh which is characterized by an excessive granulation in wounds and ulcers.

provitamin, a substance such as ergosterol that can form a vitamin when acted upon by the body.

proximal, nearest to the point of reference.

pruritogenic, causing itching or pruritus.

pruritus, an intense, chronic itching, as in the anal region.

pseudesthesia, a subjective sensation which occurs without an appropriate stimulus, such as a pain felt in an amputated limb.

pseudocyesis, false pregnancy.

pseudoplegia, paralysis due to hysteria.

pseudopregnancy, a condition in which all symptoms of pregnancy appear to be present but without being substantiated; false pregnancy; pseudocyesis.

psilocybin, a hallucinogen derived from the mushroom Psilocybe mexicana.

psittacosis, an infectious viral disease occurring in birds that may be transmitted to humans that causes pulmonary disorders, chills followed by fever, headache, nausea, constipation, and epistaxis; parrot fever.

psoriasis, a chronic skin disease of various characteristics such as the formation of red scaly patches or flat-topped papules that cause itching.

psychasthenia, an emotional disorder marked by obsessions, compulsions, anxiety, doubts, feelings of inadequacy, and phobias.

psyche, the mind and all its mental processes both conscious and subconscious.

psychedelic, pertaining to any of several drugs that induce hallucinations, intensification of perception of the senses, psychotic states, and heightened awareness. The most commonly used psychedelics are LSD, marijuana, mescaline, psilocybin, and morning-glory seeds.

psychiatric, pertaining to psychiatry.

psychiatrist, a physician who specializes in the treatment of mental disorders, or psychiatry.

psychiatry, the medical science concerned with the origin, diagnosis, treatment and prevention of mental illness.

psychic, pertaining to the mind.

psychoanalysis, a psychologic method or theory of human development and behavior originated by Sigmund Freud that provides a system of psychotherapy which analyzes the subconscious thoughts in order to determine and eliminate physical and mental disorders.

psychoanalyst, a psychiatrist who has training in psychoanalysis.

psychoanalytic, pertaining to psychoanalysis.

psychobiology, the science concerned with the interaction between the mind and body as being an integrated unit in the formation and functioning of the personality.

psychodrama, a technique of group psychotherapy in which individuals dramatize roles enabling them to increase awareness of their emotional problems.

psychodramatic, pertaining to psychodrama.

psychodynamics, a systemized theory of human behavior and the role of unconscious motivation.

psychogenesis, the origin and development of the mind; the causation of a symptom or illness by mental or psychic factors as opposed to organic ones.

psychogenetic, pertaining to a disease which has its origin in the mind.

psychogenic, of mental origin; having a psychological origin.

psychokinesis, the alteration of motion directed by thought processes.

psycholepsy, sudden alteration of moods.

psychological, pertaining to the study of the mind.

psychologist, one who specializes in psychology.

psychology, the science concerned with mental processes and the behavior in man and animals.

psychometry, the science dealing in testing and measuring psychologic ability, efficiency, potential, and functioning.

psychomotor, pertaining to motor effects of the cerebral or psychologic functioning; causing voluntary movement.

psychoneurosis, a neurosis of a functional nature characterized by anxiety, phobias, compulsions, obsessions, and physical complaints without physical cause; neurosis.

psychoneurotic, one suffering from psychoneurosis.

psychoparesis, weakness of the mind.

psychopath, one lacking moral sensibility, but possessing normal intelligence; a mentally unstable person.

psychopathic, pertaining to a mental disorder; relating to treatment of mental disorders; abnormal.

psychopathology, the study of the causes and processes of mental disease or abnormal behavior.

psychopathy, any mental disease, especially one characterized by a defective personality.

psychopharmacology, the science of drugs as they relate to mental and behavioral effects on emotional states; the use of drugs to modify psychological symptoms.

psychophysics, the study of mental processes in relation to physical processes; the study of the relation between stimuli and the effects they produce.

psychophysiology, the physiology of the mind; the correlation between the body and mind.

phychosis, a major mental disorder of organic or emotional origin, often characterized by regressive behavior, inappropriate mood, lack of impulse control, delusions, hallucinations, loss of contact with reality, and a disintegration of personality.

psychosomatic, referring to illnesses in which bodily symptoms are of mental or emotional manifestation.

psychosomatic medicine, the branch of medical science emphasizing mental factors as the cause of functional and structural changes in disease processes.

psychosurgery, surgery of the brain to relieve certain symptoms in mental illness, as a lobotomy.

psychotherapeutic, pertaining to psychotherapy.

psychotherapist, one trained in psychotherapy.

psychotherapy, a treatment or method based primarily upon the verbal and non-verbal aspects of communication with a patient, as distinguished from the use of drugs or other measures of treatment.

psychotic, pertaining to psychosis; one exhibiting psychosis.

psychotropic, a term applied to drugs that have a special action upon the mind or psyche.

psychrophobia, an abnormal fear or sensitivity to cold.

psychrotherapy, treatment of disease by application of cold.

ptamic, that which causes sneezing.

ptarmus, spasmodic sneezing.

pterygoid, shaped like a wing; pertaining to the two large processes of the sphenoid at the base of the skull.

ptilosis, the loss of eyelashes.

ptomaine, any of a class of nitrogenous organic bases which become toxic resulting from the action of putrefactive bacteria produced in animal and vegetable matter.

ptosis, a drooping of the upper eyelid caused by paralysis of the levator muscle; the prolapse of any organ of the body.

ptotic, pertaining to ptosis.

ptyalism, excessive secretion of saliva; salivation.

ptyaloith, a salivary concretion or stone.

puberal, concerning puberty.

puberty, the period in life during which the secondary sex characteristics begin to develop and either sex becomes capable of sexual reproduction.

pubes, the pubic region; the anterior region of the innominate bone covered with pubic hair; os pubis.

pubescence, one arriving at puberty; the covering of fine hair on the body.

pubescent, reaching puberty.

pubic, pertaining to the pubes.

pubis, pubic bone, or the innominate bone.

pudendal, relating to the external female genitalia, or genitals. pudendum, external female genitals; vulva.

puerile, childlike.

puerilism, childish behavior exhibited by an adult; immature behavior.

puerperal, pertaining to puerperium.

puerperal fever, septicema following childbirth.

puerperium, the state of a woman immediately following childbirth, usually a period of 3 to 6 weeks.

pulmometry, determination of the capacity of the lungs with a pulmometer.

pulmonary, pertaining to the lungs.

pulmonary artery, an artery which conveys venous blood directly from the heart to the lungs.

pulmonary vein, any of four veins conveying oxygenated blood directly from the lungs to the heart.

pulmonectomy, surgical removal of part or all of a lung's tissue; pneumonectomy.

pulmonic, pertaining to the lungs.

pulmonitis, inflammation of the lung; pneumonia.

pulmotor, a mechanical apparatus for inducing artificial respiration by forcing oxygen into the lungs or to expel the lung contents, as in asphyxiation or drowning.

pulp, the soft part of an organ; referring to dental pulp in the interior of a tooth.

pulpy, resembling pulp.

pulsation, the process of rhythmic beat, as in the heart and blood vessels; pulse.

pulse, the rate or rhythm of the heart contractions causing the arteries to contract and expand at regularly throbbing intervals; the pulsation of the radial artery at the wrist.

pulsimeter, an instrument for measuring the frequency and force of a pulse; sphygmometer.

pulverization, the crushing of any substance into tiny particles. pulverulent, resembling powder; fine powder; dusty.

pulvis, a powder.

pump, an apparatus used to transfer or to remove fluids or gases by suction or pressure.

puncture, a hole or wound made by a sharp pointed device; to make a hole with a pointed instrument.

pupil, the round contractile orifice or opening at the center of the iris.

pupillary, concerning the pupil of the eye.

purgative, a substance that evacuates the bowels; a cathartic.

purge, a drug that causes evacuation of the bowels; to evacuate the bowels by means of a purgative.

purpura, a condition of the skin marked by purple or livid spots caused by tiny hemorrhages that invade the tissues.

purpuric, pertaining to purpura.

purulent, consisting of matter or pus; resembling pus.

pus, a yellowish-white product of inflammation composed of a thin albuminous fluid and leukocytes or particles of their remains.

pustulant, causing pustules or blisters; a pustulant medication or agent.

pustular, pertaining to or having the nature of a pustule; covered with pustules.

pustulation, the formation of pustules.

pustule, a small, elevated pus-containing lesion of the skin; any circumscribed, flat, or rounded protuberance found on the skin resembling a pimple or blister with an inflammed base and containing pus.

putrefaction, the process of putrefying; the enzymatic decomposition of animal or vegetable matter, producing a foul- smelling compound.

putrefy, to undergo putrefaction.

putrescence, the process of undergoing putrefaction; becoming putrid.

putrescine, a polyamine found in decaying meat products.

putrid, decayed or rotten; putrefied.

pyelitis, inflammation of the renal pelvis.

pyelocystitis, inflammation of the renal pelvis and the bladder.

pyelogram, the x-ray film produced by pyelography.

pyelography, a radiography of the kidneys and ureter after an injection of a contrast solution or dye.

pyelonephritis, inflammation of the whole kidney due to a bacterial infection.

pyelonephrosis, any disease of the kidney and its pelvis.

pyelotomy, surgical incision of the kidney.

pyemia, septicemia or blood poisoning caused by pyogenic bacteria.

pyknic, having a shorot, thick, and stocky body build.

pyknometer, an apparatus for determining the specific gravity of fluids.

pylephlebitis, inflammation of the portal vein.

pylic, pertaining to the portal vein.

pyloric, pertaining to the pylorus.

pylorus, the opening between the stomach and the duodenum; used to refer to the pyloric part of the stomach.

pyoderma, any purulent disease of the skin.

pyogenic, producing pus; pertaining to the formation of pus.

pyorrhea, a bacterial gum infection with a copious discharge of pus.

pyostatic, a drug that arrests suppuration.

pyothorax, an accumulation of pus in the pleural cavity; empyema.

pyramidal, pertaining to drugs which have an accumulative effect; resembling a pyramid; see extrapyramidal.

pyretic, pertaining to fever.

pyrexia, a fever; a febrile condition.

Pyridium, a brick-red powder used to treat infections of the genitourinary tract; trademark for phenazopyridine hydrochloride.

pyridoxine, one of the forms of Vitamine B6 used in its salt form to treat a deficiency of B6 in the body; sometimes used in treatment of myasthenia gravis.

pyromania, an obsessive preoccupation with fires or the compulsion to set them.

pyrosis, heartburn.

pyrotic, caustic; burning.

pyuria, the presence of pus in the urine.

Q

Q-fever, an acute infectious disease marked by fever, headache, muscular pains, chills, and loss of appetite, caused by rickettsia and transmitted by inhaling infected dust or drinking contaminated milk. Common among those who handle hides and animal products; Queensland fever.

q-sort, an assessment of personality in which the subject (or one who observes) indicates the degree to which a standardized set of descriptive statements are representative of the subject.

quack, one who pretends to have experience in medicine, as in diagnosis and treatment of disease; charlatan.

quackery, the methods used by a quack.

quadrant, a fourth of a circle; the four regions of the abdomen which are divided for diagnostic purposes.

quadriceps, having four heads, as in the large quadriceps muscle in front of the thigh.

quadripara, a woman who has produced four viable offspring.

quadripartite, having four parts.

quadriplegia, paralysis affecting all four limbs.

quadroon, the offspring of a white person and a mulatto; an individual having one-quarter Negro heritage.

quadruplet, being one of four children born to the same mother and of one birth.

quarantine, a period of detention or isolation to prevent the spread of a communicable disease.

quartan, recurring every fourth day, as in quartan fever.

Queensland fever, see Q-fever.

quenching, to suppress or extinguish by immersing in water.

querulent, fretful or complaining.

quickening, the first noticeable movement of the fetus in utero.

quinidine, a crystalline alkaloid isomer of quinine used to treat abnormal cardiac arrythmias.

quinine, a bitter-tasting alkaloid, obtained from the bark of cinchona trees, used in its salt form to treat malaria; quinine is used as an analgesic, antipyretic, oxytocic, cardiac depressant, and for other various treatments.

quinsy, an inflammation of the tonsils and the formation of abscess of the peritonsillar tissue.

quintipara, a woman who has had five viable offspring.

quintuplet, one of five offspring produced at one labor.

quotidian, occurring daily; recurring daily fever.

quotient, a number derived at by division.

Q-wave, a downward wave of an electrocardiogram that is associated with the contractions of the heart ventricles.

R

rabbetting, interlocking of the splintered edges of a bone fracture.

rabbit fever, Tularemia.

rabic, pertaining to rabies.

rabid, being affected with rabies; relating to rabies.

rabies, an acute viral disease that produces infection of the central nervous system marked by paralysis of the muscle of deglutition, glottal spasm, manic behavior, convulsions, tetany, and respiratory paralysis. May be communicated by a bite of a rabid animal, often fatal to man without proper treatment.

racemose, resembling a cluster or bunch of follicles which are divided and subdivided, as in a gland.

rachialgia, pain in the spine.

rachianesthesia, spinal anesthesia.

rachicentesis, lumbar puncture to determine the pressure of fluid and to obtain fluid for examination.

rachidial, rachidian, pertaining to the spinal column.

rachigraph, a device that outlines the curves of the spine.

rachiometer, a device that measures spinal curvatures.

rachiopathy, any disease of the spine.

rachioplegia, spinal paralysis.

rachiotome, an instrument used to divide the vertebrae.

rachiotomy, surgical incision of the vertebral column.

rachis, vertebral or spinal column.

rachitis, rickets.

radectomy, surgical excision of the root of a tooth.

radial, pertaining to the radius bone of the arm.

radiate, to spread from a common center.

radiation, emission of rays from a central point; a treatment for certain disease using a radioactive substance.

radiation syndrome, an illness due to exposure of a body part to ionizing radiations from radioactive substances marked by anorexia, headache, nausea, vomiting, and diarrhea.

radical, directed to the origin to eliminate the cause of a disease; treatment by surgical excision, usually by the total eradication of diseased tissues.

radicle, the smallest branches of a nerve or blood and lymph vessels.

radicular, pertaining to a root or radicle.

radiculitis, inflammation of the spinal nerve roots.

radioactive, pertaining to radioactivity.

radioactivity, the ability of a substance to emit alpha rays, beta rays, and gamma rays that undergo spontaneous disintegration.

radiobiologist, a specialist in radiobiology.

radiobiology, the scientific study concerned with the effects of radiant energy or radioactive material on living tissue or organisms.

radiocystitis, inflammation of the bladder following roentgen rays or radium treatment.

radiodermatitis, inflammation of the skin caused by roentgen rays or radium treatment.

radiodiagnosis, the use of x-ray in diagnosis.

radioelement, an element possessing radioactive power.

radiograph, a film produced by radiography.

radiography, the production of film records of internal structures of the body for diagnostic purposes; roentgenography.

radioisotopes, radioactive forms of chemicals used in research and in the diagnosis and treatment of certain diseases; radioactive isotopes.

radiologist, one specializing in radiology.

radiology, the branch of science concerned with roentgen rays, radium rays, and other forms of radiation and their medical uses; the process of photographing organs or bones for diagnostic purposes.

radiolucency, the quality of being partly or wholly permeable to radiant energy.

radionecrosis, disintegration of tissue exposed to radium or x-rays.

radioneuritis, neuritis caused by exposure to radiant energy.

radioresistance, resistance to radiation by certain tumors or tissues.

radiosensitive, the ability to be destroyed by radiation, as a tumor by x-rays.

radiosurgery, the use of high-energy radioactive particles in treating cancer or other diseased tissues.

radiotherapist, one who specializes in radiotherapy.

radiotherapy, treatment of disease by radioactive elements such as radium or thorium.

radiothermy, short-wave diathermy.

radioulnar, pertaining to the radius and ulna.

radium, a radioactive element found in minerals used in radiography for treating cancer.

radius, a bone in the forearm on the thumb side; a line from the center of a circle to a point on its circumference.

radix, root, as of a spinal or cranial nerve.

rage, being violently angry.

ragocyte, a cell often found in the joints of one suffering from rheumatoid arthritis.

rale, an abnormal respiratory sound heard on auscultation indicating a pathologic condition; death rattle.

ramification, a branching.

ramiform, branchlike; having the form of a branch; ramal.

ramose, having many branches.

ramulose, having many tiny branches.

ramus, a branch of an artery, nerve, or vein.

ranula, a tumor or cyst beneath the tongue, caused by obstruction and subsequent swelling of a glandular duct.

ranular, pertaining to a ranula.

rape, sexual intercourse with a female without her consent; stupration.

raphe, the line of union or seam of the two symmetrical parts or halves of an organ.

rarefaction, a condition of becoming less dense.

rash, a temporary eruption on the skin which may be in the form of red spots or patches.

raspatory, a file or rasp used in surgery.

ratbite fever, an infectious disease transmitted to humans by the bite of an infected rat, marked by recurring fever, skin eruptions, and muscular pain; sodoky.

ratio, proportion.

ration, a fixed allowance of food and drink for a certain period of time.

rational, having a sound mind; logical or reasonable; sane.

rauwolfia, any group of trees or shrubs from the genus Rauwolfia from which numerous alkaloids are derived for medicine, such as reserpine which is used as an antihypertensive and sedative.

rave, irrational verbalization; to talk irrationally, as in delirium; to be furious or raging.

reaction, a response of an organism to a stimulus; counterreaction; the specific effect caused by the action of chemical agents; a chemical transformation of one substance into another substance; the emotional state that is manifested in a particular situation.

reaction formation, a defense mechanism by which a person assumes an attitude or behavior that is the opposite of the impulse harbored, usually operating unconsciously.

reactivation, the act of causing something to become active again, especially the reactivating of an immune serum which has lost its potency.

reactive, the ability to respond to a stimulus.

reagent, a substance used to produce a chemical reaction in order to detect, measure, or produce other substances.

reagin, an antibody.

recall, to remember; the act of bringing a memory into consciousness.

rebound, the act of rebounding; resilience.

receptor, the ending of an afferent neuron that is sensitive to stimuli.

recess, a small cavity or indentation.

recessive, a tendency to recede; a hidden trait or recessive character, as opposed to a dominant character.

recidivation, recurrence of a disease; relapse; the repetition of a crime or offense.

recidivist, one who tends to relapse or return to crime; a mentally ill patient who has repeated relapses.

recipe, a prescription of a physician.

recrement, secretions, such as saliva, which are reabsorbed into the blood stream.

recrudescence, the recurrence of disease after abatement or remission.

rectal, pertaining to the rectum.

rectalgia, proctalgia; pain in the rectum.

rectectomy, surgical excision of the rectum or anus; proctectomy.

rectitis, an inflammation of the rectum; proctitis.

rectocele, the protrusion of the posterior wall of the vagina with the anterior wall of the rectum into the vagina.

rectocolitis, inflammation of the rectum and colon.

rectoscope, proctoscope.

rectostenosis, a narrowing or stricture of the rectum.

rectum, the lower portion of the large intestine between the sigmoid flexure and the anal canal.

rectus, any straight muscle.

recumbent, lying down or reclining position.

recuperate, to be restored to normal health; to recover.

recuperation, the restoration to normal health.

recurrence, the return of symptoms of an illness or disease.

recurrent, returning at intervals, as a fever; relapse.

red blood cell, a blood corpuscle containing hemoglobin; erythrocyte.

reduce, to restore to a normal place, as the ends of a fractured bone; to lose weight.

reduction, the process of restoring a dislocated bone to its normal place.

reflector, an apparatus which reflects light or sound waves.

reflex, a reflected action, or an involuntary response to a stimulus, such as a movement.

reflex arc, impulses which travel from receptors to effectors between the point of stimulation and the responding organ in a reflex action; neural pathway.

reflexogenic, producing or causing a reflex action.

reflexograph, an instrument for charting a reflex.

reflexophil, characterized by exaggerated reflex activity.

reflux, a backward flow; regurgitation.

refraction, the bending of a light ray as it passes from a medium of one density to another of different density.

refractory, stubborn or obstinate; resistant to ordinary treatment, as in some diseases; resisting stimulation.

regeneration, regrowth, repair, or restoration of part of the body or of damaged tissues.

regimen, a method of therapy to improve or restore health.

region, a particular division or area of the body.

regional, pertaining to particular regions or areas of the body.

registered nurse, a professional nurse who receives a license to practice nursing after completing a training period of 3-5 years depending on the school of nursing and passing an examination by a state or provincial board of examiners. Specialization usually requires a master's degree which prepares a nurse for teaching, supervision, or administration.

regression, reverting to an earlier or more infantile pattern of behavior; returning to a prior status in physical or mental illness.

regurgitate, to pour forth; to vomit.

regurgitation, the act of regurgitating; a backflow of blood through a defective valve of the heart.

rehabilitation, the process of restoring to health or activity, as one physically handicapped.

rehalation, a rebreathing process sometimes employed in anesthesia.

rehydration, replacement of the water or fluid content to a body or a substance that has undergone dehydration.

reimplantation, replacement of a structure or tissue in the original site from which it was previously lost.

reinfection, a recurrence of an infection by the same agent or bacteria.

reinforcement, strengthening; in behavioral science, the presentation of a stimulus (either a reward or punishment) which elicits a response.

reinforcer, that which produces reinforcement, such as a stimulus.

reinoculation, a repeated inoculation with the same organism.

relapse, recurrence of an illness or disease; to slip or slide back.

relapsing fever, a tropical disease resulting from spirochetal infections transmitted by head lice, body lice, and ticks marked by intermittent attacks of high fever.

relaxant, an agent that relaxes tension, especially in muscles.

relaxation, a reduction of tension; the act of relaxing.

relief, the removal of distressing or painful symptoms.

REM, rapid eye movements, the dream phase during the sleep cycle.

remediable, capable of being remedied.

remedial, curative; intended to improve certain skills.

remedy, anything that cures a disease or illness; a curative medication, application, or treatment; to restore to the natural state or condition.

remission, an abatement of symptoms of a disease or pain.

remit, to abate or relax.

remittent, a temporary easing; having periods of abatement and returning.

renal, pertaining to the kidneys.

reniform, having a kidney-shaped form or structure.

renin, a proteolytic enzyme secreted by the juxtaglomerular cells of the kidney, which is a powerful vasoconstrictor.

renopathy, any disease of the kidney.

reposit, to replace surgically.

repositor, an instrument used in surgery to return a displaced organ to its original position.

repress, to reject or force out of consciousness, as impulses or fears.

repressed, affected by repression; marked by repression.

repression, the act of repressing, restraining, or inhibiting; a defense mechanism in which one banishes unacceptable ideas or impulses from conscious awareness.

resect, to surgically excise a portion of an organ or a structure.

resection, surgical excision of a segment of a structure or a portion of an organ.

reserpine, an alkaloid of rauwolfia which acts centrally on the vasomotor center to decrease peripheral vasoconstriction, used as an antihypertensive and as a tranquilizer for extremely agitated patients.

residual, pertaining to that which is left as a residue; that which remains behind; an aftereffect of experience which influences later behavior.

residue, remainder; that which remains after removal of another substance.

resilience, having the quality to bounce back; elasticity; flexibility.

resilient, elastic; rebounding; coming back to original shape.

resolution, disappearance of a disease, inflammation, or tumor.

resolve, to return to normal.

resolvent, an agent that causes dispersion of inflammation.

resonance, the act of resounding; the sound produced by tapping the chest or by percussion of a body cavity.

resonant, pertaining to resonance.

respiration, the act of respiring; breathing; inspiration and expiration in exchange of oxygen and carbon dioxide.

respirator, a mechanical apparatus used to aid breathing; a device for giving artificial respiration or promoting pulmonary ventilation.

respiratory, pertaining to respiration.

respiratory system, includes the lungs, pleura, bronchi, pharynx, larynx, tonsils, and the nose.

respirometer, a device that determines the nature of respiration.

response, a reaction resulting from a stimulus.

rest, refreshing repose of the body due to sleep; the freedom from activity or bodily exertion; a remnant of embryonic tissue that persists in the adult organism.

restiform, twisted or shaped like a rope.

restitution, returning to an original position or to a former state; the spontaneous turning of the fetal head either to the left or right after it has extended through the vagina.

restorative, causing a return to health or to consciousness; a remedy or substance that is effective in the regaining of health or strength.

restore, to bring back to health, or consciousness.

restraint, to forcibly control; state of being hindered.

resuscitate, to restore life to one apparently dead.

resuscitation, the process of restoring life to one who has stopped breathing; the act of bringing one back to full consciousness. CPR or cardiopulmonary resuscitation, in which the heart and lung action is reestablished after cardiac arrest or apparent death or loss of consciousness resulting from electric shock, drowning, respiratory obstruction, and various other causes. The two important components of CPR are artificial ventilation and cardiac massage.

resuscitator, one who initiates resuscitation; a device used for producing respiration in persons who have stopped breathing.

retardation, delayed development; subnormal general intellectual and physical activity due to impairment of social adjustment or of maturation, or both; mental retardation.

retarded, one who exhibits retardation.

retch, to strain, as in vomiting.

retching, an involuntary effort to vomit.

rete, a network of blood vessels.

retention, the process of holding back or retaining in the body materials which are normally excreted, such as urine.

retial, pertaining to a rete.

reticular, having a netlike structure; resembling a net.

reticulation, formation of a network.

reticulocyte, an immature red blood corpuscle containing a network of granules; a young erythrocyte or red blood cell.

reticulocytosis, an excessive amount of reticulocytes in the peripheral blood.

reticulum, a small network of protoplasmic cells or structures.

retiform, reticular.

retina, the innermost coat of the eyeball which receives images formed by the lens, and transmits these images to the brain by the optic nerve.

retinal, pertaining to the retina.

retinene, an orange-yellow pigment formed in the retina resulting from the action of light on rhodopsin (visual purple pigment) used in dark adaptation.

retinitis, inflammation of the retina.

retinoscope, an apparatus used for measuring refractory errors.

retinoscopy, an examination of the retina to determine refractory errors.

retinosis, any noninflammatory, degenerative condition of the retina.

retractile, able to be drawn back.

retractility, the capability of retraction.

retraction, drawing back; the condition of being drawn back.

retractor, an instrument for holding open the edges of a wound; a muscle that retracts.

retral, posterior; at the back.

retrobuccal, pertaining to the back part of the mouth.

retrocedent, returning or going backward.

retroflex, to bend backward.

retroflexion, a bending backward of an organ.

retrograde, going backward; decline or deterioration; catabolic.

retrogress, to revert.

retrogression, return to an earlier and less complex state; degeneration; decline or deterioration.

retrogressive, degenerative changes; changes to a lower complexity, such as atrophy, degeneration, or necrosis.

retroinfection, the infection of a mother communicated by the fetus in the uterus.

retrolental, behind the lens of the eye.

retrolingual, behind the tongue.

retromammary gland, behind the mammary gland.

retromandibular, behind the lower jaw.

retromastoid, behind the mastoid process.

retronasal, concerning the back of the nose.

retroocular, behind the eye.

retroparotid, behind the parotid gland.

retroperitoneal, behind the peritoneum.

retroperitoneum, the space behind the peritoneum.

retroperitonitis, inflammation of the retroperitoneal space.

retropharyngeal, behind the pharynx.

retropharyngitis, inflammation of the posterior region of the pharynx.

retroplasia, degeneration of tissues into a more primitive structure.

restrospect, to reflect, or look back in thought.

retrospection, by thought, to look back into the past; a survey of past experiences.

retrospective falsification, an unconscious distortion of past experiences to conform to the emotional needs of the present.

retrosternal, behind the sternum.

retrovaccination, vaccination with a virus obtained from a calf inoculated with a smallpox virus which was first obtained from a human.

retroversion, a state of being turned back; bending backward, as part of an organ, especially the uterus.

reversion, return to a previously existing form or condition; the expression of traits possessed by a remote ancestor; atavism.

revulsion, the act of drawing blood from one part of the body to another in diverting disease; counterirritant.

revulsive, an agent causing revulsion; a counterirritant.

rhagades, painful fissures appearing at the corner of the mouth or anus, caused by movement or infection.

rhegma, a rupture, or fracture.

rheum, a catarrhal or watery discharge.

rheumatic, pertaining to rheumatism.

rheumatic fever, a systemic inflammatory disease which varies in severity, duration, and frequently followed by heart disease, usually occurring in young adults or children.

rheumatism, pain, swelling, and deformity of joints causing stiffness, or limitation of motion.

rheumatoid, resembling rheumatism.

rheumatoid arthritis, an inflammation of the joints causing stiffness, swelling, pain, and cartilaginous hypertrophy.

rheumic, pertaining to rheum.

rhexis, the rupture of a blood vessel, or an organ.

Rh factor, Rhesus factor, first detected in the blood of Rhesus monkeys; inherited antigens in red blood cells of most humans who have a Rh positive blood type and, due to a blood transfusion or pregnancy, are capable of destroying red blood cells in one who is typed Rh negative, such as a newborn infant.

rhinal, pertaining to the nose; nasal.

rhinalgia, pain in the nose; nasal neuralgia.

rhinencephalon, the portion of the brain concerned with olfactory impulses.

rhinitis, inflammation of the nasal mucous membranes.

rhinolaryngology, the branch of science concerned with the structures and diseases of the nose and larynx.

rhinologist, one who specializes in the diseases of the nose.

rhinology, the study of the nose and its diseases.

rhinopathy, any disease of the nose.

rhinophonia, having a nasal tone in speaking.

rhinoplasty, plastic surgery of the nose.

rhinopolyp, a polyp of the nose.

rhinopolypus, a nasal polyp.

rhinorrhagia, a nosebleed; epistaxis.

rhinorrhea, a thin, watery discharge from the nose.

rhinoscope, a speculum used in nasal examination.

rhinoscopy, an examination of the nasal passages with a rhinoscope.

rhizomelic, concerning the roots of the extremities, such as the hips and shoulders in man.

rhizotomy, the surgical section of a root, as a nerve or tooth.

rhodogenesis, the formation or regeneration of visual purple that has been bleached by light.

rhodophylaxis, the ability of the retina to form or regenerate rhodopsin (visual purple).

rhodopsin, visual purple, a photosensitive red pigment in the outer segment of retinal rods important to night vision.

rhombencephalon, a primary division of the embryonic brain from which the metencephalon and myelencephalon are formed.

rhoncal, rhonchial, pertaining to rhoncus or rattle in the throat.

rhonchus, a rale or rattling in the throat; a snoring sound; a dry, coarse rale that occurs in the bronchial tubes because of a partial obstruction.

rhubarb, an extract made from roots and rhizome of Rheum officinale (rhubarb), used as a cathartic and astringent.

rhypophagy, eating of filth.

rhypophobia, a morbid disgust to the act of defecation or filth.

rhythm, a measured time or movement which occurs at regular intervals, as the action of the heartbeat.

rhythmic, pertaining to a rhythm; rhythmical.

rhytidectomy, plastic surgery for the excision of wrinkles.

rhytidosis, wrinkling of the skin; wrinkling of the cornea.

rib, a bone or cartilage that forms the chest cavity and protects certain vital organs.

riboflavin, a water-soluble vitamin of the B complex family found in milk, muscle, liver, kidney, eggs, malt, and algae, essential to man; Vitamin B_2.

ribonucleic acid, RNA which is a nucleic acid containing ribose found in cytoplasm in all cells.

ribose, a monosaccharide sugar present in ribonucleic acid (RNA).

ribosome, a large particle containing RNA and protein present in the cytoplasm of cells.

ricin, a poisonous white powdery substance made from the castor bean used in medicine as an agglutinin.

ricinoleic acid, an organic acid found in castor oil in the form of glyceride which is used as a laxative.

ricinus, the castor oil plant from which ricin and castor oil are derived used as a cathartic or lubricant.

rickets, a disease occurring in infancy and childhood due to a deficiency of Vitamin D, marked by bone distortion and softening, muscle pain, and sweating of the head.

rickettsia, a genus of the Rickettsiaceae which is transmitted by lice, ticks, fleas, and mites to humans from animals causing diseases, as typhus.

ridge, a narrow, elevated edge or border.

rigidity, stiffness; immovability; inability to bend.

rigor, chill preceding a fever; a state of stiffness as in a muscle.

rigor mortis, stiffening of muscles of a dead body.

rima, a slit, fissure, or crack.

rimose, filled with fissures or cracks.

rimula, a minute fissure or slit, especially of the brain or spinal column.

ring, a round organ or band which encircles an opening.

Ringer's solution, an aqueous solution used intravenously in conditions of dehydration and for improving circulation.

ringworm, a disease caused by fungi which appears in ring formations or patches on various parts of the body, especially on the scalp.

risus, laughter.

risus sardonicus, a peculiar grin caused by muscle spasms, as seen in tetanus.

R.N., registered nurse.

RNA, ribonucleic acid.

roborant, a tonic; strengthening.

Rocky Mountain spotted fever, an infectious disease caused by a parasite, Rickettsia rickettsii, which is transmitted to man by a wood tick, resulting in fever; pain in the bones and muscles, prostration, skin eruptions, and chills.

roentgen, the unit of measurement of radiation that is used internationally, pertaining most commonly to x-rays.

roentgenogram, the film made by x-rays.

roentgenography, the x-ray pictures of internal body structures.

roentgenologic, pertaining to roentgenology.

roentgenologist, one who specializes in roentgenology.

roentgenology, the study of x-rays and technical application to medical diagnosis and therapy.

roentgenoscope, an apparatus which has a fluorescent viewing screen; fluoroscope.

roentgenoscopy, examination by means of roentgen rays.

roentgenotherapy, treatment of a disease by roentgen rays.

rongeur, a surgical instrument for cutting or removing small fragments of bone or tissue.

root, proximal end of a nerve; that portion of an organ that is implanted in tissues, such as a tooth, hair, or nail.

Rorschach test, a projective technique which seeks to determine personality traits and emotional conflicts by an analysis of subjective responses to a standard series of ten ink blots.

rosacea, a chronic disease of the skin, usually involving the nose, cheeks, and forehead, marked by flushing, papules, and acne-like pustules.

rose fever, rose cold, an allergy attributed to inhalation of rose pollen in the early part of summer.

roseola, a rose-colored rash from various causes.

rotation, the process of turning on an axis; in obstetrics, the twisting or turning of the fetal head as it follows the curves of the birth canal as it descends.

roughage, indigestible, rough material such as fibers, and cellulose which are found in certain fruits and cereals that stimulate peristalsis.

rouleau, a grouping of red blood cells arranged like a roll of coins.

roundworm, a nematode which is a parasite that thrives in the intestines.

rubedo, blushing; a temporary redness of the skin, especially the face.

rubefacient, an agent that reddens the skin; causing reddening of the skin.

rubella, German measles; an acute viral infection that resembles measles, but runs a shorter course, marked by a pink macular rash, fever, lymph node enlargement, and sometimes, a sore throat and drowsiness may occur.

rubeola, measles, rubella.

rubescent, growing red, or reddish; ruddy.

rubor, redness due to inflammation.

rudimentary, undeveloped; imperfectly developed.

ruga, a ridge, crest, or fold, especially of mucous membrane.

rugose, marked by wrinkles; ridged.

rumination, the casting up of food, or regurgitation, to be chewed the second time, as in cattle; preoccupation of the mind.

rump, the buttock; gluteal region.

rupia, a skin eruption marked by large cutaneous elevations, usually occurs in the third stage of syphilis.

rupophobia, morbid aversion to dirt or filth.

rupture, hernia; a tearing apart, as of an organ.

rutilizm, red-headedness.

Rx, symbol; a simple method for writing "take", "recipe", or prescription; treatment.

rytidosis, the contraction of the cornea preceding death which causes wrinkling of its surface.

S

sabulous, sandy or gritty.

sac, a baglike structure or organ; a pouch.

saccate, having the form of a pouch or sac; contained within a sac.

saccharide, one of the carbohydrates containing sugar; a sugar substitute.

sacchariferous, yielding sugar.

saccharification, the conversion into sugar.

saccharin, a white, crystalline compound which is several hundred times sweeter than sucrose, used as a non-nutritive sweetener.

saccharine, resembling sugar; sugary consistency.

saccharolysis, chemical splitting up of sugar.

saccharolytic, pertaining to saccharometer.

saccharometer, saccharimeter, an optical instrument used to determine the strength of sugar solutions by measuring a plane of polarized light rotations after it passes through a sugar solution.

saccharomycetes, a genus of yeasts, including brewers' yeast, used in the fermentation of sugar.

saccharomycetic, pertaining to yeast fungi.

saccharomycosis, any of several diseases caused by yeast fungi.

saccharum, sugar.

sacciform, shaped like a pouch or sac.

saccular, resembling a sac.

sacculate, having saclike expansions; containing saccules.

saccule, a little sac; applied to the smaller of two sacs in the membranous labyrinth of the ear.

sacculocochlear, relating to both the saccule and cochlea.

sacculus, a saccule.

sacrad, toward the sacrum.

sacral, pertaining to the sacrum.

sacralgia, pain in the sacrum.

sacrectomy, surgical removal of part of the sacrum.

sacrocoxitis, inflammation of sacroiliac joint.

sacrodnia, pain in the sacrum region.

sacroiliac, pertaining to the sacrum and the ilium; relating to the juncture of the hipbone and the lower spine.

sacrolumbar, pertaining to the sacrum and the loins.

sacrosciatic, pertaining to the sacrum and the ischium.

sacrospinal, pertaining to the sacrum and the spinal column.

sacrospinalis, pertaining to the large muscle on either side of the spinal column which extends from the sacrum to the head.

sacrotomy, surgical removal of part of the sacrum.

sacrouterine, pertaining to the sacrum and uterus.

sacrum, part of the vertebral column between the lumbar and coccygeal regions.

sadism, a pathological condition in which pleasure is derived from inflicting physical or psychological pain on others; a perversion or sexual deviation when it is necessary to inflict pain upon another in order to obtain sexual gratification.

sadist, one who finds pleasure in inflicting pain on others.

sadistic, pertaining to sadism.

sadomasochism, the derivation of pleasure from inflicting physical or mental pain upon others or on oneself.

sagittal, resembling an arrow; pertaining to the suture that unites the parietal bones of the skull; referring to a plane that divides a body into two halves.

Saint Vitus's dance, involuntary muscular movements; chorea.

salacious, lustful.

salicylate, a salt of salicylic acid.

salicylic acid, a powder which is soluble in water, used as a food preservative, and in medicine as an analgesic and an antipyretic. Salicylic acid is too irritating internally to be used by itself, but is widely used in the preparation of acetylsalicylic acid (aspirin).

salify, combining an acid with a base to form a salt; to infuse with a salt.

saline, consisting of salt; containing chemical salt, as an alkali metal; salty.

saline solution, sodium chloride and distilled water in a solution; an isotonic solution.

salinometer, an instrument that measures the amount of salt present in a solution.

saliva, the slightly acid fluid secreted by the glands of the mouth that serves as the first digestive enzyme, ptyalin. The saliva begins the digestive process of converting starches into various dextrins and to some maltose. Final hydrolysis of these products breakdown to glucose is completed in the small intestine.

salivary, pertaining to saliva.

salivary calculus, a minute stone in a salivary duct.

salivary glands, the three pairs of glands in the oral cavity that contribute to the formation of saliva: parotid glands, submaxillary glands, and sublingual glands.

salivation, the process of secreting saliva; ptyalism.

salivatory, producing the secretion of saliva.

Salk vaccine, a vaccine against poliomyelitis produced from inactivated poliomyelitis virus, given by injection or orally on a sugar cube.

Salmonella, any rod-shaped bacteria belonging to the family Enterobacteriaceae that cause food poisoning, intestinal inflammation, or genital-tract diseases.

salmonellosis, infestation with Salmonella bacteria which cause food poisoning.

salpingectomy, surgical removal of a fallopian tube.

salpingemphraxis, an obstruction of an eustachian tube; an obstruction of a fallopian tube.

salpingian, concerning the eustachian tube, or an oviduct.

salpingitis, an inflammation of a fallopian tube, or eustachian tube.

salpingocele, a herniated protrusion of an oviduct.

salpingocyesis, a pregnancy in an oviduct; tubal pregnancy.

salpinx, pertaining to the fallopian or eustachian tube.

salsoda, a crystalline sodium carbonate which is used as a cleaning agent, or water softener.

salsalate, an analgesic and anti-inflammatory agent.

salt, sodium chloride; common table salt.

saltation, leaping, jumping, or dancing, as in chorea; conduction along myelinated nerves; in genetics, a mutation.

saltatory, characterized by leaping, jumping, or dancing.

salt-free diet, a diet with no more than two grams of salt.

salubrious, healthful; promoting good health; wholesome.

salutary, healthful; curative; promoting health.

Salvarsan, a yellowish arsenical powder used in treatment of syphilis; trademark; rarely used since the development of penicillin.

salve, a thick, soothing ointment or cerate.

sanative, having a healing quality; curative.

sanatorium, sanitarium, an institution for the treatment of diseases, for convalescents, or patients with mental disorders.

sanatory, healing; hygienic; conducive to health.

sand-blind, having imperfect eyesight.

sandfly, flies of the family Psychodidae, a biting fly inhabiting the seashore; a fly of the genus Phlebotomus which is a blood-sucking species that transmits sandfly fever and various other diseases affecting the skin, nasal cavity, or visceral organs such as the liver or spleen.

sandfly fever, usually a three-day fever produced by a mild virus transmitted by the sandfly from the genus Phlebotomus papatasii, similar to dengue fever.

sane, of sound mind; able to anticipate and judge one's action; having reason; rational.

sanguicolous, a parasite inhabiting the blood.

sanguifacient, making blood, or forming blood.

sanguiferous, conducting blood, as the circulatory system.

sanguine, abounding in blood; pertaining to blood; hopeful.

sanguineous, bloody; abounding in blood; relating to blood.

sanguinolent, tinged with blood; containing blood.

sanies, a fetid serous discharge from a wound or ulcer, containing pus tinged with blood.

sanious, pertaining to sanies.

sanitarian, a person skilled in public health science and sanitation.

sanitary, promoting health; clean; healthful.

sanitation, the use of measures to promote conditions favorable to health.

sanitization, the process of being made sanitary.

sanitize, to disinfect, or to sterilize.

sanity, rationality; soundness of mind; reasonableness.

sap, any fluid of a living structure essential to life.

saphena, small saphenous or the great saphenous veins of the leg.

saphenous, pertaining to certain arteries, nerves, or veins.

saphenous nerve, a branch of the femoral nerve that follows the long saphenous vein in the lower leg.

sapid, savory or very tasty.

sapiens, referring to modern man, Homo sapiens.

sapor, that which affects the sense of taste.

saporific, imparting a taste; pertaining to sapor.

sapphism, lesbianism.

sapremia, a toxic condition of the blood produced by putrefactive bacteria.

saprodontia, tooth decay.

saprogen, any bacteria produced by putrefaction, or causing it.

saprogenic, resulting from putrefaction or causing it.

saprophilous, living on decaying substances, such as bacteria.

saprophyte, any organism living upon decaying matter.

saprophytic, relating to a saprophyte.

sarcitis, inflammation of muscle tissue.

sarcoid, tuberculoid; resembling a sarcoma tumor; sarcoidosis.

sarcoidosis, a chronic, progressive granulomatous reticulosis of any organ or tissue marked by the presence of tubercle-like lesions, generally affecting the skin, lymph nodes, lungs, and bone marrow.

sarcology, the branch of medicine concerned with the study of soft body tissues.

sarcoma, a malignant tumor originating in connective tissue, bone, or muscle.

sarcomatoid, resembling a sarcoma.

sarcomatosis, a condition in which many sarcomas develop at various sites in the body; sarcomatous degeneration.

sarcous, belonging to flesh or muscle.

sardonic laugh, sardonic grin, a spasmodic affectation of the muscles of the face, giving the impression of laughter; risus sardonicus.

sartorius, a narrow, ribbon-shaped muscle of the thigh, the longest muscle in the body which aids in flexing the knee, and in rotating the leg to a cross-legged position.

satiable, capable of being satisfied.

satiety, a fullness or gratification; completely satisfied.

saturated, unable to hold any more in solution of a given substance; referring to an organic compound in which only single bonds exist between carbon atoms.

saturation, the state of being saturated.

saturnine, morose or gloomy; pertaining to the absorption of lead, as in lead poisoning.

saturnism, lead poisoning.

satyriasis, an exaggerated sexual desire in males.

saxitoxin, a neurotoxin produced by poisonous mussels, clams, and plankton; gonyaulax poison.

scab, a crust formation of a superficial sore or wound.

scabicide, a substance lethal to Sarcoptes scabiei.

scabies, a contagious skin disease caused by the itch mite, Sarcoptes scabiei, resulting in intense itching and eczema.

scabious, pertaining to scabies.

scabrities, a condition of the skin marked by a roughened and scaly appearance; a sand-like roughness of the inner surface of the eyelids.

scala, a ladder-like structure, as the spiral passages of the cochlea.

scald, a burn to the flesh or skin caused by hot liquid or steam.

scalene, pertaining to the scalenus.

scalenus, one of the three muscles located in the vertebrae of the neck and attached to the first two ribs; known as scalenus anterior, medius, and posterior.

scall, a scalp disease marked by scaly eruptions.

scalp, the skin covering the cranium; hairy integument of the upper part of the head.

scalpel, a straight, small, sharp-bladed surgical knife used in dissection and surgical procedures.

scaly, resembling scales.

scan, an image produced by a sweeping beam of radiation.

scanner, an apparatus that inspects and detects certain conditions of the body, as in ultrasonography.

scanning speech, pronunciation of words in syllables in a slow and hesitating manner, usually a symptom of disease involving the nervous system.

scaphocephalic, having a deformed head, resembling a boat's keel.

scaphoid, the boat-shaped bone of the carpus on the radial side; navicular bone.

scaphoiditis, inflammation of the scaphoid bone.

scapula, the large, flat bone of the shoulder; shoulder blade.

scapulalgia, pain in the shoulder blade region.

scapular, pertaining to the shoulder blade.

scapulectomy, surgical removal of part or all of the shoulder blade.

scar, the mark left on the skin by a healing wound or sore.

scarification, having many small superficial punctures or scratches in the skin over a part, as for introduction of vaccine.

scarificator, scarifier, an instrument with many sharp points.

scarlatina, mild form of scarlet fever.

scarlatiniform, resembling scarlet fever.

scarlet fever, a contagious disease characterized by sore throat, fever, rash, and rapid pulse, usually occurring in children.

scatacratia, fecal incontinence.

scatemia, intestinal toxemia in which chemical poisons are absorbed from retained fecal matter.

scatology, the study and analysis of waste products for diagnostic purposes.

scatophagy, the eating of feces.

Schick test, test for susceptibility to diphtheria.

Schiller's test, a test for superficial cancer of the cervix.

schistoprosopia, congenital fissure of the face.

Schistosoma, a genus of blood flukes which cause infection in man by penetration of the skin while coming in contact with infected waters; schistosomiasis.

schistosomiasis, infection with Schistosoma.

schistothorax, congenital fissure of the chest or thorax.

schizogenesis, reproduction by fission.

schizoid, resembling schizophrenia; referring to a person with a schizoid personality.

schizomycete, an organism of the class of Schizomycetes, a group of plant organisms belonging to fungi.

schizomycetous, pertaining to schizomycetes.

schizont, a stage in the development of the malarial parasite following the trophozoite in which its nucleus divides into smaller nuclei.

schizonychia, splitting of fingernails and toenails.

schizophasia, muttered or disordered speech of the schizophrenic.

schizophrenia, any of a large group of severe emotional disorders, usually of psychotic proportion, characterized by disturbances of thought, mood, and behavior, such as misinterpretation of reality, delusions and hallucinations, ambivalence, inappropriate affect, and withdrawn, bizarre, or regressive behavior.

schizophrenic, one afflicted with schizophrenia.

schizotrichia, splitting of the hair at the ends.

sciatic, pertaining to the ischium or hip.

sciatic nerve, the largest nerve in the body extending from the sacral plexus on either side of the body down the back of the thigh and leg.

sciatica, inflammation of or injury to the sciatic nerve and its branches; severe pain in the leg along the course of the sciatic nerve.

scirrhoid, pertaining to a hard scirrhus or carcinoma.

scirrhoma, a hard tumor or carcinoma; scirrhus.

scirrhous, hard like a scirrhus; knotty.

scirrhus, a hard, cancerous tumor caused by an overgrowth of fibrous tissue.

scissor leg, an abnormal crossing of both legs in walking due to adduction of both hips.

sclera, the white outer coat of the eye which extends from the optic nerve to the cornea; sclerotica.

scleradenitis, inflammation and hardening of a gland.

scleral, pertaining to the sclera.

sclerectasia, a protrusion of the sclera.

sclerectoiridectomy, surgical removal of part of the sclera and iris as a treatment for glaucoma.

sclerencephalia, sclerosis of the brain.

scleriasis, progressive hardening of the skin.

scleritis, inflammation of the sclera.

scleroderma, a disease that causes the skin to become hard and rigid.

sclerodermatitis, a skin inflammation accompanied by thickening and hardening.

scleroid, having a hard texture.

scleroma, sclerosis; a hardened patch or induration of nasal or laryngeal mucous membranes.

sclerose, to become hardened.

sclerosis, a hardening of tissue or a part, due to excessive growth of fibrous connective tissue.

sclerotic, pertaining to the sclera of the eye; affected with or pertaining to sclerosis.

sclerous, hard; indurated; bony.

scolex, the round, attachment organ of a tapeworm; the larva of a tapeworm.

scoliosiometry, measurement of spinal curvature.

scoliorachitic, relating to scoliosis or rickets.

scoliosis, a lateral curvature of the spine.

scoliotic, pertaining to scoliosis.

scoop, a surgical spoon-shaped instrument used in extracting the contents of cysts or cavities.

scopolamine, an anticholinergic alkaloid obtained from the Scopolia carniolica plant, used as a sedative, mydriatic, cycloplegic.

scopophobia, a morbid fear of being seen.

scorbutic, pertaining to or affected with scurvy.

scorbutus, a disease casued by a deficiency of vitamin C; scurvy.

scotodinia, vertigo accompanied by faintness and black spots before the eyes.

scotoma, a blind gap in the visual field.

scotomatous, pertaining to scotoma.

scotometer, an instrument for diagnosing and measuring areas of depressed vision in the visual field.

scotophobia, an aversion or fear of the dark.

scotopia, night vision; the adaptation of the eye to the dark.

scotopsin, a protein that combines with retinene to form rhodopsin, important to the adjustment of vision for darkness.

scratch, a superficial injury or mark on the skin produced by scraping with a fingernail or a rough or sharp surface.

screen, a structure used in fluoroscopy on which light rays are projected for diagnostic purposes.

screening, an examination of a large segment of a population to detect a particular disease.

screwworm, the larva of a two-winged fly that deposits its eggs in wounds or in the nose; the larva, then, thrives upon the tissue of the host.

scrobiculate, marked with furrows or pits.

scrobiculus, a small groove, furrow, or pit.

scrofula, a condition of primary tuberculosis of the lymph glands of the neck characterized by swelling and degeneration.

scrofuloderma, a skin disease characterized by suppurating abscesses on the chest, neck, and in the axilla and groin area. The condition responds to ultraviolet light and chemotherapy.

scrofulous, pertaining to scrofula.

scrotal, pertaining to the scrotum.

scrotectomy, surgical excision of part of the scrotum.

scrotitis, inflammation of the scrotum.

scrotocele, hernia of the scrotum.

scrotum, the external double pouch that contains the testicles.

scruple, 20 grains of the apothecaries' unit of weight; one-third of a dram.

scurf, a desquamation of the skin, or a flaking of dry scales resembling dandruff.

scurvy, a deficiency disease due to the lack of vitamin C, marked by anemia, swollen and bleeding gums, livid skin patches and exhaustion.

scutiform, shaped like a shield.

scutulum, shoulder blade; scapula.

scutum, any shield-shaped bone; thyroid cartilage.

scyphoid, shaped like a cup.

seasickness, motion sickness; nausea, and vomiting due to unusual motion.

sebaceous, pertaining to or secreting sebum.

sebaceous cyst, a swelling formed beneath the skin due to a blockage of a duct or gland filled with sebaceous material.

sebaceous gland, an oil-secreting gland of the skin.

sebiferous, producing fatty or sebaceous matter.

sebiparous, secreting or producing sebum.

seborrhea, a functional disease of the sebaceous glands marked by an excessive increase of sebaceous secretion.

seborrheic, pertaining to seborrhea.

sebum, the fatty secretion of the sebaceous glands of the skin.

secobarbital, a short-acting barbiturate used as an hypnotic and sedative prior to anesthesia; also used to control convulsions; trademark name, Seconal.

secondary sex characteristic, any manifest characteristic due to the effect of gonadal secretions of hormones, such as the development of beards in males, and the development of mammary glands in females at puberty.

second-degree burn, a burn marked by blistering and redness without destruction of the epidermis.

secretagogue, an agent that causes secretion of glands; stimulating secretion.

secrete, to separate from the blood; to produce secretion.

secretin, a hormone secreted by the duodenal and jejunal mucosa which aids digestion; it also stimulates secretion of pancreatic juice and bile.

secretion, the cellular process of releasing a specific product; any substance produced by secretion of glands.

secretory, pertaining to secretion; a secretory organ or gland.

section, the act of separating by cutting, as in surgery; a segment of material for microscopic examination.

sector, a separate part; an area of the body.

secudines, afterbirth.

sedation, the act of alleviating distress, pain, or tension by administering a sedative.

sedative, a tranquilizer; an agent allaying irritability or excitement; quieting.

sedentary, habitually sitting; inactive; staying in one locale.

sediment, the material settling at bottom of a liquid.

sedimentation, a formation of sediment; settling out of sediment.

sedimentator, a centrifuge apparatus for separating sediment from urine.

segment, a part of a whole, especially of an organ; a division or section.

segmental, pertaining to a portion; resembling segments.

segmentation, a division into parts that are similar.

segregation, separating; in genetics, the separation of paired genes into different gametes during meiosis.

seismotherapy, sismotherapy, treatment of disease by vibratory or mechanical massage.

seizure, a sudden attack of a disease or of a symptom; a convulsion, or epileptic attack, heart attack, or a stroke.

selectivity, the degree to which a single dose of medicine produces the desired effect.

self-antigen, the ability of the body's tissues to stimulate autoimmunity.

self-destruction, the destruction of oneself, as in suicide.

self-hypnosis, self-induced hypnosis, often used to overcome bad habits or to accomplish a specific feat.

self-limited, influenced by one's own peculiarities; a disease that runs a precisely limited course.

self-tolerance, individual tolerance of immunity to self-antigens.

semeilogy, the study of symptoms; symptomatology.

semeiotic, pertaining to symptoms or signs; symptomatic.

semen, the viscous secretion at ejaculation in the male containing spermatozoa.

semicanal, a passage or channel open at one end.

semicircular canals, three small tubular canals in the labyrinth of the ear responsible for maintaining equilibrium.

semilunar, resembling a half-moon, or a crescent shape.

semilunar bone, crescent shaped bone of the carpus or wrist.

semilunar valves, the valves of the aorta and pulmonary artery.

seminal, pertaining to semen.

seminal vesicle, one of two sac-like glands lying in back of the bladder of the male, which join the ductus deferens on each side.

semination, insemination; introduction of semen into the vagina.

seminiferous, producing or carrying semen.

semipermeable, permeable only to certain molecules, as a membrane that permits passage of a solvent but not the solute.

semisynthetic, produced by chemical manipulation of substances that occur naturally.

senescence, the process of aging, or growing old.

senile, pertaining to old age; decline of mental faculties.

senilism, premature aging, or old age.

senility, the physical and mental deterioration that accompanies old age.

senna, any of various leguminous herbs, shrubs, or trees of the genus Cassia, the dried leaves of which are used as a cathartic.

senopia, an improvement of vision in the aged usually a sign of incipient cataract.

sensation, an impression produced by impulses through the sense organs; the power of feeling or sensing; an awareness of stimulus to the nervous system.

sense, perceived through the nervous system or a sense organ; the normal power of understanding.

sense organ, any organ of the body that transmits impulses to the brain, such as the nose, ear, eye, and skin; receptor.

sensibility, an ability to feel or perceive; sensitivity.

sensitive, able to respond to stimuli; unusually responsive to stimulation; reacting quickly.

sensitivity, the quality of being sensitive; the state of being acutely affected by the action of a chemical or other agents.

sensitization, a condition of being made sensitive to certain stimulus; the exposure of a person to a specific antigen by repeated injections of it, as a serum; anaphylaxis.

sensorimotor, being both sensory and motor.

sensorineural, pertaining to a sensory nerve.

sensorium, the sensory nerve center in the cerebral cortex that receives and coordinates impulses sent to individual nerve centers; the special sensory perceptive powers and their integration in the brain; having a clear, accurate memory together with a correct orientation for time, place, and person; consciousness.

sensory, pertaining to sensation.

sensuous, pertaining to the senses; appealing to the senses; readily affected through the senses or susceptible to influence.

sentient, capable of sensation.

sepsis, the presence of pathological microorganisms or their toxins in the blood; a state of poisoning of the system caused by the spread of infection through the blood.

septal, pertaining to a septum.

septate, divided by a septum.

septectomy, surgical removal of a septum or part of it.

septic, pertaining to sepsis.

septicemia, blood poisoning, or a systemic disease caused by the presence of pathological microorganisms or their toxins in the bloodstream.

septicemic, pertaining to septicemia.

septic sore throat, an inflammation of the throat caused by streptococcus bacteria, accompanied by fever and prostration.

septicophlebitis, septic inflammation of a vein.

septimetritis, septic inflammation of the uterus.

septometer, an instrument that measures the width of the nasal septum.

septonasal, pertaining to the nasal septum.

septotome, an instrument used for surgical cutting of a section of the nasal septum.

septotomy, surgical incision of the nasal septum.

septum, a dividing membrane or partition; a partition of tissue.

septuplet, one of seven children born of one pregnancy.

sequel, sequela, the consequence of an illness or disease; a morbid condition occurring as a consequence of another condition.

sequestration, the formation of sequestrum; isolation of a patient.

sequestrectomy, surgical excision of a sequestrum.

sequestrum, a portion of dead bone which has separated from sound bone due to necrosis.

sera, plural of serum.

seroalbuminuria, the presence of serum albumin in the urine.

serocolitis, inflammation of the serous coat of the colon.

seroculture, bacterial culture on blood serum.

seroenteritis, inflammation of the serous coat of the intestine.

serohepatitis, inflammation of the peritoneal covering of the liver.

serologist, one who specializes in serology.

serology, the science concerned with the nature and reactions of blood serum.

serolysin, a bacterial substance occurring in blood serum.

serosa, serous membrane, as peritoneum, pleura, and pericardium.

serositis, inflammation of a serous membrane.

serotherapy, therapeutic measure in treatment of disease by injecting blood serum, either human or animal, containing antibodies.

serotonin, a hormone and neurotransmitter found in certain cells that causes muscle contraction and vasoconstriction.

serous, resembling serum; producing or containing serum.

serous membrane, any thin membrane lining a serous cavity such as the peritoneum.

serpiginous, creeping; having a wavy border.

serpigo, a creeping eruption, especially ringworm.

serum, any serous fluid that moistens the surfaces of serous membranes; the fluid portion of the blood after coagulation; serum from the blood of an animal that has been rendered immune to some disease, given by inoculation as an antitoxin; consisting of plasma minus fibrogen.

serum albumin, a simple protein found in blood serum.

serum globulin, a plasma protein that may be separated into three blood fractions, alpha, beta, and gamma globulin responsible for the body's resistance to certain infections.

serum sickness, an eruption of purpuric spots accompanied by pain in the limbs and joints following a serum injection.

sesamoid, a small nodular bone that is embedded in a tendon or joint capsule; sesamoid bone, resembling a sesame seed.

setaceous, bristle-like; resembling a bristle; bristly, or hairy.

seventh cranial nerve, the facial nerve.

sex, the distinctive characteristics which differentiate between males and females; activities related to sexual attraction; sexual reproduction; sexual intercourse.

sex chromosome, a chromosome that carries sex-linked traits, as determined by the presence of the XX (female) or XY (male) genotype in somatic cells.

sex hormone, a hormone that affects the growth or function of the sexual organs and the development of secondary sex characteristics in males and females.

sex-linked, transmitted by a gene which is located on the X chromosome.

sexological, pertaining to sexology.

sexologist, one specializing in sexology.

sexology, the study of sexual behavior in humans.

sextuplet, one of six children born at the same birth.

sexual, pertaining to sex.

sexual intercourse, copulation; coitus; sexual relations.

sexuality, state of having sex; the collective characteristics differentiating between the male and female; the constitution of a person relating to sexual behavior and attitudes.

sexual organs, genitalia; genitals.

shaft, the long slender portion of a long bone.

shakes, shivering due to a chill; fine vibrations of the hands, often seen in chronic alcoholics.

shaking palsy, a basal ganglion disease marked by progressive rigid tremulousness, affected gait, muscular contraction and weakness, often seen in Parkinson's disease.

shank, leg, or shin; tibia.

sheath, a tubular encasement or enveloping structure.

shedding, loss of deciduous teeth; casting off the top layer of the epidermis or skin.

shell shock, a form of psychoneurosis, often seen during military service and in training camps; war neurosis.

shield, a protective covering.

Shigella, a genus of nonmotile, gram-negative rods belonging to the family Enterobacteriaceae, which produce digestive disturbances ranging from mild diarrhea to dysentery.

shin, the anterior edge of the tibia or leg, between the ankle and the knee; shinbone.

shingles, a viral infection involving the central nervous system causing eruption of acute, inflammatory vesicles or blisters on the skin along peripheral nerves which are painful; herpes zoster.

shiver, slight tremor; involuntary shaking, as with cold, fear, or excitement.

shivering, an involuntary shaking or tremor of the body, as with cold.

shock, a sudden debilitating disturbance of bodily functions resulting from acute peripheral circulatory failure due to hemorrhage, severe trauma, burns, dehydration, infection, surgery, or drug toxicity. Outstanding symptoms of shock are: prostration, pallor, perspiration, rapid pulse, pulmonary deficiency, coldness of skin, and often anxiety.

shock therapy, a treatment in mental illness involving three different types: electric shock therapy, insulin shock therapy, or metrazol shock therapy.

shortsightedness, unable to see distant objects clearly; myopia, or nearsightedness.

shoulder, joining of the clavicle and scapula, where the arm joins the trunk.

shoulder-blade, scapula.

shoulder dislocation, displacement of the shoulder joint caused by falling on an outstretched arm.

shoulder girdle, the bony semicircular band which forms an arch, serving as supporting structure for the upper extremities.

show, appearance of a discharge of blood prior to labor; menstruation.

shudder, temporary convulsive shaking of the body resulting from fright, fear, or anxiety; tremor.

shunt, to turn to one side or to bypass; a passage between two blood vessels or between two sides of the heart that has an abnormal opening in its wall partition; a surgical creation of an anastomosis.

sialaden, a salivary gland.

sialadenitis, inflammation of a salivary gland.

sialadenocus, tumor of a salivary gland.

sialagogic, pertaining to sialagogue.

sialagogue, an agent that increases the flow of saliva.

sialaporia, a deficiency in saliva secretion.

sialemesis, vomiting caused by excessive secretion of saliva.

sialine, concerning saliva.

sialism, sialismus, excessive secretion of saliva; ptyalism.

sialoadenectomy, surgical removal of a salivary gland.

sialoadenitis, an inflammation of a salivary gland; sialadenitis.

sialoaerophagia, swallowing of saliva and air.

sialoangitis, inflammation of a salivary duct.

sialocele, a salivary cyst.

sialolith, a salivary calculus, or stone.

sialolithiasis, formation of several salivary calculi, or stones.

sialoncus, a tumor under the tongue caused by obstruction of a salivary duct.

sialorrhea, ptyalism.

sialosis, the flow of saliva; ptyalism.

Siamese twins, any twins born joined together, usually at the hips or buttocks; twins congenitally united.

sib, a blood relative; kinsman descended from a common ancestor; sibling.

sibilant, hissing or whistling.

sibling, offspring of the same parents; a brother or sister.

sibship, brothers and sisters of the same family group.

siccus, dry.

sick, not well; affected by disease; nauseous.

sickle cell, an abnormal crescent-shaped red blood cell.

sickle cell anemia, a hereditary form of anemia in which the presence of crescent-shaped red blood cells causes a crystallization of the hemoglobin within the cells, resulting in the clogging of blood vessels. This disease affects about 1 in 500 American Negroes and is marked by severe anemia, jaundice, abdominal, muscular, and joint pains, skin ulcerations, formation of bilirubin gallstones, and many other complications.

sicklemia, sickle cell anemia.

sickly, not robust; habitually indisposed; in poor health.

sickness, state of being affected with disease; illness.

side effect, an unintended secondary reaction to medication; an effect that is aside from the desired effect of a treatment.

siderocyte, a red blood corpuscle that contains iron in a form other than hematin.

sideroderma, a disorder of iron metabolism that causes a bronze discoloration of the skin.

sideropenia, iron deficiency in the blood or the body.

sideropenic, pertaining to sideropenia.

sideroscope, a device used to find metal particles in the eye.

siderosis, a form of pneumoconiosis caused by dust or fumes containing iron particles being inhaled, as in occupations such as arc-welding.

siderous, pertaining to or containing iron.

sigh, deep inspiration preceded by an audible, slower expiration; suspirium.

sight, the act of seeing; having the faculty of vision.

sightless, blind.

sigmoid, shaped like the letter S; pertaining to the sigmoid colon.

sigmoidectomy, surgical excision of all or part of the sigmoid colon.

sigmoid flexure, the lower segment of the descending colon between the crest and the rectum, shaped like the letter S.

sigmoiditis, inflammation of the sigmoid colon.

sigmoidoscope, an endoscope with an illuminated end used for examination of the sigmoid flexure.

sigmoidoscopy, examination of the sigmoid colon with a sigmoidoscope.

sigmoidostomy, a surgical creation of an artificial opening from the sigmoid colon to the body surface.

sign, any existing evidence of an abnormal nature in the body or of an organ.

signa, meaning "mark", used in writing prescriptions; designated "S" or "sig".

signature, that part of a prescription which gives instructions for use of medication.

sign language, hand signs or gestures used as a substitute for speech by the deaf.

silicon, a nonmetallic element found in soil which occurs in traces in skeletal structures such as teeth and bone.

silicone, any organic compound in which all or part of the carbon has been replaced by silicon, used in preparations of oils, greases, synthetic rubber, and resins.

silicosis, a lung condition caused by inhalation of dust of stone, sand, or flint containing silica, resulting in nodular, fibrotic changes in the lungs.

silicotic, pertaining to silicosis.

silver nitrate, a chemical element which is used as a local anti-infective, or prophylaxis of opthalmia neonatorum, a purulent conjunctivitis in the newborn.

silver protein, silver made colloidal in combination with protein, used in solutions as an active germicide.

simple, not complex; something not mixed or compounded; being deficient in intellect; a medicinal herb, or plant.

simple fracture, fracture without torn ligaments or broken skin; bone fracture without complications.

simulate, to feign illness or disease.

simulation, feigning disease or symptoms of a disease.

simulator, one who simulates; malingerer; something that simulates.

sinapism, a mustard plaster.

sincipital, pertaining to the sinciput.

sinciput, upper and front portion of the head.

Sinequan, trademark for doxepin hydrochloride used in treatment of psychoneurosis to alleviate symptoms of anxiety, tension, depression, sleep disturbances, guilt, fear, apprehension, worry, and lack of energy.

sinew, a tendon of a muscle.

singuitus, hiccup.

sinister, on the left side; left.

sinistral, pertaining to the left side; left-handed.

sinistraural, hearing better with the left ear.

sinistrocardia, a displacement of the heart to the left side of the medial line of the body.

sinistrocerebral, pertaining to or situated in the left cerebral hemisphere.

sinistrocular, having stronger vision in the left eye.

sinistromanual, left-handed.

sinistropedal, using the left foot more than the right; left-footed.

sinistrotorsion, a turning or twisting to the left, as of the eye.

sinuitis, sinusitis; inflammation of a sinus.

sinuous, winding or bending in and out.

sinus, a cavity, recess, or passage, as in bone; dilated channel or vessel for venous blood; any cavity having a narrow opening leading to an abscess.

sinusal, pertaining to a sinus.

sinusitis, inflammation of a sinus, especially of a paranasal sinus.

sinusoid, resembling a sinus.

sinusotomy, surgical incision of a sinus.

sitiergia, hysterical refusal to take food, probably related to anorexia nervosa.

sitiology, the science of nutrition; dietetics.

sitomania, periodic bulimia; excessive hunger, or abnormal craving for food.

sitophobia, an abnormal repugnance to food, either generally or to certain selective dishes.

sitosterol, any of a group of sterols from closely related plants used in varying combinations as an anticholesterolemic substance in the synthetic production of steroid hormone drugs.

sitotherapy, treatment by diet.

situs, a position, or the site of a body part or organ.

sitz bath, a bath in which to sit with water covering the hips; hip bath.

skeletal, pertaining to the skeleton.

skeleton, the bones of the body collectively, forming the framework. The human body consists of 206 bones.

Skene's glands, glands which lie inside of the posterior floor of the urethra in the female.

skenitis, inflammation of the Skene's glands or paraurethral ducts.

skiagram, an X-ray picture; roentgenograph.

skiagraph, an object made visible by a shadowed outline; a radiograph.

skiagraphy, the process of taking pictures with roentgen rays; radiography.

skiameter, an apparatus that determines differences in density and penetration of roentgen rays.

skiascope, an apparatus that examines by fluoroscope errors of refraction in the eye by observing movement of shadow and light; retinoscope.

skiascopy, shadow test of the eye to determine the refractive error; fluoroscopic examination of the body.

skin, the external covering of the body consisting of two layers, the epidermis and the corium. In the skin of the palms of the hands and soles of the feet there are five layers of epidermis.

skin graft, a viable section of skin transplanted in skin grafting.

skin grafting, the grafting of skin from another part of the body, or from a donor, to repair a defect or to replace skin that has been destroyed, as by burns.

skleriasis, progressive patches of hardened skin; scleroderma.

skin test, injected substances beneath the skin or applied to the surface of the skin to determine allergic sensitivity; scratch test; Schick test.

skull, the cranium; bony framework of the head.

sleep, a periodic and normal loss of consciousness in which bodily functions are reduced since the body and mind are at rest.

sleeping sickness, an infectious disease, usually fatal, marked by fever, drowsiness, increased lethargy, muscular weakness, weight loss, and cerebral symptoms caused by a parasitic protozoan, Trypanosoma gambiense, introduced into the blood by the bite of a tsetse fly; encephalitis lethargica.

sleep walking, walking in one's sleep; somnambulism.

sling, a support, usually out of a triangular cotton cloth or material, for an injured upper extremity.

slipped disk, a displaced vertebral disk that causes pressure on the spinal nerve, creating extreme pain.

slough, to cast off or shed; necrotic (dead) matter separated from living tissue.

sloughing, formation of slough or dead matter; the separating of necrosed tissue from living tissue.

slow, mentally dull; having a retarded pulse; bradycardia.

smallpox, an acute viral disease marked by fever, macules and papules that leave small depressed scars on the skin; variola.

smear, a specimen prepared on a slide for microscopic study.

smegma, a cheesy secretion of sebaceous glands, consisting of desquamated epithelial cells found under the labia minora and the foreskin.

smegmatic, pertaining to the smegma.

smegmolith, a calcareous mass in the smegma.

smell, to perceive by stimulation of the olfactory nerves or olfactory sense; to render an offensive or pleasant odor.

smelling salts, ammonium carbonate used for resuscitation and stimulation.

snapping hip, a hip joint that slips with a snap due to displacement over the great trochanter of a tendinous band.

snare, a surgical device for excision of polyps, tumors, and other growths by encircling them at the base with a wire loop and closing the loop.

sneeze, to emit air forcibly through the mouth and nose by involuntary spasmodic contractions of muscles of expiration, due to irritation of nasal mucosa.

Snellen's chart, used to test visual acuity.

snore, noisy breathing during sleep through the mouth which causes a vibration of the uvula and soft palate.

snoring rale, a sonorous, low-pitched rale resembling a snore.

snow blindness, an irritation to the conjunctiva of the eye caused by reflection of the sun on the snow.

snuffles, catarrhal discharge from nasal mucous membranes while breathing, especially in infants with congenital syphilis.

soap, a chemical compound formed by an alkali acting on fatty acid, used for cleansing purposes.

SOAP, a process of recording progress notes in a problem-oriented assessment of data obtained subjectively from a patient.

sob, to weep with convulsive movements of the throat, involving a sudden inspiration accompanied by spasmodic closure of the glottis, resulting in a wail-like cry.

socialization, the process by which society integrates the individual and the way in which one learns to behave in a socially acceptable way.

sociobiology, the study that proposes that all human behavior has a biological basis and is controlled by the genes.

sociogenic, imposed by society.

sociologist, one who specializes in sociology.

sociology, the scientific study concerned with social relationships, social organization, and group behavior in contrast to individual behavior.

sociometry, the study of measurement of human social behavior.

sociopath, an individual with an antisocial personality; a psychopath.

socket, a hollow or cavity into which a correspondent part fits.

soda, usually applied to sodium bicarbonate, sodium hydroxide, or sodium carbonate.

soda lime, combined mixture of sodium hydroxide or caustic soda and calcium hydroxide or slaked lime, used in the production of ammonia and the absorption of moisture; combined mixture of calcium hydroxide with sodium or potassium, or both, used as an absorbent of carbon dioxide in equipment, such as in oxygen therapy.

sodium bicarbonate, used in the production of baking powder and as an antacid.

sodium chloride, common table salt.

sodium citrate, used as an anticoagulant in blood transfusions.

sodium iodide, used in preparation of a compound resembling potassium iodide.

sodium salicylate, a compound powder used as an analgesic and antipyretic.

sodium sulfate, used as a mild cathartic and diuretic; Glauber's salts.

sodomy, unnatural sexual intercourse; anal intercourse; bestiality; fellatio.

soft palate, soft part of the palate.

solar, pertaining to the sun.

solar plexus, a network of nerves behind the stomach and situated at the upper part of the abdomen in front of the aorta from which sympathetic fibers pass to the visceral organs.

sole, the undersurface or bottom part of the foot.

soleprint, a footprint used in hospitals to identify newborn infants.

solution, process of dissolving; a homogeneous mixture of one or more substances; a rupture or separation; termination of an illness.

solvent, any substance which has a dissolving effect upon another substance.

soma, the body as distinguished from the mind or psyche; body tissues distinguished from germinal tissues.

somatic, pertaining to the body, as somatic symptoms.

somatic cells, any of the body cells that compose various organs and tissue except reproductive cells or germ cells.

somatogenic, originating in the body.

somatology, the study of anatomy and physiology; the study of the structure, functions, and development of the human body.

somatopathy, bodily dysfunction as distinguished from mental dysfunction.

somatoplasm, the protoplasm of the body cells as distinguished from that of germ plasm.

somatopleure, the embryonic layer formed by ectoderm and somatic mesoderm.

somatopsychic, pertaining to both body and mind; relating to a physical disorder which manifests mental symptoms.

somatopsychosis, any mental dysfunction symptomatic of bodily disease.

somatotherapy, treatment focused at relieving or curing bodily ills.

somatotrophic, influencing body cells and stimulating growth.

somatotype, a particular body build based on a theory that certain types of body build are associated with personality types, such as endomorphy, mesomorphy, actomorphy.

somesthetic, sensibility to bodily sensations.

somite, any embryonic segment alongside the neural tube, forming the vertebral column and various organs.

somitic, pertaining to a somite.

somnambulate, walking while asleep.

somnambulism, the state of walking during sleep; a hypnotic state in which the individual has full possession of the senses but no subsequent memory.

somnambulist, one subject to somnambulism.

somniferous, producing or inducing sleep, as a narcotic or soporific.

somniloquism, habitual talking in one's sleep.

somnolence, unusual drowsiness; sleepiness.

somnolentia, inclined to sleep; drowsiness, or somnolence; a lack of natural sleep with disorientation and anxiety.

sonorous, a deep resonant sound.

sonovox, an electronic device used for transmitting sounds to be emitted through the mouth by a person whose larynx has been removed.

sopor, a very deep sleep; stupor.

soporiferous, producing sleep; soporific.

soporose, soporous, pertaining to profound sleep; coma.

sordes, undigested food in the stomach.

sore, any lesion of the skin or mucous membranes; tender or painful.

sore throat, inflammation of the pharynx; laryngitis; pharyngitis; tonsillitis.

souffle, a soft, blowing sound heard through a stethoscope in auscultation, as any cardiac or vascular murmur.

sound, the effect produced in the auditory organs by sound waves or certain vibrations; a noise, which is normal or abnormal, heard within the body; an instrument for exploring and detecting by sound any foreign body within a cavity.

space, an area, region, or cavity of the body; delimited area; the universe beyond earth.

Spanish fly, a blister beetle used in medicine as a counter-irritant or diuretic.

sparganosis, infestation with a variety of Sparganum.

Sparganum, the larva of tapeworms, especially of the genus Dibothriocephalus.

spargosis, distention of the female mammary glands with milk; swelling and thickening of the skin; elephantiasis.

spasm, a sudden, abnormal, involuntary muscular contraction; a transitory constriction of a passage or orifice; spasms may be clonic, described as alternating contraction and relaxation of involuntary muscles, or they may be tonic, described as sustained involuntary muscle contraction.

spasmodic, occurring in spasms; relating to the nature of a spasm.

spastic, characterized by spasms; a hypertonic state of muscles producing rigidity and awkward movements; an individual exhibiting spasticity, as occurs in cerebral palsy.

spasticity, hypertension of the muscles, or sustained increased muscular tension.

spay, to remove female sex glands, usually said of animals.

specialist, a medical practitioner who limits his practice to a particular branch of medicine or surgery.

specialty, the specific field of a specialist.

specific, pertaining to a species; restricted in application or effect to a particular function or structure; a drug indicated for a particular disease; pertaining to special affinity of an antigen for its corresponding antibody.

specimen, a small sample to determine the nature of the whole, as a small quantity of urine for diagnostic purposes or a segment of tissue for microscopic examination.

spectacles, a pair of lenses to aid defective vision or to protect the eyes from light rays or dust particles.

spectroscope, an instrument used for developing and analyzing spectra.

spectrum, a series of wavelengths of electromagnetic radiation obtained by refraction and diffraction of a ray of white light. The visible spectrum consists of the colors red, orange, yellow, green, blue, indigo and violet. The invisible spectrum includes rays such as X-ray, infrared, ultraviolet, cosmic, etc.; a measurable range of activity of bacteria which are affected by an antibiotic.

speculum, an instrument for examining canals or for opening a body orifice to permit visual inspection.

speech, the power to express thoughts and ideas by articulated vocal sounds and words.

sperm, semen; spermatozoon; reproductive seminal fluid in males.

spermacrasia, lack of spermatozoa in the semen.

spermatemphraxis, an obstruction that prevents the discharge of seminal fluid.

spermatic, pertaining to the semen; seminal.

spermatic cord, the cord suspending the testis within the scrotum, and which contains the blood vessels, lymphatics, nerves, and ductus deferens.

spermatid, a cell developed from a spermatocyte which becomes a mature reproductive cell or spermatozoon.

spermatism, the ejaculation of semen, voluntary or involuntary.

spermatocele, a cystic tumor of the epididymis which contains spermatozoa.

spermatocyte, a primary male germ cell that develops from the division of a spermatogonium and then itself divides into spermatids which give rise to spermatozoa.

spermatogenesis, the formation of mature spermatozoa.

spermatogenic, pertaining to the origin and development of spermatozoa.

spermatogonium, a primitive germ cell that gives rise to the spermatocyte.

spermatoid, resembling spermatozoa.

spermatology, the study of seminal fluid.

spermatolysis, the destruction of spermatozoa.

spermatopathy, any disease of sperm cells or their secreting glands or ducts.

spermatorrhea, involuntary discharge of semen without orgasm.

spermatozoic, pertaining to spermatozoa.

spermatozoon, the mature germ cell which is formed in the seminiferous tubules of the testes.

spermaturia, discharge of semen with urine.

spermiogenesis, the second stage in the formation of spermatozoa, in which the spermatids are transformed into functional spermatozoa.

sphenoid, wedge-shaped or cuneiform.

sphenoid bone, the large bone at the base of the skull which is wedge-shaped.

spherocyte, an erythrocyte which is spheroid in shape but more fragile, occurring in certain hemolytic anemias.

spheroid, having a body shaped like a sphere.

spheroidal, resembling a sphere.

sphincter, a ringlike, or circular muscle which closes a natural passage, as the anus.

sphincteral, pertaining to a sphincter.

sphincteralgia, pain in the anal sphincter muscles; pain in a sphincter muscle.

sphincterectomy, surgical excision of a sphincter.

sphincteritis, inflammation of a sphincter.

sphincterotomy, surgical incision of a sphincter.

sphygmogram, tracing of the pulse produced by a sphygmograph.

sphygmograph, an instrument which records differences of pulse in disease and health.

sphygmoid, resembling the pulse.

sphygmomanometer, an instrument for determining the blood pressure in an artery.

sphygmomanometric, pertaining to the blood pressure in an artery.

sphygmometer, an instrument that measures the pulse rate; sphymograph.

sphygmophone, an instrument which makes the pulse beat audible.

sphygmoscope, an instrument which makes the pulse beat visible.

sphygmotonometer, an instrument which measures the elasticity of arterial walls.

sphygmous, pertaining to the pulse.

sphygmus, a pulse.

spica, a reverse spiral bandage with turns crossing each other, resembling a spike of wheat.

spicule, a tiny, needle-shaped body.

spiculum, a sharp, small spike.

spiloma, a mole or skin discoloration; nevus.

spina bifida, the protrusion of the spinal membranes due to a defective closure of the bony encasement of the spinal cord which is a developmental anomaly.

spinal, pertaining to the backbone or spine.

spinal column, the vertebral column which encloses the spinal cord, consisting of thirty-two bones.

spinal cord, the ovoid column of nervous tissue extending through the spinal canal which serves as a center for spinal reflexes and a conducting pathway of impulses to and from the brain.

spine, the vertebral column.

spinobulbar, pertaining to the spinal cord and the medulla oblongata.

spinocerebellar, pertaining to the spinal cord and the cerebellum.

spinose, spinous, pertaining to the spine; spinelike.

spinous process, the prominence at the posterior part of each vertebra.

spireme, the continuous threadlike figure formed by the chromosome material during prophase of meiosis.

spirillemia, the condition caused by the presence of spirilla bacteria in the blood from the genus Spirillum.

Spirillum, a genus of gramnegative bacteria that causes fever in man resulting from a rat-bite.

spirit, any volatile liquor or a solution of volatile liquid in alcohol; alcohol.

spirochete, a slender threadlike bacteria which is spiral in shape that is from the genus Spirocheta causing diseases, as syphilis and yaws.

spirochetosis, infection caused by spirochetes.

spirograph, an instrument for recording respiratory movements.

spiroid, resembling a spiral.

spirometer, an instrument that determines the air capacity of the lungs; pneometer, pneumatometer.

spirometry, measurement of the air capacity of the lungs.

spirophore, a device used for artificial respiration; iron lung.

spit, saliva; to expectorate spittle; expectoration; sputum.

spittle, saliva; digestive fluid of the mouth.

splanchna, intestines or viscera.

splanchnemphraxis, obstruction of any internal organ, such as intestines.

splanchnic, pertaining to viscera or intestines.

splanchnicectomy, surgical excision of part of a splanchnic nerve.

splanchnic nerves, three nerves from the thoracic sympathetic ganglia that control the viscera.

splanchnicotomy, surgical procedure of incising a splanchnic nerve.

splanchnology, the branch of medicine concerned with the study of the viscera or intestines.

splanchnopathy, any diseased condition of the viscera.

splayfoot, flatfoot; talis valgus.

spleen, a spongy, glandlike organ situated in the upper part of the abdomen posterior and inferior to the stomach, important to blood formation, blood storage, blood filtration, and formation of antibodies.

splenadenoma, enlargement of the spleen due to hyperplasia of its pulp.

splenalgia, pain in the spleen.

splenectasis, enlargement of the spleen.

splenectomy, surgical removal of the spleen.

splenectopia, displacement of the spleen; floating spleen.

splenic, pertaining to the spleen.

splenitis, inflammation of the spleen.

splenius, a compress or bandage; a broad, flat, band-like muscle of the upper dorsal region and the back and side of the neck, which serves in rotating the head and neck.

splenocele, hernia of the spleen.

splenoma, a tumor of the spleen.

splenomegaly, an abnormal growth of the spleen; enlargement of the spleen.

splint, a rigid appliance made of bone, wood, metal, or plaster used to fixate a fractured or dislocated bone or to protect an injured part of the body.

splinting, application of a splint to fixate a fractured or dislocated bone; in dentistry, a fixed restoration of two or more teeth into a rigid unit; rigidity of muscles which occurs as a means of avoiding pain caused by movement.

spondylalgia, pain in the vertebrae.

spondylitis, inflammation of the vertebrae.

spondylopathy, any disorder of the vertebrae.

spondylosyndesis, a surgical formation of joining two vertebrae.

spondylotomy, surgical removal of part of the vertebral column.

sponge, a porous, absorbent mass of gauze or cotton surrounded by gauze used in surgery to mop up fluids; an elastic fibrous skeleton of certain marine animals.

spontaneity, the quality of being spontaneous; behavior or activity that is spontaneous.

spontaneous, occurring voluntarily, as arising from one's own impulses.

spontaneous fracture, fracture resulting from the state of the bone and causing little or no injury.

sporadic, intermittent; occurring singly and widely scattered.

spore, an oval, refractile body formed within bacteria, as in Bacillus and Clostridium, which is resistant to environmental changes and difficult to destroy.

spot, a small blemish or macula; scar; birthmark.

spotted fever, any various eruptive fevers: Typhus, Tick fever, Cerebrospinal meningitis, or Rocky Mountain spotted fever.

sprain, the wrenching of a joint without producing dislocation.

sprue, a chronic malabsorption syndrome applied to three closely related conditions: namely, tropical sprue, idiopathic steatorrhea (nontropical), and celiac. Tropical sprue and nontropical sprue affect adults. Celiac disease is limited to children, but all three conditions involve the mucosa of the small intestine -resulting in impaired food absorption. Symptoms are diarrhea, bulky and foul stools which are usually greyish in color, weakness, loss of weight, and other conditions.

spud, a spadelike bladed surgical instrument used to dislodge foreign substances.

spur, a sharply pointed bony projection; calcar.

sputum, spittle; any mixed matter with saliva that is expectorated through the mouth.

squama, a thin, scaly plate-like structure.

squint, strabismus; to partly close the eyes, as in excess light.

stabile, resistant to change; stable; fixed.

stability, the quality of being stable.

stable, fixed; resistant to change; steady.

staccato speech, jerky pronunciation of words and syllables; scanning speech.

stage, a time period in the course of disease.

stagnation, the cessation of motion; stasis.

stain, a dye or reagent used in staining specimen for microscopic examination.

stamina, endurance; having strength to endure conditions resulting from disease, fatigue, or privation.

stammer, speech disorder marked by involuntary pauses while speaking; stuttering.

standard, an established measurement or model of authority to which other similar things should conform.

stanch, to stop the flow of blood from a wound.

stapedectomy, surgical removal of the stapes in the ear.

stapedial, pertaining to the stapes.

stapes, the stirrup, one of the three small bones in the middle ear.

staphyle, the fleshy mass hanging from the soft palate; uvula.

staphylectomy, surgical excision of the uvula; staphylotomy.

staphylitis, inflammation of the uvula, or staphyle.

staphylococcus, any organism of the genus Staphylococcus causing body infection.

Staphylococcus aureus, a species commonly present on the skin and mucous membranes of the nose and mouth that causes inflammation and suppurative conditions such as boils, carbuncles, and internal abscesses.

staphylohemia, the presence of staphylococci in the blood.

staphylorrhaphy, suture of a cleft palate.

starch, any of a group of polysaccharides found in plants that are able to be hydrolized by water in the body into maltose and then into glucose which provide heat and energy for humans.

stasis, stoppage of the flow of blood, urine, or the contents of the intestines due to illness, or disease.

stasophobia, abnormal fear of standing up.

stat, at once.

state, condition of a patient; situation.

statistics, numerical facts pertaining to a certain subject, such as vital statistics which present human natality, morbidity, and mortality in a given population.

status, a condition or state.

statutory rape, sexual intercourse with a female under legal age of consent.

steapsin, a fat-splitting enzyme of the pancreatic juice; lipase.

stearate, salt or ester of stearic acid.

stearic acid, a fatty acid found in solid animal fats and in a few vegetable fats used in producing lubricants, cosmetics, and medicine preparations.

steariform, resembling fat.

stearodermia, a disease of the sebaceous glands of the skin.

stearrhea, an excessive secretion of sebum or fat.

steatitis, inflammation of adipose tissue.

steatoma, a lipoma; a fatty mass found within a sebaceous gland.

steatopathy, disease of the sebaceous glands of the skin.

steatopygia, abnormal fat accumulation of the buttocks.

steatorrhea, excessive secretion of sebaceous glands; fatty stools caused by pancreatic diseases.

stegnosis, checking an excess secretion or discharge; closing a passageway; constipation.

stellate, star-shaped; radiating from a center.

stenocephaly, an abnormal narrowness of the head.

stenosed, narrowed or constricted.

stenosis, narrowing of a body opening or passage.

stenotic, pertaining to stenosis.

stereoarthrolysis, surgical formation of a new movable joint in cases of bony ankylosis.

stereognosis, having the ability to recognize the form and nature of objects by touch.

sterile, barren; not fertile; aseptic; free from living microorganisms.

sterility, state of being sterile.

sterilization, complete destruction of all microorganisms; any procedure rendering an individual incapable of reproduction.

sterilizer, an appliance for sterilizing especially medical instruments, such as an autoclave or steam-pressure cooker.

sternal, pertaining to the sternum.

sternalgia, pain in the sternum.

sternocostal, pertaining to the sternum and ribs.

sternohyoid, pertaining to the sternum and hyoid bone.

sternoid, resembling the sternum.

sternum, the narrow, flat bone in the median line of the thorax; breastbone.

sternutatory, an agent that causes sneezing; inducing sneezing.

steroid, a group of fat-soluble organic compounds which includes many hormones, cardiac aglycones, bile acids, and sterols.

sterol, any of a group of substances which are related to fats and belong to the lipids found in animals or plants.

stertor, laborious breathing or snoring due to obstruction of the air passages.

stertorous, pertaining to laborious breathing or sonorous respiration; a snoring sound.

stethoscope, an instrument used in auscultation of sounds produced in the body, which consists of rubber tubing in a Y shape.

stethoscopic, pertaining to a stethoscope.

stethoscopy, examination by menas of the stethoscope.

sthenia, normal strength.

sthenic, active, vigorous, and strong.

stigma, a mark or pupuric lesion on the skin; any mental or physical peculiarity that helps to identify or diagnose a specific disease or condition.

stigmatic, pertaining to a stigma; marked with a stigma.

stigmatism, marked by the presence of stigmata; a condition of the eyes in which the rays of light are accurately focused on the retina.

stilbestrol, diethylstilbestrol, a synthetic estrogen.

stilet, stilette, a very small, sharp-pointed instrument used for probing; a wire used to pass through a flexible catheter.

stillbirth, the birth of a dead fetus.

stillborn, dead at birth.

stimulant, any agent that produces a transient surge of energy and strength of activity.

stimulate, to increase functional activity.

stimulation, the act of stimulating or that of being stimulated.

stimulus, any agent that produces functional or tropic reaction in a receptor, organ, or irritable tissue.

sting, a sharp sensation due to a prick, wound, astringent, or tiny pointed organ of bees, wasps, and certain other insects.

stirrup, stapes in the middle ear.

stitch, a sudden, temporary pain; a suture.

stoma, a mouthlike opening which is kept open to allow drainage.

stomach, the large musculo-membranous pouch which is the principal organ of digestion extending from the esophagus to the duodenum, and consisting of a fundus, or cardiac part, a body, and a pyloric part.

stomachalgia, pain in the stomach.

stomachic, a medicine which aids functional activity of the stomach.

stomatitis, inflammation of the mouth.

stomatology, the branch of medicine concerned with diseases and treatments of the mouth.

stomatomycosis, any disease of the mouth caused by fungi.

stomatopathy, any disorder of the mouth.

stomatoplasty, plastic repair of the mouth.

stomodeum, the ectodermal depression in the embryo which becomes the front part of the mouth.

stone, a calculus.

stool, fecal discharge from the bowels.

strabismus, a squint; a disorder of vision due to the turning of one or both eyes so that both cannot be directed at the same point at the same time; cross-eyed.

strabometer, a device for measuring the degree of strabismus.

strabotomy, section of an ocular tendon, a surgical procedure used in treatment of strabismus.

strain, to overexercise; overexertion or overstretching of musculature; to filter.

strangulated, congestion by restriction, or hernial stricture.

strangulation, a choking or arrest of respiration by an obstruction of the air passages.

strangury, a condition in urination marked by slow and painful discharge of urine.

stratification, an arrangement in layers.

stratum, a layer.

Streptobacillus, a genus of gram-negative bacteria which are grouped together to form a chain, the causative agent of Haverhill fever.

streptococcus, spherical bacteria from the genus Streptococcus, usually resembling long chains which are nonmotile, some of which are dangerous pathogens of man causing infection.

streptokinase, a proteolytic enzyme present in hemolytic streptococci which break down blood clots and fibrinous material.

streptomycin, an antibiotic derived from soil fungus.

streptosepticemia, septicemia resulting from infection by streptococci.

stress, a forcibly exerted influence or pressure; any adverse stimulus that tends to disturb the homeostasis of an organism, such as a physical, mental, or emotional stressor.

stressor, an agent or condition capable of producing stress.

stria, a streak line, or ridge; a narrow band or stripe; in anatomy, the longitudinal collections of nerve fibers found in the brain.

stria atrohica, fine pinkish or purplish, scarlike lesions that later become white found on the skin of the abdomen, breasts, thighs, and buttocks, caused by weakening of elastic tissues associated with obesity, tumor, or pregnancy (striae gravidarum).

stricture, an abnormal contraction or narrowing of a passage, or duct; stenosis.

stridor, a harsh or high-pitched respiratory sound, caused by an obstruction of the air passages.

stroke, a sudden attack or affliction, such as apoplexy or paralysis.

stroma, supporting tissue or matrix around an organ.

Strongylus, a genus of nematode parasites which inhabit man and many animals producing serious pathological conditions.

strophanthin, a white, crystalline glucoside obtained from the dogbane plant family, used as a stimulant in certain heart diseases.

struma, an enlargement of the thyroid gland; goiter.

strychnine, a poisonous alkaloid derived from plants.

strychninism, chronic strychnine poisoning induced by overdosing.

stump, the distal part of a limb after amputation.

stupe, a hot, wet cloth for external application which may be medicated.

stupefactive, an agent that produces stupor.

stupor, partial or complete unconsciousness, or deadened sensibility, mental apathy, or reduced responsiveness.

stuporous, affected with stupor, or reduced responsiveness.

stuttering, a speech disorder marked by spasmodic repetition of sounds, especially consonants.

sty, stye, an inflammatory enlargement of a sebaceous gland on the eyelid near the edge.

stylet, a wire placed into a catheter or cannula to render it stiff, used as a probe to remove debris.

styloid, resembling a pillar; pertaining to the styloid process of the temporal bone.

stype, a tampon of cotton.

styptic, contracting a blood vessel; an astringent that checks a hemorrhage; hemostat; astringent.

subacute, somewhat acute; between acute and chronic, but having some acute features.

subarachnoid, between the arachnoid and the pia mater.

subcartilaginous, below the cartilage.

subclavian, below the clavicle.

subclavian artery, the main artery of the arm at the base of the neck beneath the clavicle.

subclavian vein, the main vein beneath the clavicle leading to the arm.

subclinical, pertaining to disorders without clinical manifestations.

subconscious, not clearly conscious; existing beyond consciousness.

subcortex, the substance of the brain underlying the cortex.

subculture, pertaining to a culture of bacteria derived from another culture; a culture derived from another culture.

subcutaneous, beneath the skin; an injection introduced beneath the skin.

subduct, to draw downward.

subfebrile, somewhat feverish, less than 101°F.

subglossal, below the tongue.

subiliac, below the ilium.

subject, an individual or animal subjected to treatment, observation, or experiment; a corpse for dissection.

subjective, perceived only by the subject or person, and not by the examiner.

sublatio retinae, detachment of the retina.

sublimation, a defense mechanism operating outside of conscious awareness in which unacceptable instinctual drives are exhibited in a personal and social acceptable way.

subliminal, below the threshold of sensation; subconscious.

sublingual, situated beneath the tongue.

submaxilla, mandible.

submaxillary, below the maxilla or lower jaw.

submaxillary gland, a salivary gland.

submicroscopic, a size too small to be seen with a microscope.

subnormal, less than normal intelligence.

subocular, situated beneath the eye.

suborbital, beneath the orbit of the eye.

subpharyngeal, beneath the pharynx.

subphrenic, below the diaphragm.

subscapular, below the scapula.

subscription, the directions for compounding ingredients in a prescription.

subsidence, gradual abatement of symptoms of a disease.

substantia alba, the white substance of the brain.

substantia cinerea, the gray matter of the brain and spinal cord.

succorrhea, an excessive flow of any body secretion or of a digestive fluid.

succus, fluid produced by a living tissue.

succussion, shaking of a patient to determine the presence of either fluid or gas in a body cavity.

suckle, to nurse from a breast.

sucrase, an enzyme in the intestinal juice.$ sucrose, a crystalline compound obtained from sugar cane, sugar beet and other sources which is hydrolyzed in the intestine to glucose and fructose.

sudation, sweating.

sudatorium, a hot-air bath to induce sweating.

sudor, perspiration, or sweating.

sudoriferous, conveying or producing sweat; secretion of perspiration.

sudorific, a drug that causes sweating.

suffocate, to asphyxiate; to smother; to choke by stopping respiration.

suffocation, the stoppage of respiration; asphyxiation.

sugar, a sweet carbohydrate belonging to one of two groups, either diasaccharides or monosaccharides; sucrose.

suggestibility, being susceptible to suggestion.

suggestion, an idea that is introduced to an individual from without.

suicidal, pertaining to or suggesting suicide.

suicide, taking one's own life; one who intentionally takes his own life.

sulcate, sulcated, furrowed or grooved.

sulcus, a slight depression or fissure, as of the brain.

sulfa drugs, any of the sulfonamide group which possesses bacteriostatic properties; sulfonamides.

sulfanilamide, a crystalline compound derived from sulfanilic acid, used for its potent antibacterial action.

sulfur, a colorless chemical element existing in several forms, used most commonly in pharmaceutical preparations and, in a dry form, as an insecticide and rodenticide.

sunburn, dermatitis caused by prolonged exposure to the sun's rays; to be affected with sunburn; actinodermatitis.

sunstroke, a condition due to excessive exposure to rays of the sun or extreme heat.

superciliary, pertaining to the eyebrow.

supercilium, the eyebrow.

superego, that part of the personality associated with morals, standards, ethics, and self-criticism; part of the psyche which is derived from the id and the ego that acts as a mediator of the ego; the conscience.

superfecundation, fertilization of two or more ova during the same menstrual cycle by two separate acts of coitus.

superfetation, the occurrence of a second conception after one already existing, resulting in two fetuses in the womb at the same time, but of different ages.

superficial, situated on or near the surface of the skin.

superficies, an outer surface.

superinduce, to bring on in addition to something that already exists.

supernormal, beyond what is normal; beyond average human intellect.

supernumerary, in excess of a normal number.

supersaturate, to saturate more of an ingredient than can be contained in a solution.

supinate, to turn the hand so that the palm faces upward; to rotate the foot and leg outward; to assume a position of supination.

supination, turning of the palm or foot upward; lying flat upon the back.

supinator, a muscle that produces the motion of turning the palm and hand upward.

supplemental, adding something to supply a need.

suppository, a semi-solid mass in the form of a cone for introduction into the rectum, vagina, or urethra where it dissolves; a vehicle for medicine to be absorbed.

suppress, to conceal; to restrain from course of action.

suppression, the act of suppressing; conscious effort to conceal unacceptable impulses, thoughts or feelings.

suppurant, the production of pus; any agent that causes the formation of pus.

suppuration, the formation of pus.

suppurative, producing the generation of pus; a drug that produces pus formation.

supraliminal, above the threshold of consciousness; conscious.

supramaxilla, the upper jawbone.

supraorbital, located above the orbit of the eye.

suprarenal, above the kidney; pertaining to an adrenal gland.

suprascapular, situated above the scapula or shoulder blade.

sura, the calf of the leg.

sural, pertaining to the calf of the leg.

surdity, deafness.

surdomute, a deaf-mute; one who is deaf and dumb.

surface, the exterior of the body.

surgeon, a specialist in surgery.

surgery, the branch of medicine concerned with operative procedures for correction of deformities, repair of injuries, diagnosis and cure of diseases, and the relief of suffering and prolongation of life in humans; a room where surgery is performed.

surrogate, a substitute; a thing or person who takes the place of something or someone.

susceptibility, the quality of being susceptible; capacity for feeling emotions; sensitiveness.

suspend, to cease temporarily.

suspension, a condition of cessation, as of animation or pain or of any vital process; a treatment of spinal disorders by suspending a patient by supporting the chin and shoulders.

suspensory ligament, any of a number of ligaments that support anatomical parts, such as the ring-shaped fibrous tissue which holds the lens of the eye.

suspiration, a sigh; the act of sighing.

sustentacular, supporting or sustaining.

sustentation, sustenance, or support of life.

susurrus, a soft murmuring sound; whisper; murmur.

suture, a stitch or stitches that unite the edges of a wound; the material used in stitching a wound; the line of union between the skull bones.

swab, a small bit of cotton or gauze applied to one end of a slender stick which is used for wiping or cleansing or as an applicator for medication.

sweat, perspiration; the substance secreted by the sweat glands.

sweat glands, tubular glands found on all surfaces of the body except the lips, glans penis, and inner surface of prepuce.

sweating, the process of excreting sweat.

swelling, a temporary enlargement of a body part; an abnormal protuberance; a tumor.

swoon, to faint.

sycoma, a large, soft wart.

sycosis, an inflammation of hair follicles of the beard and scalp.

syllepsis, impregnation; pregnancy or conception.

sylvian aqueduct, a narrow passage from the 3rd to 4th ventricle; aqueduct of Sylvius.

symbion, symbiont, an organism which lives with another in a state of symbiosis.

symbiosis, the living together of two different organisms in a close association with both benefiting from the relationship.

symbolia, having the ability to recognize the nature of objects through the sense of touch.

symbolism, a condition in which everything that occurs is interpreted as a symbol of the patient's own thoughts.

symmelus, a fetus with fused legs and one to three feet, or no feet.

symmetrical, pertaining to symmetry.

symmetry, correspondence in arrangement, form, and size of parts found on the opposite side of an axis.

sympathectomy, resection or interruption of some part of the sympathetic nervous system.

sympathetic nervous system, autonomic nervous system which stimulates the heartbeat, dilates the pupils, and contracts the blood vessels, and, in general, functions in opposition of the parasympathetic nervous system.

sympathin, a neurohormonal mediator of nerve impulses at the synapses of sympathetic nerves.

symphysion, most anterior point of the alveolar process of the lower jaw.

symphysis, line of fusion of two bones which are separate in early development, such as the mandible.

symptom, a condition that results or accompanies an illness or a disease from which a diagnosis may be made.

symptomatic, relating to a symptom or symptoms.

symptomatology, the branch of medicine concerned with symptoms; all of the symptoms of a given disease.

synapse, the junction where neural impulses are transmitted, either between two neurons or a neuron and an effector by the release of a chemical neurotransmitter, as acetylcholine or norepinephrine.

synapsis, a stage in meiosis in which homologous chromosomes from the male and female pronuclei pair off.

synaptic, pertaining to a synapse or synapsis.

synarthrosis, a fibrous joint in which two bones that unite cannot move freely; fixed articulation.

synchilia, congenital joining of the lips.

synclonus, a successive clonic contraction of various muscle groups; muscular tremors.

syncope, loss of consciousness; faint; generalized cerebral ischemia causing temporary unconsciousness.

syncytium, a multinucleated mass of protoplasm which is not divided into definite cell structures.

syndactyl, a fusion between adjacent digits of the hand or foot, so that they are more or less webbed together.

syndesis, synapsis; arthrodesis.

syndesmosis, connection of bones by ligaments formed by fibrous connective tissue other than a joint articulation.

syndesmotomy, surgical incision of a ligament.

syndesmus, a ligament.

syndrome, symptoms that occur together; complexus of symptoms.

syneresis, the contraction of a gel causing it to separate from the liquid, as a shrinkage of fibrin from a colloidal gel.

synergetic, cooperative action of muscles working together.

synergism, any cooperative action of two agents that produce more effective results which neither alone could produce, such as two drugs.

synergy, combined action of two or more organs or muscles; coordinated action.

synesthesia, a sensation in one area of the body from a stimulus applied to another area; a subjective sensation of another sense than the specific one being stimulated, as a sound which produces a visual sensation of color.

syngamy, sexual reproduction; the union of female and male gametes to form a zygote in fertilization.

synostosis, union between adjacent bones by the formation of osseous material.

synovia, the transparent lubricating fluid secreted by the synovial membranes present in joints, cavities, bursae, and tendon sheaths.

synovitis, inflammation of the synovial membrane.

synthesis, the process which involves the formation of a complex substance from a simpler compound, as in the synthesis of protein from an amino acid.

synthetic, artificially prepared; relating to synthesis.

syphilis, a venereal disease caused by Treponema pallidium, transmitted by direct sexual contact or in utero, marked by lesions which involve any body organ. The disease usually has three degenerative stages that occur over the course of many years; leus venera.

syphilogy, the study of syphilis and its treatment.

syringe, a small, tubular device for injecting fluids or withdrawing them from a blood vessel or cavity.

syringitis, inflammation of the eustachian tube.

syringomyelia, a disease of the spinal cord in which fluid accumulates in the cavities, replacing the nerve tissue and causing muscle atrophy and spasticity.

syringotome, a surgical instrument used in operating, as an incision of a fistula.

syssarcosis, muscular articulation of bones, as of the hyoid and patella.

systaltic, contracting and dilating of the heart alternately; pulsating.

system, organized grouping of related structures that act together for a common purpose; a method of practice based on specific principles; the human body as an anatomical whole.

systemic, pertaining to a specific system of parts; affecting the entire bodily system or the body as a whole.

systole, the period of contraction of the heart, especially of the ventricles; opposed to diastole.

systolic, pertaining to systole.

systremma, cramp in the calf muscles of the leg.

syzygium, a partial fusion of two structures.

syzygy, the fusion of two organs with each remaining distinct.

T

tabella, medicated material that is formed into a small disk; lozenge, tablet, or troche.

tabes, a gradual wasting or emaciation in any chronic disease.

tabes dorsalis, a late form of syphilis involving the degeneration of the spinal cord and sensory nerve trunks, causing muscular incoordination, intense pain, disturbances in sensation, and eventual paralysis.

tabetic, pertaining to or afflicted with tabes or tabes dorsalis.

tablature, separation or division of the cranial bones into inner and outer tables.

tablet, a small disk containing a solid dose of medicine.

taboparesis, general paralysis associated with tabes.

tache, a blemish, spot, or freckle on the skin.

tachistoscope, an apparatus used to test visual perception by exposing an object or group of objects to view for a selected brief period of time.

tachography, a recording of the movement and speed of the blood flow.

tachyarrhythmia, tachycardia associated with irregularity of normal heart rhythm.

tachycardia, an abnormal rapid heart rate, usually between 160-190 per minute.

tachylalia, speaking extremely rapidly.

tachyphagia, rapid eating.

tachyphrasia, extreme volubility of speech, often accompanying a mental disorder.

tachyphrenia, mental hyperactivity.

tachypnea, extremely rapid respiration.

tactile, pertaining to the sense of touch; touch.

tactile corpuscles, numerous elongated bodies that enclose the endings of afferent nerve fibers which serve as receptors for touch or for slight pressure beneath the epidermis of the finger tips, toes, soles, palms, lips, nipples, and tip of the tongue.

tactometer, a device that measures tactile sensibility.

tactus, touch.

taenia, a bandlike structure; a tapeworm.

taeniacide, an agent that is lethal to tapeworms.

taeniasis, infestation with tapeworms of the genus Taenia.

Tagement, trademark for cimetidine. used to decrease gastric acid secretion.

talalgia, pain in the heel or ankle.

talc, talcum powder, used as a dusting powder.

talipea, a congenital deformity of the foot; clubfoot.

talipomanus, clubhand.

talocalcaneal, pertaining to the talus and calcaneus.

talofibular, pertaining to the talus and fibula.

talpa, mole.

talus, the anklebone; the ankle.

Talwin, trademark for pentazocine used as an analgesic, anti-inflammatory, and antipyretic agent.

tampon, a pack, pad, or plug of cotton used in surgery to control hemorrhage or to absorb secretions, as produced in the nose or vagina; to plug with a tampon.

tannin, an acid substance found in the bark of certain plants and trees and in coffee and tea, used as an astringent, for burns, as an antidote for various poisons, and as a hemostatic; tannic acid.

tantalum, a noncorrosive chemical element used in replacement of cranial defects, for prosthetic appliances, and for fine sutures.

tantrum, a violent outburst of temper, anger, or rage.

tap, to drain of body accumulations of fluid by paracentesis.

tapeinocephaly, a flattening of the top of the skull or head.

tapetum, a layer of cells which cover a structure; a stratum in the human brain which is composed of fibers; a membranous layer, as in the retina.

tapeworm, a parasitic intestinal worm belonging to the class Cestoda, having a flat or bandlike form, characterized by having larval and adult stages in separate hosts.

taphophobia, a morbid fear of being buried alive.

tarantism, a nervous affection marked by manic or hysterical fits of dancing, melancholy, or stupor, believed to be attributed to the bite of a tarantula.

tarantula, a large, venomous spider feared by many, but relatively harmless.

tardive, late or tardy.

tardive dyskinesia, a serious side effect of antipsychotic drugs marked by grimacing, choreiform movements of the arms, fingers, ankles, and toes, and tonic contractions of the muscles of the neck and back, usually irreversible.

target, an area or an object toward which something is directed.

tarsal, pertaining to the tarsus of the foot.

tarsalgia, pain in the tarsus.

tarsalia, referring to the tarsal bones.

tarsectomy, surgical excision of the tarsus or tarsal bone.

tarsectopia, dislocation of the tarsus.

tarsitis, inflammation of the tarsus; inflammation of the upper eyelid.

tarsometatarsal, pertaining to the tarsus and metatarsus.

tarsoplasty, plastic surgery of an eyelid.

tarsotibial, pertaining to the tarsus and the tibia.

tarsotomy, surgical incision of the tarsal cartilage of an eyelid, or the tarsus of the foot.

tarsus, the proximal part of the foot; instep; the collection of bones between the tibia and metatarsus; the connective tissue plate along the edge of the eyelid.

tartar, the hard yallowish substance deposited on the teeth, mainly composed of calcium phosphate.

tastant, any salt capable of gustatory excitation that stimulates the sense of taste.

taste, the ability to distinguish flavor by the sense of taste; taste sensation occurs through stimulation of gustatory nerve endings in the tongue. Four distinguished qualities are: sweet, sour, salty, and bitter.

taste bud, a tiny end organ located on the surface of the tongue which mediates the sensation of taste.

taxis, the replacement of a displaced structure; reduction of a herniated tumor by manipulation, not by incision; the response of a mobile organism to a stimulus.

taxonomy, an orderly classification of organisms into categories according to correct or suitable names.

Tay-Sachs disease, an inherited disease that destroys the nervous system, caused by a lipid metabolism disorder which is always fatal. Tay-Sachs disease results from the absence of the enzyme hexosaminidase which is responsible for the breakdown of fat.

tears, a saline fluid secreted by the lacrimal glands that moistens the surface and cleanses the eyes of foreign particles.

tease, to pull apart or separate gently with very fine needles before microscopic examination.

teat, the nipple of a mammary gland.

technic, technique; expertness in performing the details of a procedure or operation.

technician, one skilled in specific technical procedures.

technologist, a technician who is highly trained and certified.

tectocephaly, having a roof-shaped cranium.

tectum, a roof-shaped structure.

teeth, hard, bony projections in the jaw. There are 32 permanent teeth, 16 in each jaw.

teething, the process of eruption of the teeth.

tegmen, a covering or integument.

tegmental, pertaining to the tegmentum.

tegmentum, a covering or roof; referring to the cerebral peduncle dorsal, a portion of the midbrain.

tegument, a natural covering of skin.

tegumental, pertaining to the skin.

teichopsia, attacks of temporary blindness, marked by zigzag lines appearing in the visual field, sometimes accompanying headache and mental or physical strain.

tela, a weblike structure.

telalgia, pain felt at a distance from its stimulus; pain referred.

telangiectasis, dilatation of the capillaries and other small blood vessels which cause an angioma of macular appearance, such as a birthmark in young children, or as caused by alcoholism, exposure to cold weather, diseases, and infections. May occur on the face, thighs, or nose.

telangitis, inflammation of the capillaries.

telencephalic, pertaining to the telencephalon.

telencephalon, endbrain; the anterior division of the forebrain.

teleneuron, a nerve ending.

teleopsia, a disturbance in vision in which objects appear to be farther away than they actually are.

telepathy, the communication of thought by means of extrasensory perception.

telesthesia, telepathy; the ability to respond to a stimulus beyond the usual range of perception.

telesystolic, pertaining to the termination of cardiac systole.

telolemma, the membrane covering the motor end plate in a striated muscle fiber.

telomere, pertaining to the ends of the chromosomes which have specific properties, such as having polarity that prevents reunion with any fragments after the chromosome has been broken.

telophase, the last of four stages of mitosis, and of two divisions of meiosis.

temperament, the combination of qualities, physical and mental, that determine personality.

temperature, heat or cold expressed in terms of a specific scale. Normal body temperature is 98.6° F or 37° C.

temple, the flattened area on either side of the forehead.

temporal, pertaining to the temple; pertaining to time; temporary.

temporal bone, one of the two bones on either side of the head.

temporalis, a muscle in the depression of the temporal bone which elevates the mandible.

temulence, intoxication; drunkenness.

tenaculum, a hooklike instrument used to grasp and hold parts in surgery or dissection.

tenalgia, pain in a tendon.

tenderness, sensitiveness to pain when pressure is applied to the skin.

tendinitis, inflammation of a tendon.

tendinous, resembling tendons; composed of tendons.

tendon, a fibrous cord of connective tissue by which a muscle is attached to a bone or cartilage.

tenesmus, painful straining in defecating or urinating.

tenia, taenia, a flat band of soft tissue; a tapeworm of the genus Taenia.

teniacide, an agent that is lethal to tapeworms.

teniafuge, an agent that expels tapeworms.

tennis elbow, radiohumeral bursitis; epicondylitis; pain caused by overexertion of the arm.

tenodesis, surgical fixation of the end of a tendon to a bone.

Tenon's capsule, a thin connective tissue that envelops the eyeball behind the conjunctiva.

tenontitis, inflammation of Tenon's capsule; tendinitis.

tenophyte, a growth in a tendon.

tenotomy, surgical section of a tendon.

tensile, pertaining to tension; capable of being stretched.

tension, the act of stretching or being stretched or strained.

tensor, any muscle that stretches or tightens a body part.

tent, a fabric covering placed over a patient's head for administering oxygen or vaporized medication.

tentative, a diagnosis which is subject to change because of insufficient data; experimental.

tenth nerve, vagus nerve.

tentum, the penis.

tenuity, the condition of being thin.

tenuous, slender or thin.

tephromyelitis, inflammation of the gray matter of the spinal cord.

teras, a deformed fetus; a monster.

teratology, the science dealing with monstrosities and malfomations of fetuses.

teratoma, congenital tumor that contains embryonic elements of the three primary germ layers, as teeth or hair; dermoid.

teratoid, resembling a monster.

terebration, the act of boring; boring pain; trephining.

teres, round and smooth; long and cylindrical.

term, parturition; a definite period; the normal nine months of pregnancy.

terminal, pertaining to an end; a termination, or ending.

terminology, the vocabulary of a science; nomenclature.

Terramycin, trademark for the oxy derivative of tetracycline, used as an antibiotic effective against rickettsias and some viruses.

tertiary syphilis, the third stage of syphilis and the most advanced stage.

test, an examination or trial; a chemical reaction; reagent.

testectomy, surgical removal of a testicle.

testicle, one of two oval-shaped glands of reproduction in the male; testis.

testicular, pertaining to the testis.

testitis, inflammation of the testicle or testicles.

testosterone, the principal male hormone responsible for secondary male sex characteristics.

tetanic, pertaining to tetanus.

tetanoid, resembling tetanus.

tetanus, an infectious disease, often fatal, caused by the neurotoxin of Clostridium tetani, marked by painful spasms of the voluntary muscles, especially those of the lower jaw and neck; lockjaw.

tetany, a condition characterized by painful muscle spasms, which are irregular and intermittent, usually occurring in the extremities due to an inability to utilize calcium salts.

tetracycline, a drug obtained naturally from certain soil bacilli of the genus Streptomyces or produced synthetically, used as an antibiotic.

tetrad, an arrangement of four chromosomes during meiosis by splitting off paired chromosomes.

tetralogy of Fallot, a congenital malformation of the heart involving pulmonic stenosis. As the infant grows, the pulmonary blood flow cannot increase causing right ventricular hypertrophy and shunting of blood from the right to the left ventricle, producing cyanosis. Growth of the child is poor, symptoms of fatigue, polycythemia and clubbing of the hands appear at the time cyanosis, a blue discoloration to the skin from lack of oxygen, becomes evident; a series of four congenital heart defects.

tetraparesis, muscular weakness present in all four extremities.

tetraplegia, quadriplegia.

tetraploidy, having four sets of chromosomes.

tetter, any of many cutaneous diseases, as impetigo, herpes, ringworm, and eczema.

textural, pertaining to the structure of tissues.

thalamencephalon, the part of the brain containing the optic thalami and the pineal gland.

thalamus, the region of the brain concerned with many bodily functions which lies between the hypothalamus and epithalamus, the center for sensory impulses to the cerebral cortex.

thalidomide, a sedative and hypnotic that causes serious congenital anomalies in the fetus when taken during early pregnancy.

thanatoid, resembling death.

thanatology, the science concerned with death and dying.

thanatophoric, lethal or deadly.

thanatos, in psychoanalysis, death instinct.

theca, a caselike structure or sheath.

thecal, pertaining to a sheath.

thecitis, inflammation of the sheath of a tendon.

thelalgia, pain in the nipples.

theleplasty, plastic surgery on a nipple.

thelitis, inflammation of a nipple.

thelium, a nipple or papilla.

thenar, the fleshy part of the hand below the thumb; palm.

theobromine, an alkaloid found in cacao seeds which have properties similar to caffeine, used as a smooth muscle relaxant, a diuretic, and as a myocardial stimulant and vasodilator.

theophobia, a morbid fear of God.

therapeutic, pertaining to therapeutics; curative.

therapeutics, the science of healing; scientific treatment of diseases and the application of remedies.

therapeutist, one skilled in therapeutics; a therapist.

therapy, the treatment of disease or a pathological condition.

therm, a unit of heat.

thermal, pertaining to heat.

thermoanesthesia, inability to distinguish between heat and cold.

thermocauterectomy, excision by thermocautery.

thermocautery, cautery by a heated wire or point.

thermogenesis, the production of heat within the body.

thermogram, a graphic record of variations of temperature.

thermograph, an instrument used for recording variations of temperature.

thermolabile, changed easily by heat; unstable.

thermolysis, a heat loss from the body due to evaporation; a chemical dissociation caused by heat.

thermomassage, the use of heat in massage.

thermometer, an instrument to measure heat.

thermophile, an organism that thrives in elevated temperatures.

thermophore, an apparatus for retaining heat.

thermoplegia, sunstroke; heatstroke.

thermostable, not destroyed by heat.

thermotaxis, the regulation and normal adjustment of the body to temperature; the movement of an organism toward or away from the stimulation of temperature or heat source.

thermotherapy, the therapeutic use of heat in treatment of disease.

thermotropism, the property within organisms to respond to heat stimulus.

thiamine, a B-complex vitamin compound found in animal and plant foods, dry yeast, and wheat germ which are the richest natural resources, essential to man for normal metabolism of both fats and carbohydrates; vitamin B_1.

thigh, that part of the leg between the knee and the hip.

thighbone, femur.

thigmesthesia, sense of touch; tactile sensibility.

thimerosal, used as a germicide and an antiseptic.

thinking, the process of forming concepts and images in one's mind.

thiopental, a short- acting barbiturate used in its salt form intravenously or rectally to induce general anesthesia.

thiouracil, an antithyroid drug used in treatment of hyperthyroidism, thyroiditis, and thyrotoxicosis which reduces the production of thyroid gland hormones.

third cranial nerve, regulates eye movements.

third-degree burn, implies a destruction of the full thickness of the skin, often of underlying fat, muscles and even bone, giving a pale white or charred appearance to the skin.

thirst, a craving for fluids, especially water.

thoracentesis, a puncture through the chest wall for tapping or removal of fluids; pleurocentesis.

thoracic, pertaining to the chest.

thoracic duct, the main lymphatic vessel of the body, which originates at the cisterna chyli on the abdomen.

thoracostomy, an opening of the chest wall for drainage or for an enlarged heart.

thoracotomy, surgical cutting into the chest wall.

thorax, the area between the base of the neck and the diaphragm.

Thorazine, trademark for chlorpromazine, a major tranquilizer used to treat severely excited psychiatric patients.

threadworm, term commonly applied to the pinworm which inhabits the intestines.

three-day fever, a viral disease which resembles dengue, transmitted by the sandfly.

threonine, one of the essential amino acids.

threshold, that point at which an effect is produced by a stimulus.

thrill, a vibration felt on palpation; to produce a sensation of tingling, as in excitement.

throat, the passage that extends from the nose and mouth to the lungs; pharynx; fauces.

throb, pulsating movement, as a heart beat,; palpitation.

throbbing, a pulsation, beating, or rhythmic movement.

throe, a severe pain, especially the sharp pain in childbirth.

thrombin, the enzyme that produces coagulation of the blood, resulting from the activation of prothrombin; a preparation used as a topical hemostatic that controls capillary bleeding.

thromboangitis, inflammation of a blood vessel.

thrombocyte, a blood platelet which aids in coagulation.

thromboembolism, an embolism carried by the blood from the site of origin to block another vessel.

thrombogenesis, clot formation.

thrombolysis, dissolution or breaking up of a thrombus.

thrombophlebitis, inflammation of a vein caused by a thrombus formation.

thromboplastic, acceleration of the formation of clots in the blood.

thromboplastin, a lipoprotein that promotes the conversion of prothrombin to thrombin.

thrombosis, formation of a thrombus.

thrombotic, pertaining to thrombosis.

thrombus, a blood clot that obstructs a blood vessel or a cavity of the heart.

thrush, a disease of the oral mucous membranes that forms whitish patches which become ulcerated, usually in infants and young children, caused by Candida albicans.

thumb, the first digit of the hand on the radial side.

thylacitis, inflammation of the sebaceous glands of the skin.

thymectomy, surgical removal of the thymus gland.

thymic, pertaining to the thymus gland.

thymion, a wart.

thymin, a hormone-like substance secreted by the thymus gland that impairs neuromuscular transmission.

thymine, a pyrimidine base found in DNA.

thymitis, inflammation of the thymus gland.

thymocyte, a lymphocyte produced by the thymus gland.

thymolysis, dissolution of thymus tissue.

thymolytic, thymus tissue destruction.

thymoma, a tumor arising from lymphoid or epithelial tissues of the thymus gland.

thymus, a ductless gland situated in the upper thoracic cavity, necessary in early life for the development of immunological functions, and which undergoes involution in adults.

thyroadenitis, inflammation of the thyroid gland.

thyrocele, a goiter.

thyrochondrotomy, surgical incision of the thyroid cartilage.

thyroid, a gland, in the neck, that partially surrounds the thyroid cartilage and upper rings of the trachea; thyroid secretions consist of two hormones, thyroxine and triiodothyronine, which help to regulate the metabolic rate, the growth process, and tissue differentiation. Thyroid extract is composed of dried thyroid glands of ox and sheep.

thyroid cartilage, the principal cartilage of the larynx which forms a v-shaped structure known as the Adam's apple.

thyroidectomy, surgical removal of part or all of the thyroid gland.

thyroiditis, inflammation of the thyroid gland.

thyroptosis, a displaced thyroid gland, partially or completely into the thorax.

thyrotome, a surgical instrument for excising the thyroid cartilage.

thyrotoxicosis, a disorder caused by an overactive thyroid gland; Graves' disease.

thyroxine, an iodine-containing hormone that is secreted by the thyroid gland responsible for increasing the rate of cell metabolism.

tibia, shinbone.

tibial, pertaining to the tibia.

tic, an involuntary, repetitive, compulsive movement of certain muscles of the face and shoulders.

tic douloureux, facial neuralgia accompanied by convulsive twitching.

tick, a parasitic mite or acarid of the genus Ixodes which buries its head into the skin of the host to suck blood, often transmitting diseases.

tick fever, an infectious disease transmitted by the bite of a woodtick; Rocky Mountain spotted fever.

tilmus, picking at bedsores in delirious patients.

tincture, diluted alcoholic solution used in preparation of a drug or a chemical substance, such as ginger, benzoin, guaiac, and others.

tinea, any of many different superficial fungal infections of the skin; ringworm.

tinnitus, a ringing or buzzing sound in the ear.

tissue, a grouping of similarly specialized cells that perform certain specific functions.

titillation, sensation produced by tickling, as in the throat; state of being tickled.

titubation, a staggering walk with shaking of the head and trunk, usually due to cerebellar diseases.

tocology, obstetrics.

toe, a digit of the foot.

Tofranil, trademark for imipramine preparations used to alleviate depression associated with specific mental conditions.

toilet, the cleansing and dressing of a wound.

tolbutamide, an oral hypoglycemic drug used to control uncomplicated, mild, stable diabetes mellitus in those who have some functioning islet cells; trademark name, Orinase.

tolerance, having the ability to endure without injury or effect.

tolerate, to resist the action of drugs or toxins.

tolmentum, a network of blood vessels found within the cortex of the brain and the cerebral surface of the pia mater.

tomography, a method of producing images of cross-sections of the body.

tonaphasia, the loss of recall of a tune due to cerebral lesions.

tone, having normal tension and vigor in muscles; tonus; a quality of sound or vocal production.

tone deafness, inability to distinguish musical pitch.

tongue, the freely moving muscular organ situated in the floor of the mouth which functions in mastication of food, taste, and in speech production.

tongue tie, a congenital shortening of the frenum which restricts tongue movement.

tonic, restoration of normal muscle tone; characterized by tension or contraction; an agent or remedy.

tonicity, the normal elastic tension of living muscles, arteries, etc.; in body fluid physiology, the effective osmotic pressure equivalent; tone.

tonography, recording the changes in intraocular pressure due to sustained pressure on the eyeball.

tonometer, a physiological instrument that measures the tension of the eyeball.

tonometric, pertaining to a tonometer or tonometry.

tonometry, measurement of tension of the eyeball.

tonsil, a rounded mass of lymphoid tissue, one on either side of the pharynx, which acts as a filter to protect the body from infection or invasion of bacteria.

tonsillar, pertaining to a tonsil.

tonsillectomy, surgical excision of a tonsil.

tonsillitis, inflammation of the tonsils.

tonus, the normal state of tension in muscles; a continuous contraction of a muscle.

tooth, one of the hard processes situated in the jaw which serves for biting and mastication of food.

toothache, pain in a tooth or area around the tooth.

tophus, a deposit of sodium biurate formed in the fibrous tissue near a joint, especially in gout.

topical, pertaining to a definite area; applied to a particular part of the body.

topography, a description of a specific part of the body.

tormen, a twisting or griping pain in the intestines.

torpor, sluggishness; abnormal inactivity; apathy.

torporific, causing torpor.

torque, rotary force; in dentistry, the rotation of a tooth on its axis by use of an orthodontic instrument.

torsion, the act of twisting, or state of being twisted.

torso, the trunk of the body, which excludes the head and limbs.

torticollis, wryneck; torsion of the neck caused by the contracted state of cervical muscles.

tortuous, full of many twists and turns.

torulus, a papilla or small elevation in the skin.

torus, a rounded swelling; a bulging or protuberant part.

touch, tactile sense; palpation by touching with the fingers.

tourniquet, a band that is placed tightly around a limb for the temporary arrest of circulation or hemorrhaging in the distal region.

toxalbumin, poisonous albumin or protein.

toxanemia, toxemia.

toxemia, the spread of bacterial toxins by the bloodstream, marked by fever, diarrhea, vomiting, quickened or depressed pulse and respirations, prostration.

toxemia of pregnancy, a specific hypertensive disease of pregnancy or of early puerperium (six week period after childbirth).

toxic, pertaining to a toxin or poison; poisonous.

toxicant, any toxic agent, or poison.

toxicity, having a toxic or poisonous quality; state of being toxic.

toxicoderma, a skin disease caused by poison.

toxicogenic, producing toxic or poisonous products.

toxicologist, one who specializes in the field of poisons and treatments.

toxicology, the science concerned with poisons, their effects, and antidotes.

toxicosis, any abnormal diseased condition due to poisoning or toxic action.

toxin, any organic poison of animal or plant origin; any poisonous substances produced by pathogenic organisms that cause disease in other living organisms.

toxin-antitoxin, a nearly neutral mixture of diphtheria toxin with an antitoxin, used for immunization against diphtheria.

toxinic, pertaining to a toxin.

toxipathy, any disease due to a poison.

toxiphobia, morbid fear of being poisoned.

toxoid, toxic properties of a toxin destroyed by a chemical agent, but still capable of inducing the formation of antibodies.

toxoplasmosis, a disease of the nervous system caused by Toxoplasma gondii, a parasitic protozoan, of which there is a congenital form and an acquired form.

trabecula, a supportive strand of connective tissue, which resembles a small beam extending from a structural part, as from a capsule into the enclosed organ.

trabecular, pertaining to a trabecula.

trachea, the windpipe; the membranous tube extending from the larynx to the bronchi.

tracheal, pertaining to the trachea.

tracheitis, inflammation of the trachea.

tracheobronchial, related to both the bronchi and the trachea.

tracheobronchoscopy, inspection of the trachea and bronchi with a bronchoscope.

tracheoscopy, inspection of the interior of the trachea with a laryngoscope.

tracheostomy, an incision of the trachea for the creation of an opening through the neck; used also for the insertion of a tube to relieve obstruction of the upper airway and to facilitate breathing or ventilation.

tracheotome, a surgical instrument for incising the trachea.

tracheotomy, surgical incision of the trachea.

trachitis, tracheitis, inflammation of the trachea.

trachoma, a contagious disease involving the conjunctiva and cornea of the eyes caused by Chlamydia trachomatis, marked by formation of granulations or tiny rounded growths.

trachomatous, pertaining to or affected with trachoma.

tract, a specific area of the body, especially of a system of related organs; a bundle of nerve fibers within the brain or spinal cord which compose a functional unit.

traction, the act of pulling or drawing.

tractus, a path or tract.

tragus, a cartilaginous projection in front of the external meatus of the ear.

trait, a distinguishing quality of an individual; a characteristic.

trance, an unconscious or hypnotic condition or state.

tranquilize, to render tranquil.

tranquilizer, drugs used in treatment of anxiety states, mental disorders, and neuroses.

transcription, synthesis of RNA using a DNA template.

transect, to cut across or divide.

transection, cross section.

transference, the unconscious transfer of attitudes and feelings to others that once were associated with parents, siblings, or significant others in forgotten childhood experiences; in psychiatry, the patient shifts any affect from one idea to another, or from one person to another by unconscious identification. Transference in the patient-physician relationship may be negative or positive.

transformation, the change of one tissue into another; degeneration.

transfuse, to transfer blood or blood components from one person into another directly into the blood stream.

transfusion, the process of transfusing.

transillumination, examination of a cavity or organ by the passage of a strong light through a body structure.

translocation, in genetics, the attachment of a fragment of one chromosome to another that is nonhomologous.

transmigration, the process of passing across or through, especially passage of white blood cells through the capillary membranes into the surrounding tissues; the passage of an ovum from the ovary to the uterus.

transmission, the transfer of disease from one individual to another; transfer of hereditary characteristics or traits.

transmutation, the process of evolution in which one species changes into another; change of properties of one substance into another.

transpiration, the discharge of moisture, air, or vapor through the skin or a membrane; perspiration.

transpire, to excrete perspiration through the pores in the skin.

transplant, a transfer of tissue in a graft to be transplanted from another person or from one body part to another site.

transplantation, the grafting of tissue or an organ from one person to another; grafting from one part of the body to another part.

transudation, a substance that has transuded; a fluid that has extruded from a tissue.

transude, to ooze through the pores of a membrane.

transverse, extending from side to side; lying crosswise.

transverse colon, that part of the colon that extends crosswise the abdominal cavity.

transversectomy, surgical removal of the transverse vertebral process.

transverse process, the right and left lateral projections from the posterior part of vertebra.

transvestism, the condition of finding sexual pleasure by wearing clothing appropriate to the opposite sex.

transvestite, one who has an uncontrollable compulsion to dress in clothing appropriate to the opposite sex.

trapezium, a bone in the wrist which is the first bone in the distal row of eight carpal bones.

trapezius, a large, flat triangular muscle that covers the posterior surface of the neck and shoulder serving to raise and lower the shoulder.

trauma, an injury or wound; an emotional shock causing injury to the subconscious which may have a lifelong effect.

traumatic, pertaining to trauma.

traumatism, an abnormal condition of the system produced by an injury or trauma.

treatment, the care and management of a patient; the application of medicinal remedies or surgery in combating disease or pathological conditions; therapy.

tremble, involuntary shaking or quivering.

tremor, involuntary quivering or shaking from fear, fever, or general weakness.

tremulous, marked by shaking, quivering, or trembling.

trench fever, recurrent fever caused by Rickettsia pediculi spread by body lice.

trench foot, a condition of the feet resembling frostbite, due to exposure to wet and cold for long periods, seen in trench warfare.

trench mouth, infection involving the tonsils and floor of the mouth caused by Vincent's bacillus, marked by inflammation, painful swelling, and ulceration; Vincent's angina.

trepan, to trephine.

trephine, a form of surgical trepan for removing a circular disk of skull bone; an instrument for removing a circular portion of cornea.

trepidation, trembling involuntary movements of the limbs due to fear or anxiety.

treponema, a spirochete of the genus Treponema, some of which are pathogenic and parasitic for man, as the organism that causes syphilis.

triceps, having three heads, as a triceps muscle that extends the lower arm.

trichiasis, an inversion of eyelashes that causes irritation by rubbing against the cornea of the eyeball.

trichina, a parasitic worm sometimes present in the muscular tissues of man as an encysted larva of the genus Trichinella.

trichinosis, a disease caused by Trichinella spiralis which is ingested into the system through eating pork insufficiently cooked. Symptoms include diarrhea, pain, nausea, fever, and later swelling of muscles, edema, stiffness, and many other conditions.

trichinous, infected with trichinae.

trichoid, resembling hair; hairlike.

trichologia, the pulling out of hair by some patients.

trichomadesis, abnormally premature loss of hair on the scalp.

trichome, a hairlike structure.

trichomegaly, a congenital condition marked by excessive hair growth of eyelashes and eyebrows associated with dwarfism, mental retardation, and degeneration of retina pigmentation.

trichomoniasis, an infection caused by Trichomonas vaginalis resulting in vaginitis and urethritis, marked by inflammation and persistent discharge with pruritus.

trichoptilosis, a splitting of the ends of hairs.

trichorrhea, an abnormally rapid falling of hair.

trichromatic, normal color vision in which one is able to see the three primary colors.

trichromic, able to distinguish only three colors of the spectrum of seven colors.

tricrotic, pertaining to three sphygmographic waves to one beat of the pulse.

tricuspid, having three cusps, as a tooth having three points or cusps; the tricuspid valve of the heart.

tricuspid valve, serving to prevent the back flow of blood from the right auricle into the right ventricle.

trifacial, pertaining to the 5th pair of cranial nerves; trigeminal.

trigeminal neuralgia, facial neuralgia; tic douloureux.

trigone, referring to the triangular space at the base of the bladder.

triorchidism, having three testes.

triplegia, paralysis involving three extremities.

triplet, one of three children produced at one birth.

trismus, a motor disturbance affecting the trigeminal nerve causing spasms of the masticatory muscles and difficulty in opening the mouth; an early symptom of tetanus.

trisomy, having an additional chromosome of one type in a diploid cell.

trituration, a reduction to a powdery substance by grinding or by friction, especially in a mixture of a medicinal preparation.

trocar, a surgical instrument with a sharp-tipped rod used to insert a cannula that serves to draw off body fluid from a cavity.

trochanter, a prominence on the upper part of the femur.

troche, a medicinal preparation that dissolves in the mouth.

trochlea, a pulley- shaped structure that provides a smooth surface over which tendons pass or with which other structures articulate.

trochlear, resembling a trochlea; pulleylike.

trochoides, a pivot joint.

trombiculiasis, being infested with mites of the genus Trombicula.

trophic, pertaining to nutrition.

trophoblast, the outer edge of cells of the blastocyst that attaches the fertilized ovum to the uterine wall, and develops into the placenta and membranes serving to nourish and protect the developing embryo.

tropic, having to do with a turning or a change.

true ribs, the upper seven ribs on each side that articulate directly with the sternum attached by cartilages.

trunk, truncus, the main part of the body to which the head and limbs are attached.

truss, a device for retaining a reduced hernia which may be composed of elastic, canvas, or metallic material.

truth serum, a drug such as scopolamine, used to induce a state in which a patient or subject will talk unrestrainedly.

trypanosoma, a genus of parasitic flagellate protozoa present in the blood of man and other vertebrates, transmitted by insect vectors causing serious diseases, as sleeping sickness.

trypanosomiasis, any of the several diseases caused by a species of Trypanosoma; sleeping sickness.

trypsin, a proteolytic enzyme formed in the intestine from the action of enterokinase on trypsinogen which is secreted by the pancreas capable of converting proteins into proteoses, peptones, and polypeptides.

trypsinogen, a pancreatic juice converted into trypsin by enzyme action.

tryptic, relating to trypsin.

tryptophan, an amino acid in proteins necessary for tissue growth and repair; an essential amino acid necessary for human metabolism.

tsetse, a fly of Africa, genus Glossina, which transmits diseases, as sleeping sickness in man and domestic animals.

tubal, pertaining to a tube, especially the fallopian tube.

tubal pregnancy, a pregnancy occurring in one of the oviducts.

tube, any hollow, cylindrical organ or vessel.

tubercle, a minute rounded elevation on a bone; pertaining to a small rounded nodule of the skin; pertaining to tuberculosis.

tuberculation, the formation of many tubercles.

tuberculin, a sterile substance prepared from tubercle bacillus, used to determine the presence of a tuberculosis infection.

tuberculin test, a test to determine the presence of tuberculous infection based on a positive reaction to tuberculin.

tuberculosis, an infectious disease due to Mycobacterium, marked by the formation of tubercles and caseous necrosis in the tissues of an organ. The lung is the major site of the infection in man.

tuberculous, pertaining to or being affected with tuberculosis.

tuberosity, a protuberance or elevation of a bone.

tubule, tubular, a small tube.

tubulus, a tubule, or minute canal.

tularemia, a disease of rodents which is transmitted to man, by handling infected animals or by insects, causing intermittent fever and swelling of the lymph nodes.

tumescence, swelling; being swollen.

tumis, swollen; edematous.

tumor, an abnormal swelling, usually from inflammation; morbid enlargement; neoplasm; an uncontrolled new tissue growth in which the cells multiply or proliferate rapidly.

tunic, a coat or covering.

tunica, a tunic; a membrane covering or lining a body part or organ.

turbidity, a cloudiness or sedimentation in a solution.

turbinal, scroll-like structure; a turbinate bone.

turbinate, having a shape like a top; the spongy turbinate bone of the nasal concha.

turbinectomy, surgical excision of the turbinate bone.

turgescence, a swelling or distention of a part.

turgescent, growing turgid or swollen.

turgid, distended or swollen.

turgor, a condition of being turgid; normal fullness.

twelfth cranial nerve, one of a pair of cranial nerves extending to the base of the tongue; hypoglossal nerve.

twilight sleep, a state of partial anesthesia in which pain sensation is greatly reduced.

twin, one of two offspring born at the same birth.

twinge, afflicted with sudden, sharp pain or pains.

twitch, a spasmodic muscle contraction producing a jerking action; a brief contraction of muscles that is involuntary.

tyloma, a callosity.

tympanectomy, surgical excision of the tympanic membrane.

tympanic, pertaining to the tympanum; bell-like; resonant.

tympanic membrane, a membrane separating the tympanum or middle ear from the external ear; eardrum.

tympanites, distention or swelling of the abdomen resulting from a collection of air or gas in the peritoneal cavity.

tympanitis, pertaining to tympanites; bell-like quality.

tympanum, the middle ear cavity in the temporal bone.

tympany, a tympanic or bell-like percussion sound.

type, the general or prevailing character of a disease, a person, or a substance.

typhlology, the study of blindness, its causes and treatment.

typhoid, an infectious disease caused by the bacillus Salmonella typhosa, marked by intestinal inflammation and ulceration, usually acquired through ingestion of food or drink; typhoid fever; resembling typhus.

typhomania, delirium present with typhoid fever.

typhus, an acute infectious disease marked by high fever, severe nervous symptoms, macular eruptions of reddish spots, and severe headache, caused by Rickettsia prowazeki and transmitted to man by body lice; typhus fever.

tyrosinase, ferment that acts on tyrosine.

tyrosine, naturally occurring amino acid found in most proteins; a product of phenylalanine metabolism which is a precursor of thyroid hormones.

tyrosinuria, the presence of tyrosine in the urine.

tyrosis, the curdling of milk; the cheesy vomitus of infants; tyromatosis.

U

uaterium, a medicinal preparation for the ear.

uberous, fertile; prolific.

ualgia, pain in the gums.

ulatropia, recession or shrinking of the gums.

ulcer, an open lesion of the skin or mucous membrane produced by the casting off of necrotic tissue, sometimes accompanied by pus formation.

ulcerate, to become ulcerous.

ulceration, the process of ulcerating.

ulcerous, pertaining to an ulcer; marked by ulcer formations.

ulcus, an ulcer.

ulectomy, surgical removal of scar tissue; gingivectomy.

ulitis, gingivitis; inflammation of the gums.

ulna, the long bone in the forearm between the wrist and the elbow, on the side opposite to the thumb.

ulnad, toward the ulna.

ulnar, relating to the ulna, to the ulna nerve, or the ulna artery.

ulocarcinoma, carcinoma or cancer of the gums.

ulorrhagia, bleeding gums.

ulosis, the formation of scar tissue.

ulotrichous, pertaining to short, wool-like hair.

ultramicroscope, a dark field microscope having powerful side illumination.

ultrasound, pertaining to frequencies greater than 20,000 vibrations per second.

ultrastructure, that structure visible only under the ultramicroscope and electron microscope.

ultraviolet, beyond the visible spectrum at its violet end.

ultraviolet rays, extremely hot invisible rays converted into heat by the ozone layer which protects life on earth. The therapeutic effects include heat production, pigmentation of the skin, aid in production of vitamin D, bactericidal effects, and various metabolism effects.

ultravirus, any filterable virus that can be demonstrated by inoculation test.

umbilectomy, surgical removal of the navel.

umbilical, pertaining to the navel or umbilicus; located centrally, like a navel.

umbilical cord, the cord that connects the placenta with the fetus.

umbilicate, pertaining to or shaped like a navel or umbilicus.

umbilicus, navel.

unciform, hook-shaped.

unciform bone, a hook-shaped bone of the wrist.

uncinariasis, hookworm disease; ancylostomiasis.

uncinate, hooked; hook-shaped.

uncinus, shaped like a hook.

unconscious, lacking awareness of the environment; insensible; that part of personality which contains complex feelings and drives of which we are unaware, and which are not accessible to our consciousness.

unconsciousness, state of being unconscious.

unction, application of a salve or ointment; an ointment.

unctuous, having a greasy or oily quality.

uncus, any structure that has a hook-shape; the anterior end of the hippocampal gyrus of the brain that is hook-shaped.

undersized, having a stature less than normal or average.

underweight, having a weight deficiency; the weight is at least 10 percent less than the average weight for persons of the same age, sex, height, and body build.

undifferentiated, primitive.

undine, a small flask for irrigating the eye, usually made of glass.

undulation, a wavelike motion; fluctuating; pulsating.

undulatory, pertaining to undulation.

ungual, pertaining to the nails.

unguent, an ointment.

unguiculate, having nails or claws; clawlike.

unguis, a finger nail or toe nail.

unhealthy, lacking health and not vigorous of body.

uniaxial, having one axis.

unicameral, having one cavity.

unicellular, composed of a single cell, as a protozoan.

unicornous, having a single cornu.

uniglandular, affecting only one gland.

unilateral, affecting one side.

unilocular, having only one chamber.

uninucleated, mononuclear.

union, a juncture, as of broken bone.

uniovular, developed from one germ cell or ovum; monozygotic.

unipara, primipara; having one pregnancy.

uniparous, producing one ovum or one child at a time.

unipolar, having a single pole; pertaining to a nerve cell having a single process.

unipotent, pertaining to a cell having the ability to develop into only kind of structure.

unisexual, pertaining to only one sex.

unit, one portion of a whole; one of anything.

unitary, referring to a single object or person.

unmyelinated, the absence of a myelin sheath around some nerve fibers.

unsaturated, having the ability to absorb more of a solute; referring to compounds in which two or more atoms are connected by double or triple bonds.

unsex, to castrate; deprive of gonads.

unstriated, pertaining to smooth muscles which have no striations.

urachus, an epitheloid cord surrounded by fibrous tissue connecting the apex of the urinary bladder with the umbilicus.

uracil, a component of pyrimidine found in nucleic acid.

uracrasia, a disordered condition of urine; enuresis.

uraniscus, palate.

uranoplasty, surgical repair of a cleft palate.

uranoschisis, cleft palate.

urarthritis, gouty arthritis.

urate, a salt of uric acid. .

uratemia, urates in the blood.

uraturia, urates in the urine.

urea, the diamide of carbonic acid which is found in urine, blood, and lymph, and is the chief nitrogenous end-product of protein metabolism in the body.

ureapoiesis, the formation of urine.

ureameter, a device that determines the amount of urea in urine; ureometer.

urease, an enzyme which catalyzes the decomposition of urea into ammonium carbonate.

urelcosis, the ulceration of the urinary tract.

uremia, a toxic condition produced by excessive by-products of protein metabolism in the blood, causing symptoms of nausea, vomiting, vertigo, convulsions, dimness of vision, and coma.

uremic, pertaining to uremia.

uresis, the excretion of urine from the bladder; urination; voiding.

ureter, one of two tubes 10 to 12 inches long which extend from the kidneys to the posterior surface of the bladder.

ureteralgia, pain in the ureter.

ureterectasis, dilatation or stretching of the ureter.

ureterectomy, surgical excision of the ureter.

urethra, a passage which carries the urine from the bladder to the outside of the body.

urethralgia, pain in the urethra.

urethratresia, an occlusion of the urethra which prevents the passage of urine.

urethrectomy, surgical excision of the urethra.

urethremphraxis, a urethral obstruction; urethrophraxis.

urethritis, inflammation of the urethra.

urethrorrhagia, hemorrhaging from the urethra.

urethroscope, an instrument used to examine the interior of the urethra.

urethroscopy, visual inspection of the urethra by means of a urethroscope.

urgency, a sudden, involuntary need to urinate.

uric, pertaining to urine.

uric acid, a crystalline acid found in urine occurring as an end-product of purine metabolism.

urinal, a vessel used to collect urine, especially for bedridden patients.

urinalysis, a chemical analysis of urine.

urinary, pertaining to secreting or containing urine.

urinary bladder, the distensible receptacle for urine before it is voided.

urinary organs, pertaining to the structures of the urinary system, such as the kidneys, ureters, bladder, and urethra; urinary tract.

urinate, to discharge urine; void; to cast out waste material.

urination, the process of urinating.

urine, the fluid secreted from the blood by the kidneys, which is collected in the bladder and discharged by the urethra.

urinemia, uremia, the contamination of the blood with urinary constituents.

uriniferous, transporting or carrying urine.

uriniferous tubules, renal tubules extending from the Bowman's capsule of the kidney and serving to transport urine.

urinometer, an instrument that determines the specific gravity of urine.

urinous, resembling urine.

urobilin, brown-colored pigment formed by the oxidation of urobilinogen, found in stools or in urine after exposure to air.

urobilinogen, a colorless compound found in the intestines by reduction of bilirubin.

urochrome, the yellowish coloring matter in urine, closely related to urobilin.

urocyst, urinary bladder.

urocystitis, inflammation of the urinary bladder; cystitis.

urogenital, pertaining to the urinary and genital organs.

urography, X-ray of the urinary tract or part of it after the introduction of radiopaque substance.

urolith, a urinary calculus.

urologist, one who specializes in disorders of the urinary organs.

urology, the branch of science concerned with the study, diagnosis, and treatment of diseases of the urinary tract; urinology.

urometer, urinometer.

uroncus, a swelling due to retention of urine.

uropathy, any disease or condition of the urinary tract.

uropoiesis, formation of urine.

uropyoureter, an infected ureter with an accumulation of urine and pus.

urorrhagia, excessive secretion of urine; polyuria.

uroschesis, retention of urine.

urticant, producing itching or urticaria.

urticaria, hives or wheals which are either redder or paler than the surrounding area and are often attended by itching.

uteralgia, pain in the uterus.

uterine, pertaining to the uterus.

uteritis, inflammation of the uterus.

uteroplasty, plastic repair of the uterus.

uterotomy, surgical incision of the uterus.

uterus, the hollow muscular organ in females that serves the developing embryo after fertilization of the ovum; the womb.

utricle, one of two small sacs in the labyrinth of the inner ear.

utricular, pertaining to the nature of the utricle; having a utricle or utricles.

utriculitis, inflammation of the utricle.

uvea, the middle layer of the eye, composed of the ciliary muscle, the choroid, and the iris.

uveitis, inflammation of the uvea.

uvula, the small tissue projection extending from the middle of the soft palate in the throat.

uvulectomy, surgical excision of the uvula; cionectomy.

uvulitis, inflammation of the uvula.

uvulotomy, excising the uvula or part of it.

V

vaccigenous, to produce vaccine.

vaccin, pertaining to vaccine.

vaccinate, to inoculate with vaccine to provide immunity.

vaccination, the act of vaccinating with a vaccine by injection into the body.

vaccine, a suspension of killed microorganisms for prevention of infectious diseases.

vaccinia, a viral disease in cattle which is transmissible to man by inoculation of vaccinia virus used to induce antibody formation against smallpox.

vacciniform, having the nature of vaccinia or cowpox.

vacciniola, a secondary skin eruption sometimes following vaccinia.

vaccinogenous, producing vaccine.

vacuolar, possessing vacuoles.

vacuolation, the formation of vacuoles.

vacuole, a clear space within the cell protoplasm filled with air or fluid.

vacuous, empty.

vacuum, a space exhausted of its air or gaseous content.

vagal, pertaining to the vagus nerve.

vagina, a sheathlike structure; the canal within females between the vulva and the uterus.

vaginal, pertaining to the vagina, or any sheath.

vaginalitis, inflammation of the tunica of the testicles.

vaginate, to enclose in a sheath; enveloped by a sheath.

vaginectomy, surgical removal of the tunica of a testicle; excision of the vagina or part of it.

vaginismus, painful muscular spasms of the vagina.

vaginitis, inflammation of the vagina.

vaginodynia, pain in the vagina; colpopexy.

vaginoplasty, surgical repair of the vagina.

vaginoscope, an instrument used for inspecting the vagina.

vaginoscopy, visual examination of the vagina by a vaginoscope.

vaginotomy, incision of the vagina; colpotomy.

vagus, the 10th cranial nerve, a mixed nerve which has both motor and sensory functions.

valence, the degree of the combining power of an element or radical.

valeric acid, an acid extracted from the roots of the valerian plant, used in medicine.

valetudinarian, one seeking to recover health; invalid.

valgus, denoting a position, as being bent outward or twisted.

valine, an amino acid derived from the hydrolysis of proteins, essential for human metabolism.

Valium, trademark for diazepam, used for management of anxiety disorders.

vallate, rim-shaped; a rim around a depression.

vallecular, a furrow or crevice, as on the back of the tongue.

valval, pertaining to a valve.

valvate, furnished with valves; resembling a valve.

valve, a membranous fold within a hollow organ that prevents a backward flow of fluid passing through it, as the entrance to the aorta from the left ventricle of the heart.

valvotomy, surgical incision into a valve.

valvular, pertaining to a valve.

valvulitis, inflammation of a valve.

vapor, a gaseous state of a substance; medicinal substance that is administered in the form of vapor which is inhaled.

vaporization, converting a liquid or solid into a vapor for inhalation as treatment for respiratory ailments.

varicella, chicken pox.

varices, dilated veins; plural of varix.

variciform, varicose.

varicocele, a varicose enlargement of the spermatic cord veins.

varicocelectomy, surgical removal of a portion of the scrotum to remove a varicocele.

varicose, distended or swollen veins; pertaining to varices.

varicose veins, veins that are enlarged and twisted, commonly found on the leg and thigh.

varicosity, a condition of being varicose; a varix; varicose vein.

varicotomy, a condition of being varicose; a varix; varicose vein.

varicotomy, surgical removal of a varix or varicose vein.

varicula, a varix of the conjunctiva of the eye.

variola, smallpox.

variolate, resembling a smallpox lesion; to vaccinate with smallpox virus.

varioloid, resembling smallpox; a mild form of smallpox.

varix, an abnormal, tortuous dilatation of a vein; varicose vein.

varus, denoting a deformity of the bone; bent inward; bowlegged.

vas, a duct or vessel.

vascular, pertaining to blood vessels.

vascularity, the condition of being vascular.

vasculitis, inflammation of a blood vessel; angiitis.

vasculum, a very small vessel.

vas deferens, the duct which transports sperm from the testis.

vasectomy, surgical removal of all or part of the vas deferens.

Vaseline, trademark for a translucent semisolid petroleum jelly used in medicinal preparations and for other purposes.

vasifactive, forming new vessels.

vasiform, resembling a tubular structure.

vasitis, inflammation of the vas deferens.

vasoconstrictor, causing a narrowing of blood vessels; an agent that causes constriction of blood vessels.

vasodepression, the lowering of blood pressure.

vasodepressor, an agent that produces vasodepression.

vasodilatation, dilatation of small arteries and arterioles.

vasodilator, causing relaxation or widening of blood vessels; an agent or nerve that dilates the blood vessels.

vasoinhibitor, a drug that depresses vasomotor nerves.

vasoligation, a surgical procedure involving the vas deferens which renders sterility.

vasomotor nerves, those nerves distributed over muscular coats of blood vessels which cause contraction or dilation of the inner diameter.

vasoparesis, partial paralysis or weakness of vasomotor nerves.

vasopressor, an agent which stimulates the contraction of the muscular tissue of blood vessels, such as adrenalin.

vasosection, surgical cutting of a vessel, especially the vas deferens.

vasospasm, spasm of any vessel.

vasostimulant, exciting vasomotor action.

vasotomy, surgical incision of the vas deferens.

vasotrophic, concerned with the nutrition of blood vessels.

vastus, great, referring to muscles.

vector, a carrier which transfers an infective microorganism from one host to another, usually an insect or tick.

vegetarian, one who eats no animal products, but lives on food of vegetable origin.

vegetation, an abnormal fungoid growth in the nasopharynx; a morbid outgrowth on any part, especially wartlike projections.

vehicle, an inactive substance used in a medicinal preparation for transporting the active ingredient; an excipient.

vein, a vessel carrying unaerated blood to the heart, excluding the pulmonary vein.

veinlet, small vein or venule.

velamen, a covering membrane, or skin covering.

velar, pertaining to velum, or veil.

vellication, spasms or twitching of muscular fibers.

velum, a veil-like structure.

vena, a vein.

vena cava, pertaining to either of two large veins that empties into the right atrium of the heart.

venenous, poisonous.

venereal disease, (VD); any disease contracted by sexual intercourse from an infected individual.

venereologist, one who specializes in venereology.

venereology, the branch of medicine concerned with the study and treatment of venereal diseases.

venesection, phlebotomy.

venipuncture, puncture of a vein for intravenous feeding, to administer medication, or for obtaining a blood specimen.

venom, poison or a toxic substance secreted by snakes, insects, or other animals.

venomous, poisonous.

venous, pertaining to the veins.

vent, an opening in any cavity.

venter, the abdomen or belly; a hollowed cavity.

ventilation, the process of supplying a room with a continuous flow of fresh air; oxygenation of the blood; the expression of feelings and thoughts in crisis intervention; abreaction.

ventricle, a small cavity, especially one of the two lower chambers of the heart; one of the connecting cavities of the brain.

ventricose, corpulent; big-bellied or a protruding abdomen; swelled out.

ventriculus, a ventricle; hollow organ, as the stomach.

venula, a small vein; venule.

venule, any of the small vessels from the capillary plexuses that join to form veins.

vergence, turning of one eye with reference to the other; convergence or divergence.

vermicide, an agent that is lethal to intestinal parasitic worms.

vermicular, resembling a worm in appearance or movement.

vermiform, having a worm-like shape.

vermiform appendix, a small tube opening into the cecum with its other end closed, varying from three to six inches long.

vermifuge, an agent that expels parasitic intestinal worms.

vermin, an external noxious parasitic animal or insect.

verminous, pertaining to, or infested with worms or vermin.

vermis, a worm.

vernix caseosa, a sebaceous covering consisting of exfoliations of outer skin layer, lanugo, and secretions from the sebaceous glands which envelops a fetus at birth, rendering a white, cheesy appearance to the skin of the newborn, believed to have beneficial protective properties.

verruca, a wart; a wartlike elevation.

verrucose, verrucous, having little warts on the surface.

version, the spontaneous or manual turning of the fetus in the uterus at childbirth.

vertebra, any of the 33 bones composing the vertebral or spinal column, of which there are: 7 cervical, 12 thoracic, 5 lumbar, 5 sacral, and 4 coccygeal vertebrae.

vertebral, pertaining to a vertebra or the vertebrae; spinal column.

vertebrate, having a backbone or spinal column; any member of the Vertebrata, animals having a vertebral column.

vertebrectomy, surgical excision of a vertebra.

vertex, the top of the head; the crown of the head.

vertical, pertaining to the top of the head; upright.

vertigo, a condition of dizziness.

vesica, the bladder.

vesical, pertaining to the urinary bladder.

vesicant, producing blisters; a substance that produces blisters.

vesication, the process of forming blisters.

vesicle, a sac containing fluid; a bladderlike cavity; a small blister; a small bladder.

vesicocele, a hernia of the bladder.

vesicular, pertaining to vesicles; composed of small saclike bodies or blisters.

vesiculation, the formation of vesicles.

vesiculectomy, surgical excision of the complete or part of a vesicle, usually the seminal vesicle.

vesiculitis, inflammation of a vesicle.

vessel, any tube, duct, or channel conveying fluid, such as blood.

vestibular, pertaining to a vestibule.

vestibule, any cavity or channel forming an entrance to another space.

vestibulogenic, arising from a vestibule of the ear.

vestibulotomy, surgical incision of the vestibule of the ear.

vestige, a small degenerate structure which functioned in the embryo or in a past generation.

vestigial, rudimentary.

viable, capable of sustaining an individual existence; having the ability to develop and grow after birth.

vial, a small bottle, usually containing medicine for administering as an injection.

vibration, rapidly moving to and fro; oscillation.

vibrator, a device used to produce a vibrating massage.

vibratory, causing or producing vibration.

vibrissae, long coarse hairs located in the vestibule of the nose in man.

vicarious, taking the place of another.

villi, minute vascular processes on the free surface of a membrane.

villiferous, having tufts of hair or villi.

villiform, resembling villi.

villose, covered with villi.

villus, a small hairlike vascular process on a free surface of a membrane.

Vincent's angina, a painful inflammatory disease of the tonsils, pharynx, and floor of the mouth; trench mouth.

viosterol, a preparation of vitamin D made from irradiated ergosterol in vegetable oil used as a substitute for cod-liver oil.

viral, relating to a virus, or caused by a virus.

viremia, viruses found in the blood.

virile, characteristic of a man; masculine or manly; having copulative power.

virilism, relating to male secondary characteristics in a female.

virility, the state of possessing normal sex characteristics in a male.

virologist, one who specializes in virology.

virology, the branch of science concerned with viruses and virus diseases.

virucide, an agent that destroys viruses.

virulence, the degree of pathogenicity possessed by microorganisms to produce disease.

virulent, infectious or highly poisonous; having a rapid and malignant course.

viruliferous, conveying or producing a virus.

virus, a minute infectious organism that causes disease in all life forms and which depends upon a living host for its metabolism and replication.

viscera, the interior organs within the cavities of the body, especially the abdomen and thorax.

visceral, pertaining to the viscera.

visceralgia, neuralgia of any of the viscera.

viscerogenic, originating in the viscera.

viscid, adhering and thick; having a glutinous or sticky quality.

viscosimeter, a device for measuring the viscosity of fluids.

viscosity, state of being sticky and resistant to flow.

viscous, thick, sticky, or gummy; having a glutinous quality.

viscus, any interior organ of the three large body cavities, especially the abdomen.

vision, sight; seeing; faculty of sensing light and color; an imaginary sight.

visual, pertaining to vision.

visual acuity, clarity of vision; sharpness.

visual field, the total area in which objects may be seen by the fixed eye.

visual purple, purple pigment in the rods of the retina; rhodopsin.

vital, pertaining to vital functions or processes; necessary to life.

vital signs, referring to temperature, pulse, respiration (TPR).

vital statistics, pertaining to a record of births, marriages, disease, and deaths in a population.

vitamin, an organic substance which occurs in natural foods and is necessary in trace amounts for normal metabolic functioning of the body.

vitamin A, fat-soluble vitamin occurring in two forms: retinol and dehydroretinol, found in egg yolk, fish-liver oils, liver, butter, cheese and many vegetables, necessary for night vision and for protecting epithelial tissue.

vitamin B$_c$, folic acid.

vitamin B complex, an important group of water-soluble vitamins isolated from liver, yeast, and other sources which include thiamine, riboflavin, niacin, niacinamide, the vitamin B$_6$ group, biotin, pantothenic acid, folic acid and others. The vitamin B complex group affects growth, appetite, lactation, and the gastrointestinal, nervous, and endocrine systems.

vitamin B$_1$, thiamine.

vitamin B$_2$, riboflavin.

vitamin B₆, pyridoxine.

vitamin B₁₂, cyanocobalmin, extracted from liver which is essential for red blood cell formation.

vitamin C, ascorbic acid which aids in growth, weight gain, appetite, blood-building, and prevents disease, such as scurvy.

vitamin D, fat-soluble vitamins found in fish-liver oils, milk products, eggs, and ultraviolet irradiation of ergosterol, necessary for absorption of calcium and phosphorus, valuable in normal bone formation of the skeleton and teeth.

vitamin E, a fat-soluble vitamin necessary in the body for reproduction, muscular development, and resistance of red blood cells to hemolysis, found in wheat germ, cereals, egg yolk, and beef liver.

vitamin G, riboflavin.

vitamin H, biotin.

vitamin K, found in green vegetables, important for normal clotting of the blood.

vitellin, a protein found in egg yolk.

vitiligo, destruction of melanocytes which form white patches on various sites of the body.

vitreous, pertaining to the vitreous humor of the eye; vitreous body; vitreous chamber.

vitreous body, a transparent jelly-like mass that fills the vitreous chamber; vitreous humor.

vitreous chamber, the cavity of the eyeball behind the lens.

vitreous humor, the transparent gelatinous substance that fills the chamber or cavity behind the lens of the eye; vitreous body.

vivisect, to dissect the body of an animal.

vivisection, the dissection of a living animal for purposes of demonstrating or studying physiological facts or for pathological investigation of diseases.

vocal cords, either of two tissue bands projecting into the cavity of the larynx which vibrate and produce vocal sounds of speech.

voice, the sounds uttered by living beings produced by vocal cord vibrations.

void, to urinate.

vola, a hollow surface, such as the sole of a foot or palm of a hand.

volar, the palm or foot surfaces.

volaris, palmar; concerning the palm of the hand.

volition, the act of choosing, or power of willing.

volume, a space occupied by a substance; the capacity of a container.

voluntary, pertaining to or under the control of the will.

voluntary muscles, voluntary musles are attached to the skeleton and are innervated by nerves coming from the brain or spinal cord; muscles subject to being controlled by the will.

volvulus, twisting of the bowel causing intestinal obstruction.

vomer, a bone of the skull which forms a large part of the nasal septum.

vomitory, an emetic; inducing vomiting.

vomitus, the ejected matter in vomiting.

vox, the voice.

vulnerability, susceptibility to injury, or disease.

vulnerable, easily injured.

vulnus, an injury or a wound.

vulsella, vulsellum, a special forceps with claw-like hooks.

vulva, external female genitalia, including the mons pubis, labia majora and minora, clitoris, and vestibule of the vagina.

vulvectomy, surgical excision of the vulva.

vulvitis, inflammation of the vulva.

vulvovaginal, pertaining to the vulva and vagina.

vulvovaginitis, inflammation of the vulva and vagina.

W

wad, a mass of fibrous material such as cotton, used for a surgical dressing or for packing.

waist, the section between the ribs and the hips in the human body.

Waldeyer's ring, the ring of tonsillar lymphatic tissue that surrounds the nasopharynx and oropharynx.

walleye, leukoma of the cornea; strabismus; exotropia.

ward, a large hospital room containing several or many patients.

wart, epidermal tumor originating from a virus; verruca.

Wassermann test, a test which detects syphilis.

wash, a solution for cleansing or for bathing a part; eyewash, or mouthwash.

waste, gradual decay, or reduction of bodily susbtance, health, or strength; to emaciate; excrement.

wasting, enfeebling, or causing loss of bodily strength.

water, a colorless, odorless, tasteless liquid, necessary to life of humans and animals; used in preparation of medicinal substances, as an aqueous solution.

water brash, gastric burning pain; heartburn.

waters, amniotic fluid; bag of water surrounding the fetus.

water-soluble, capable of dissolving in water, as many organic compounds.

wave, any wavelike pattern.

wax, a plastic substance obtained from plants or insects; cerumen, or ear wax.

waxy, pertaining to wax, or to the degeneration of body tissue resulting from accumulations of waxlike insoluble protein; characteristic of amyloid.

weak, lacking strength.

wean, the process of discontinuing breast feeding and substituting other nourishment.

wen, a sebaceous cyst; pillar cyst.

wet-nurse, a woman who suckles other infants.

wheal, a round, localized area of edema on the skin attended by severe itching which vanishes quickly; a lesion of urticaria.

wheeze, difficult breathing with a whistling sound resulting from narrowing of the lumen of a respiratory passageway.

whelk, a wheal; a pustule, nodule, tubercle, or pimple.

whiplash, an acute cervical sprain or injury caused by a sudden jerking of the head, as in an automobile accident.

whipworm, a parasitic nematode of the genus Trichuris.

white blood cell, leukocyte; white blood corpuscle.

white matter, nerve tissue of the brain and spinal cord.

whitlow, a felon; infected finger.

W.H.O., World Health Organization.

whooping cough, an infectious disease marked by catarrh of the respiratory tract with a peculiar cough, caused by Bordetella pertussis, especially in children.

will, having the power to control one's actions or emotions.

windpipe, the trachea.

wisdom tooth, the last molar tooth on each side of the jaw which usually erupts around the 25th year.

witch hazel, used as an astringent.

withdrawal, a pathological retreat from people and the world of reality; symptoms that occur when one abstains from drugs to which one is addicted; abstention from drugs.

withdrawal symptoms, a term used to describe effects of drug withdrawal in patients who have become addicted, which include nausea, vomiting, abdominal pain, tremors, and convulsions.

wolffian body, an embryonic body on each side of the spinal column; mesonephros.

womb, uterus.

woolsorter's disease, a pulmonary form of anthrax which develops in handlers of contaminated wool.

word blindness, inability to comprehend printed or written words, a form of aphasia; alexia.

word salad, the use of a mixture of words and phrases that lack meaning or logic, commonly seen in schizophrenia.

worm, a soft-bodied elongated invertebrate without limbs.

wound, an injury to the body caused by a physical means with rupture of normal skin and flesh.

wrinkle, a small crease or fold in the skin.

wrist, the joint between the forearm and hand; carpus.

wrist drop, a paralysis of the extensor muscles of the hand and fingers.

writer's cramp, an occupational disability caused by excessive writing.

wryneck, a contracted state of one or more neck muscles, resulting in an abnormal position of the head; torticollis.

Wunderlich's curve, a typical fever curve significant in typhoid fever.

X

xanthemia, yellowish pigment in the blood.

xanthine, a nitrogenous compound, related to uric acid, present in the blood and certain tissues of the body.

xanthinuria, an excretion of xanthine in large amounts with the urine.

xanthochromia, yellowish discoloration of patches of the skin or of the spinal fluid.

xanthocyanopia, a condition in which a person cannot distinguish between red and green, but can distinguish between yellow and blue; a form of color blindness.

xanthocyte, a cell that contains yellow pigment.

xanthoderma, yellow skin.

xanthodont, yellow teeth.

xanthoma, a condition marked by small, yellow nodules of the skin, especially of the eyelids.

xanthopsia, yellow vision.

xanthosis, jaundice.

X chromosome, one of the two sex chromosomes carrying female characteristics, which occur in pairs in the female cell and zygote, and with one Y chromosome in a male cell and zygote.

xenodiagnosis, a diagnosis or means of determining parasitic disease in humans by feeding an uninfected host on material believed to be infected and observing the results.

xenogenesis, reproduction of offspring unlike either parent.

xenogenous, a condition caused by a foreign body or toxin.

xenomenia, bleeding from other sites during menstruation.

xenophobia, abnormal fear of strangers.

xenophonia, an alteration in voice production, as in lack of bodily strength.

xenopthalmia, inflammation of the eye caused by a foreign body.

xeransis, a loss of moisture of the skin causing dryness.

xerocheilia, dryness of the lips.

xeroderma, excessive dryness of the skin; a form of ichthyosis.

xerophthalmia, an abnormal condition of the eye marked by dryness and thickening of the lining membrane of the lid and eyeball due to a deficiency of vitamin A.

xerostomia, dryness of the mouth.

xiphisternum, the lower portion of the sternum or xiphoid process.

xiphoid, relating to the sword-shaped xiphisternum.

xiphoiditis, inflammation of the cartilage xiphoid process.

X-linked, sex-linked, or transmitted by genes on the X-chromosome.

X-ray, to examine by roentgen rays.

X-ray therapy, used to treat certain diseases, as cancer.

Xylocaine, trademark for lidocaine, used in medicinal preparations.

xylometazoline, used as a topical nasal decongestant.

xylose, a pentose used in diagnostic tests of intestinal absorption.

xysma, membranous material in stools of diarrhea.

xyster, a surgical instrument used in surgery to scrape bone.

Y

yaw, a primary lesion of the skin due to yaws.

yawn, an involuntary opening of the mouth with a long inhalation, due to fatigue or drowsiness.

yawning, deep inspiration with the mouth wide open, resulting from fatigue or boredom.

yaws, an infectious tropical disease, marked by eruptions of tubercles on the skin, and rheumatism, caused by the spirochete Treponema pertenue.

Y bacillus, a bacillus that causes dysentery.

Y chromosome, one of a pair of sex chromosomes, an X and Y, that carry male characteristics.

yeast, a viscid substance composed of aggregated cells of small unicellular sac fungi, used to supplement B-complex vitamins.

yellow body, the corpus luteum formed in the cavity of the graafian follicle after the expulsion of the ovum, and which persists during pregnancy.

yellow fever, an acute infectious disease marked by jaundice, vomiting, epigastric tenderness, hemorrhages, and fever, transmitted by the bite of a female mosquito.

yoke, a connecting structure.

yolk, stored in the form of protein and fat granules in the ovum, as a nutrient.

Young's rule, a children's dose of medication is determined by adding 12 to the age and dividing the result by the age, making the quotient the denominator of a fraction, the numerator of which is 1. The proportion of adult medication to be given to a child is represented by the fraction.

youth, the period of adolescence.

Z

zein, protein derived from maize or corn.

Zeiss' gland, a sebaceous gland at the free edge of the eyelid.

zelotypia, a morbid interest in any project or cause.

zero, the point on a thermometer or other scale at which the graduation begins.

zestocausis, cauterization with steam.

zinc chloride, used as an astringent, antiseptic, and escharotic.

zinc oxide, used mostly in the form of ointment and as an antiseptic and astringent.

zoanthropy, a mental condition in which one has the delusion that he is an animal.

zoetic, pertaining to life; vital.

zona, a band or girdle; herpes zoster; zone.

zonesthesia, having the sensation of constriction, as by a girdle.

zoonosis, a disease transmissible to man by animals.

zoophagous, living on animal food.

zoophobia, pathological aversion toward animals.

zooplasty, transplantation of tissue from lower animals to the human body.

zootherapeutics, veterinary medicine.

zoster, herpes zoster; shingles.

zosteriform, resembling herpes zoster.

zygapophysis, one of the articular processes of the neural arch of a vertebra, usually occurring in pairs.

zygoma, the prominence of the cheekbone.

zygomatic, pertaining to the zygoma.

zygomatic arch, the formation on each side of the cheeks composed of each malar bone articulating with the zygomatic process.

zygomatic process, a thin projection that extends from the temporal bone; that part of the malar bone which forms the zygoma.

zygote, the union of male and female gametes to produce a new single-celled individual or zygote.

zymase, an enzyme found in yeast.

zyme, a fermenting substance.

zymogen, a substance that develops into an enzyme.

zymology, the science concerned with fermentation.

zymolysis, the change produced or the fermentative action of enzymes.

zymolytic, pertaining to zymolysis.

zymose, an enzyme responsible for the changes of a disaccharide into a monosaccharide.

zymosis, fermentation; an infectious disease.

zymosthenic, increasing the functional activity of an enzyme.

zymotic, pertaining to fermentation; relating to an infectious disease.